MEDICAL RADIOLOGY
Diagnostic Imaging

Editors:
A. L. Baert, Leuven
M. F. Reiser, München
H. Hricak, New York
M. Knauth, Göttingen

D. M. Koh · H. C. Thoeny (Eds.)

Diffusion-Weighted MR Imaging

Applications in the Body

With Contributions by

Y. Amoozadeh · M. Blackledge · D. J. Collins · T. L. Chenevert · F. De Keyzer · A. Dzik-Jurasz
J. M. Froehlich · C. J. Galbán · A. Gutzeit · M. A. Haider · T. Ichikawa · K. S. Jhaveri
I. R. Kamel · D. M. Koh · T. C. Kwee · E. Liapi · A. Muhi · P. Murphy · K. Nakanishi
A. Padhani · J. Patel · A. Rehemtulla · B. D. Ross · T. Takahara · B. Taouli · H. C. Thoeny

Foreword by

A. L. Baert

With 182 Figures in 403 Separate Illustrations, 54 in Color and 26 Tables

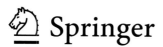 Springer

Dow-Mu Koh, MD
Royal Marsden NHS Foundation Trust
Department of Radiology
Downs Road
Sutton SM2 5PT
United Kingdom

Harriet C. Thoeny, MD
Universitätsspital Bern Inselspital
Department of Diagnostic, Interventional
and Paediatric Radiology
Freiburgstr. 10
3010 Bern
Switzerland

Medical Radiology · Diagnostic Imaging and Radiation Oncology
Series Editors:
A. L. Baert · L. W. Brady · H.-P. Heilmann · H. Hricak
M. Knauth · M. Molls · C. Nieder · M. F. Reiser

Continuation of Handbuch der medizinischen Radiologie
Encyclopedia of Medical Radiology

ISBN: 978-3-540-78575-0   e-ISBN: 978-3-540-78576-7

DOI: 10.1007/978-3-540-78576-7

Springer Heidelberg Dordrecht London New York

Medical Radiology · Diagnostic Imaging and Radiation Oncology ISSN 0942-5373

Library of Congress Control Number: 2009931696

Cover design: Publishing Services Teichmann, 69256 Mauer, Germany

Printed on acid-free paper

9 8 7 6 5 4 3 2 1

Springer is part of Springer Science+Business Media (www.springer.com)

Foreword

It is a great privilege to introduce this book devoted to the current and future roles in research and clinical practice of another exciting new development in MRI: Diffusion-weighted MR imaging.

This new, quick and non-invasive technique, which requires no contrast media or ionizing radiation, offers great potential for the detection and characterization of disease in the body as well as for the assessment of tumour response to therapy. Indeed, whereas DW-MRI is already firmly established for the study of the brain, progress in MR technology has only recently enabled its successful application in the body. Although the main focus of this book is on the role of DW-MRI in patients with malignant tumours, non-oncological emerging applications in other conditions are also discussed.

The editors of this volume, Dr. D. M. Koh and Prof. H. Thoeny, are internationally well known for their pioneering work in the field and their original contributions to the literature on DW-MRI of the body.

I am very much indebted to them for the enthusiasm and engagement with which they prepared and edited this splendid volume in a record short time for our series *Medical Radiology – Diagnostic section*.

I congratulate most sincerely the editors and the contributing authors, all well-recognized experts, on the outstanding quality of contents of this book, the highly informative text as well as the well-chosen and impeccable illustrations. This state-of-the-art volume will certainly be of immense help to all radiologists in training who want to improve their skills in MR imaging as well as to certified radiologists who will find in this book the latest advances and future trends in DW-MRI of the body. It will however also be of great interest for oncologists and oncological surgeons to assist them in the management of their patients.

I am confident that this unique book will meet great success with the readership of this series.

Leuven, Belgium   Albert L. Baert

Preface

Radiological practice often evolves in small incremental steps rather than by quantum leaps. Old techniques or ideas may be given a new lease of life through novel applications, and anecdotes of these can be drawn from oncological imaging. For example, although positron emitting radionuclear tracers have been in use since the 1950s, it is only in the last decade that the power of positron emission tomography (PET) has been widely harnessed, such that PET-CT imaging is now mainstream and indispensible for the management of a patient with cancer. By comparison, although diffusion-weighted MR imaging (DW-MRI) has been routinely employed for the evaluation of intracranial diseases for two decades, it is only in the last few years that MR technological advances have enabled the technique to be successfully implemented in the body.

DW-MRI is appealing as an imaging technique for several reasons. First, the imaging can be performed relatively quickly and thus has the potential to be widely generalized and adopted. Second, the technique does not require the administration of exogenous contrast medium, which is attractive in the light of potential serious adverse effects of gadolinium-based contrast media. Third, the technique yields both qualitative and quantitative information, the latter being of particular importance as development of quantitative imaging techniques is now acknowledged to be critical to the future of radiology.

DW-MRI yields unique information that reflects microstructural and functional alterations in tissues. Although there are still many challenges ahead, early experience with the technique has shown substantial promise. We hope that this volume will demonstrate the exciting potentials of this technique, discussing the applications of DW-MRI along broad themes of clinical practice rather than by organ systems.

The book is divided into four sections. The first describes the principles, techniques and interpretation of DW-MRI in the body. The second focuses on reviewing the non-oncological applications of DW-MRI in the body, including the evaluation of organ function. The third and largest section of the book highlights the oncological applications of DW-MRI for disease detection, disease characterization and assessment of tumour response to different therapeutic strategies. Dedicated chapters cover lymph node, bone and whole-body imaging using DW-MRI, as developments in these areas could have substantial impact on future clinical practice. Finally, the promise of multi-functional MR imaging and development of DW-MRI as a biomarker are discussed.

We are grateful to Professor Albert Baert for commissioning this project and for entrusting us to be editors of this volume. Many thanks to all our contributors who are experts in the field, for spending time to set their valuable ideas and thoughts onto paper. Special thanks to Mrs. Maureen Watts and Mrs. Janet Macdonald from the Royal Marsden Hospital (Sutton, UK) who have worked on many previous book projects and brought their vast experience to this volume, committing many hours of invaluable assistance to us to ensure its timely completion. We are also grateful to Ms. Ursula Davies and Ms. Daniela Brandt at Springer for their support.

We hope this book will stimulate, motivate and inspire radiologists working in non-academic as well as in academic institutions, to apply this novel non-invasive MR imaging technique to address critical questions in their clinical practice, making use of the unique information provided by the technique that is beyond morphological imaging.

Sutton, UK   Dow Mu Koh
Bern, Switzerland   Harriet C. Thoeny

Contents

Principles and Background

In the brain — ischaemic tissues look BRIGHTER (in ADC they are DARKER) in diffusion weighted scans.

DWI shows cytotoxic oedema patterns in the brain rather than vasogenic oedema (T$_2$ shows this well.)

intracellular water movement is restricted in cytotoxic oedema — its diffusion within cells is decreased.

Decreased water movement in tumour cells / inflammation — ↓ diffusion leads to ↑ signal in DWI + ↓ signal on ADC

= Basic principle.

Principles of Diffusion-Weighted Imaging (DW-MRI) as Applied to Body Imaging

Thomas L. Chenevert

[handwritten note:] b values - are the gradient related amplitude + duration differences i.e. the duration + amplitude of the various gradients.

CONTENTS

[handwritten note:] Low b values → problems with perfusion blood flow

[handwritten note:] High b values ↓SNR → optimise between the 2 to get the best images - varies with tissue being imaged though.

Thomas L. Chenevert, PhD
University of Michigan, 1500 East Medical Center Drive, Ann Arbor, MI 48109-0030, USA

SUMMARY

Diffusion of water molecules is the target of diffusion-weighted imaging (DW-MRI), although water mobility in biological systems is a complex process. Diffusion-weighted measurement in the body is frequently performed using Stejskal–Tanner echo-planar imaging experiment. However, in living tissues there are physiologic motions unrelated to diffusion that can mimic diffusion processes and confound in vivo measurements. In particular, the use of low b-values is sensitive to the microcapillary perfusion effects within the image voxel. Hence, accurate estimation of the apparent diffusion coefficient (ADC) of tissues in the body is dependent on the proper choice of b-values, which, in turn, is influenced by the baseline signal-to-noise and to the target tissue diffusion properties. Body tissues also exhibit true multi-exponential diffusion decay with increasing b-value that is unrelated to false multi-exponential appearance due to perfusion and/or noise. However, very high b-values (e.g. >3,000 s/mm^2) are usually required to appreciate this behaviour.

[handwritten note:] EPI technique

1.1

Introduction

Among clinical imaging modalities, MR imaging is well recognized for its broad portfolio of biophysical contrasts used to depict living tissue. A partial list includes: proton density; relaxation times (T1, T2, T2*); blood flow and vascular permeability; blood oxygen-level contrast; tissue hardness; and proton and non-proton metabolite distribution via chemical shift imaging. In practice, these contrasts are manipulated to yield exquisite anatomical detail or functional status of tissue. Certainly, diffusion-based contrast is well established in brain imaging and is rapidly becoming a mainstay for body imaging. Diffusion of water molecules is the target of diffusion-weighted imaging (DW-MRI), although water mobility in biological systems is an exceptionally complex process. Mathematical models of water mobility in tissue have been proposed, but typically, these require simplifying assumptions and/or numerical simulation methods to describe empiric observations. While the true nature of water movement in tissues is still not fully understood, the practical medical value of DW-MRI in a clinical setting is undeniable. For example, DW-MRI offers high sensitivity of acute ischaemic damage in the brain and has had a strong impact in the management of stroke. In the body, DW-MRI offers good sensitivity to detect cellular-dense lesions and may have several applications in oncological imaging. In this chapter, basic physical principles of molecular diffusion measurement are summarized along with an introduction to MR methodologies that elicit diffusion-based contrast to image the body.

1.2
Basic Diffusion Concepts

The random movement of particles suspended in a fluid or gas is referred to as Brownian motion in honour of botanist Robert Brown who first commented on the haphazard motion of pollen grains in fluid. A detailed mathematical framework of Brownian motion was published by Albert Einstein in 1905, where he established the statistical relationship between the average distance that particles move over an interval in time, as well as functional dependencies on particle size, medium viscosity and temperature. The following Einstein relationship is a good launch point (CRANK 1975)

$$< \Delta r^2 > = 6 D \Delta t, \qquad (1.1)$$

where $<\Delta r^2>$ represents the average squared displacement of a particle, or ensemble of particles, allowed to diffuse freely in three dimensions over the time interval, Δt, and D is the diffusion coefficient which incorporates temperature and media viscosity properties. When the particles and the media are the same, such as water molecules in pure water, D is also referred to

as the self-diffusion coefficient. It is instructive to consider the scale of molecular displacement over a given interval for a simple self-diffusion system. Consider, for example, pure water at body temperature (37°C) which is known to have a self-diffusion coefficient of approximately $D = 3 \times 10^{-3}$ mm²/s. If water molecules are allowed to diffuse freely in three dimensions, their root-mean-square (rms) displacement over an interval, say $\Delta t = 50$ ms, is given by the square root of (1.1), which yields 30×10^{-3} mm = 30 μm. A diffusion interval $\Delta t = 50$ ms was chosen in this example since it represents the measurement interval commonly used for in vivo diffusion imaging procedures. Now, consider the resultant rms displacement of 30 μm relative to the size of the cell, which for the sake of this argument we assume is in the order of several microns. Furthermore, consider the typical situation in tissue where the majority of water is intracellular. Since the distance water molecules migrate, *if they were free*, is much greater than cellular dimensions, it is clear the odds are very high that water molecules must encounter many cellular and subcellular impediments over this 50 ms interval. Obvious impediments that encapsulate intracellular water include cell membranes and organelles. Extracellular water will also encounter impediment presented by the tortuosity of cell packing in dense tissues (SZAFER et al. 1995; NORRIS 2001a; KAUPPINEN 2002). Lastly, water molecules are in exchange with macromolecules, thus, water transiently adopts the diffusion coefficient of the large molecule. In simple solutions of large-particle solute in small-molecule solvent, the diffusion coefficient of the large particle is inversely related to the large particle size, R, according to the Stokes–Einstein equation;

$$D_{solute} = \frac{\kappa T}{R}, \qquad (1.2)$$

where κ combines fundamental constants, media viscosity and solute surface properties, and T is the absolute temperature. Thus, water mobility is reduced secondary to its association with macromolecules. In summary, molecular water is the probe used in diffusion-sensitive MR imaging, but it is all of the non-water constituents in tissue that provides interesting contrast by virtue of reduced water mobility relative to free diffusion. The term "restricted" diffusion may be used to refer to the intracellular water, although this implies membrane confinement of the water to remain intracellular. Certainly, cell membranes are at least semi-permeable to water, thus the term "impeded" diffusion is used to describe water mobility within the cellular matrix. For some in vivo conditions, water diffusion may be effectively free such as in simple cyst, CSF, acellular necrosis, urine and other fluids.

The time-dependence of rms displacement of diffusing molecules suggests one may use time as a variable to probe cellular distance scales in tissues. That is, as one goes to much shorter Δt, the likelihood of water interaction with cellular impediments is reduced unless the impediments are tightly packed. Indeed, these studies have been performed (LATOUR et al. 1994; NIENDORF et al. 1994; PFEUFFER et al. 1999; CLARK et al. 2001; NORRIS 2001a). However, it is difficult to achieve sufficient sensitivity to diffusion effects at very short Δt (~few ms) when using human MR imaging equipment. The typical clinical MR imaging system is limited to imaging gradient strengths of around 40–80 mT/m at a slew rate of 100–200 mT/m/ms. Variable-Δt biophysics studies of cell systems on small bore MR imaging systems have been performed at gradient strengths and order-of-magnitude stronger than those available on clinical systems (LATOUR et al. 1994; PFEUFFER et al. 1999; WRIGHT et al. 2007). Given our primary interest in clinical diffusion-sensitive imaging of humans, we will only be concerned with diffusion measurements using $\Delta t \approx 50$–100 ms which is constrained to the echo-time (TE) of a spin-echo diffusion-weighted MR imaging experiment.

As previously indicated, molecular diffusion has a dependence on temperature. For pure water, the self-diffusion coefficient increases by 2.4% per °C (LE BIHAN et al. 1989). For example, the diffusion coefficient of water at 25 and 37°C is 2.29×10^{-3} and 2.96×10^{-3} mm²/s respectively. Diffusion mapping has been proposed for hyperthermia dosimetry (LE BIHAN et al. 1989), although currently, phase-based measurement of water resonance chemical shift is more commonly used over diffusion (GELLERMANN et al. 2005).

1.3

Magnetic Resonance Measurement of Diffusion

A water molecule, or spin, that migrates along trajectory path, $r(t)$, through a gradient field given by the waveform, $G(t)$, accumulates phase, ϕ, according to

$$\varphi(t) = -\gamma \int_0^t \vec{G}(t') \cdot \vec{r}(t') \mathrm{d}t', \qquad (1.3)$$

where γ is the gyromagnetic ratio ($\gamma = 42.57$ MHz/T). For the scenario where there is a large number of spins (e.g. water molecules in a voxel) having random trajectories, it is reasonable to expect there are as many positive as negative phase shifts, thus the net phase shift averaged over all spins is close to zero. So unlike coherent directional motion through a gradient field that results in measurable phase such as in flow MR imaging, a large number of randomly migrating spins yields no net phase shift, rather only spin dephasing manifest as signal attenuation. Moreover, the degree of signal attenuation increases as the breadth of the distribution of phase shifts increases. Equation 1.3 indicates phase shift (thus phase distribution width) increases with a longer integral interval, greater gradient strength, gradient duration, and/or greater migration path or mobility. This general line of logic has been applied to modify the Bloch equation to include spin diffusion along with other factors affecting magnetization evolution. The reader is referred elsewhere for a more detailed derivation of the Bloch–Torrey equation (TORREY 1956; HAACKE et al. 1999), although its solution for signal attenuation due to random spin diffusion is simply presented here as

$$S(t) = S_o e^{-D \int_0^t \vec{k}(t') \cdot \vec{k}(t') \mathrm{d}t'}, \qquad (1.4)$$

where $S(t)$ is the diffusion attenuated signal, S_o, is the signal without diffusion attenuation, D is the spin diffusion coefficient, and $k(t)$ relates to the time-integral of the gradient waveform given by

$$\vec{k}(t) = \gamma \int_0^t \vec{G}(t') \mathrm{d}t'. \qquad (1.5)$$

Equations 1.4 and 1.5 are written in general form for arbitrary gradient waveforms. Usually diffusion-sensitization gradients are incorporated within an imaging sequence, in which case the imaging and diffusion components of the gradient waveform should be included in the equations. Ignoring imaging for a moment, the simple two-pulse gradient waveform shown in Fig. 1.1, often referred to as the Stejskal-Tanner pulsed field gradient (PFG) (STEJSKAL et al. 1965), is the default diffusion sensitive sequence. Submitting the waveform of Fig. 1.1 into (1.5) and the integral in (1.4) yields the familiar result for b-value defined as (LE BIHAN et al. 1986).

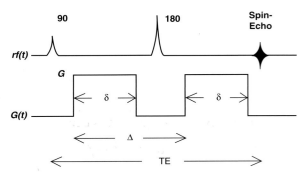

Fig. 1.1. Standard pulsed field gradient (PFG) waveform for diffusion sensitization

$$b = \int_0^{TE} \vec{k}(t') \cdot \vec{k}(t') \, dt' = (\gamma\, G\, \delta)^2 \left[\Delta - \frac{\delta}{3}\right]. \quad (1.6)$$

Frequently, only the gradient amplitude is altered to vary b-value in a diffusion imaging sequence. This leads to change in signal as a function of b-value, from which the diffusion coefficient is calculable from a minimum of two b-value settings:

$$S(b) = S_o e^{-Db} \quad or \quad D = \frac{1}{(b_2 - b_1)} \ln\left[\frac{S(b_1)}{S(b_2)}\right]. \quad (1.7)$$

Often one of the PFG gradients has zero amplitude, in which case $b_1 = 0$ and $S(b_1) = S_o$. Alternatively, more than two b-values may be acquired and the diffusion coefficient is derived by a linear fit of $\ln[S(b)]$ vs. b-value.

1.4

Anisotropic Diffusion

The formalism above only considers isotropic molecular diffusion, which is to say there is no directional dependence on how the molecules migrate. Most non-neuro tissues exhibit nearly isotropic water diffusion; although in general, one should not assume tissues are isotropic when performing quantitative diffusion imaging experiments. As indicated, neuro tissue can be highly anisotropic where the apparent water mobility varies several-fold based on relative orientation of measurement axis and myelinated white matter fibre tracts (CHENEVERT et al. 1990; MOSELEY et al. 1991; BEAULIEU 2002; MOSELEY 2002). Non-neuro tissues that exhibit diffusion anisotropy include skeletal and

cardiac muscle (KINSEY et al. 1999; SINHA et al. 2006; KARAMPINOS et al. 2007; ROHMER et al. 2007), kidney (FUKUDA et al. 2000; RIES et al. 2001; NOTOHAMIPRODJO et al. 2008) and prostate (SINHA et al. 2004; MANENTI et al. 2007; GURSES et al. 2008), although the degree of anisotropy is not as strong as in highly ordered myelinated white matter.

To allow for anisotropy while avoiding several complex mathematical issues we shall simply state without proof that for anisotropic systems the single-valued diffusion coefficient from (1.4) is generalized to a 3 × 3 second-order rank diffusion tensor (LE BIHAN et al. 2001; BASSER et al. 2002):

$$D = \begin{bmatrix} D_{xx} & D_{xy} & D_{xz} \\ D_{yx} & D_{yy} & D_{yz} \\ D_{zx} & D_{zy} & D_{zz} \end{bmatrix} \quad (1.8)$$

Moreover, generalizations of (1.6) and (1.7) are as follows

$$b_{ij} = \gamma^2 \int_0^{T_E} \left(\int_0^{t'} G_i(t'') \, dt''\right) \cdot \left(\int_0^{t'} G_j(t'') \, dt''\right) dt'. \quad (1.9)$$

and

$$\ln\left(\frac{S_o}{S_b}\right) = \sum_{i=1}^{3} \sum_{j=1}^{3} b_{ij} D_{ij}, \quad (1.10)$$

where again $b = 0$ is an isotropic measurement of S_o and i and j indices relate to any of the three gradient directions $[x, y, z]$. The b_{ij} elements of the b-matrix in (1.9) and (1.10) are the anisotropic corollary to the isotropic b-factor and are calculated for each gradient condition of a directionally sensitive diffusion acquisition. For simple gradient waveforms the b-matrix can be solved analytically (MATTIELLO et al. 1997); however, as additional gradient elements are incorporated, such as imaging pulses, numerical integration of (1.9) is preferred. The diffusion tensor is symmetric (i.e. $D_{ij} = D_{ji}$), thus it contains only six unique values. Given this, at least six non-colinear diffusion gradient directions (plus $b = 0$) are required to determine the diffusion tensor. For example, {[1,0,1]; [−1,0,1]; [0,1,1]; [0,1,−1]; [1,1,0]; and [−1,1,0]} in the $[x, y, z]$ magnet frame of reference is a reasonable set to use (BASSER et al. 1998; LE BIHAN et al. 2001). One can "over determine" the experiment and improve quality of the diffusion tensor calculation by acquisition of a larger number of non-colinear diffusion gradient directions (e.g. 9, 16, 32 directions are commonly acquired for neuro DTI) (Le Bihan et al. 2001).

Once the diffusion tensor is determined, it becomes an issue of how to efficiently summarize the information in an understandable format since there are now six unique diffusion values for each pixel in the image. For this, a tissue-based frame of reference is preferred over the magnet frame. That is, the diffusion tensor of each voxel is recast into an alternative coordinate frame that aligns with the natural architecture of the tissue as exhibited by directional diffusion values. Mathematically, this entails a linear rotation of the diffusion tensor to diagonalize it thereby setting off-diagonal elements to zero (Le Bihan et al. 2001)

$$
D = \begin{bmatrix} D_{xx} & D_{xy} & D_{xz} \\ D_{yx} & D_{yy} & D_{yz} \\ D_{zx} & D_{zy} & D_{zz} \end{bmatrix} \rightarrow \begin{bmatrix} \lambda_1 & 0 & 0 \\ 0 & \lambda_2 & 0 \\ 0 & 0 & \lambda_3 \end{bmatrix} \text{ and } [\vec{\varepsilon}_1, \vec{\varepsilon}_2, \vec{\varepsilon}_3],
$$

$$(1.11)$$

where λ_1, λ_2 and λ_3 are *eigenvalues* ($\lambda_1 \geq \lambda_2 \geq \lambda_3$) representing diffusivity along tissue-based orthogonal axes whose directions are retained in unit *eigenvectors* $[\vec{\varepsilon}_1, \vec{\varepsilon}_2, \vec{\varepsilon}_3]$. For example, λ_1 could represent the greatest diffusion value for relatively unimpeded mobility along a tissue fibre axis, denoted by direction vector $\vec{\varepsilon}_1$, and λ_2, λ_3 represent diffusion along two axes perpendicular to $\vec{\varepsilon}_1$. To further simplify diffusion, the *mean diffusivity*, D_{ave}, is most useful since it accurately summarizes mobility and is a rotationally invariant scalar (Alexander et al. 2000; Le Bihan et al. 2001). Scalar invariant quantities are highly desirable since their value is independent of relative orientation between measurement axes [x, y, z] and any potential natural tissue axes $[\vec{\varepsilon}_1, \vec{\varepsilon}_2, \vec{\varepsilon}_3]$. A fortunate feature of mean diffusivity is that it is easily derived from diffusion measurements along any three orthogonal axes, thus one does not need to generate the full diffusion tensor to produce D_{ave}.

$$
D_{ave} = \frac{\lambda_1 + \lambda_2 + \lambda_3}{3} = \frac{D_{xx} + D_{yy} + D_{zz}}{3} \quad (1.12)
$$

When a measure for the degree of anisotropy is desired, the full diffusion tensor must be determined. There are several scalar invariants available that

quantify anisotropy (Alexander et al. 2000; Hasan et al. 2001; Le Bihan et al. 2001; Westin et al. 2002; Ennis et al. 2006; Hagmann et al. 2006). A popular dimensionless index is fractional anisotropy (FA) and is calculated from the eigenvalues

$$
FA = \sqrt{\frac{3}{2}} \frac{\sqrt{\left(D_{ave} - \lambda_1\right)^2 + \left(D_{ave} - \lambda_2\right)^2 + \left(D_{ave} - \lambda_3\right)^2}}{\sqrt{\lambda_1^2 + \lambda_2^2 + \lambda_3^2}},
$$

$$(1.13)$$

where FA approaches 1 for idealized anisotropic conditions and approaches 0 for isotropic conditions. For example, in highly anisotropic human tissue, such as white matter of the corpus callosum, FA $\approx 0.7 \rightarrow 0.8$.

In summary, to quantify anisotropy, the full diffusion tensor is needed which requires at least six non-colinear diffusion gradient axes (plus $b = 0$). However to quantify mean diffusivity, diffusion measurements along at least three orthogonal axes are required. In rare instances it may be known "a priori" that the tissue of interest is isotropic, and then only one diffusion gradient direction is required, although in clinical practice, tissue architecture typically is not known; thus, measurements along at least three orthogonal axes are recommended to generate a valid mean diffusivity value.

1.5

Diffusion Measurements In Vivo

In living tissue there are physiologic motions unrelated to diffusion that can mimic diffusion processes and confound in vivo measurements. Consider, for example, blood flow through capillaries. On the voxel-size scale, perfusion through a large number of randomly oriented capillaries will appear as a hyper diffusion-like process. In addition, cardiac and respiratory motions can diminish diffusion-weighted imaging quality. Certainly cardiac and respiratory motions will not appear random over the voxel scale; however, large phase-shifts will result when diffusion-sensitization gradients are applied (Chenevert et al. 1991; Norris 2001b). Consider for example the Stejskal–Tanner PFG of Fig. 1.1 with representative clinical gradients of $G = 40$mT/m, $\delta = 20$ ms and $\Delta = 25$ ms (i.e. TE ≈ 50 ms). As designed, the resultant b-value per (1.6) for these settings would produce reasonable diffusion weighting at $b = 824$ s/mm^2.

Aside from this, however, it is interesting to calculate the phase shift per unit speed of bulk tissue motion resultant from the PFG gradients. Over the short TE interval, one can consider bulk tissue motion having constant velocity; that is, position $r(t) = r_o + v_o t$. Using this in (1.3) and the hypothetical PFG experiment ($G = 40\,\text{mT/m}$; $\delta = 20\,\text{ms}$ and $\Delta = 25\,\text{ms}$), the phase-shift per unit speed for this example is (CHENEVERT et al. 1991)

$$\frac{\varphi}{v_o} = \gamma\, G\, \delta\, \Delta = \frac{306^\circ}{\left(\text{mm}/\text{sec}\right)}. \tag{1.14}$$

According to (1.14) it is clear that even modest bulk tissue speed $\approx 1\,\text{mm/s}$ results in large phase shifts approaching 2π radians. Brain is relatively stationary compared to abdominal tissues yet intracranial tissue speeds are on the order of $1\,\text{mm/s}$ (CHENEVERT et al. 1991; ENZMANN et al. 1992; PONCELET et al. 1992). As such, bulk tissue phase shifts are apt to be very large in abdominal DW-MRI. Given such strong phase shifts due to extraneous non-diffusion-related motions, it is remarkable that diffusion-weighted imaging is able to detect differences in molecular water displacements on the order of several microns. The apparent paradox is resolved when one considers an essential element of most successful diffusion imaging sequences applied in the body. By performing all spatial encoding steps in a single shot (TURNER et al. 1991), the phase value of reconstructed pixels can be simply disregarded by retaining only the magnitude of the complex-valued pixels after two-dimensional Fourier reconstruction. Unlike conventional MR imaging where signal averaging is performed as complex values, averaging of DW-MRI data is performed on magnitude images to avoid inevitable interference of bulk motion-related phase shifts that vary from measurement to measurement. Some specialized multi-shot DW-MRI techniques based on phase corrections do work well in the brain where cardiac/respiratory motions are less severe and tissue tends to move in unison (PIPE et al. 2002). Unfortunately, these and other current multi-shot methods may not be as reliable in abdominal DW-MRI since a single phase correction value is inadequate to account for a broad range of phase shifts from elastic motion of tissues across a given slice. A variety of DW-MRI sequences have been introduced for the body, but to date most clinically successful diffusion-weighted approaches are based on the single-shot echo-planar-imaging (DW SS-EPI) sequence (TURNER et al. 1991). Even DW SS-EPI can suffer from cardiac/respiratory motion artefact when diffusion weighting and/or the spread of bulk tissue speeds that coexist in single voxels is so high that phase cancellation occurs. This form of bulk tissue motion signal loss is nearly indistinguishable from true random diffusion signal attenuation and may lead to artifact in abdominal DW-MRI such as in regions of the liver adjacent to the heart.

Thus far, our mathematical description denotes molecular mobility by simple diffusion coefficients D, D_{ij}, and D_{ave}; although we realize water movement through cellular tissues is highly complex and our results depend on empiric settings such as measurement interval. Perfusion and other bulk tissue motions further complicate the in vivo situation such that diffusion measurements of tissue are qualified as an "apparent diffusion coefficient" (ADC) in recognition of all these issues. Dimensionally, "D" and "ADC" are equivalent and without further justification we freely substitute ADC for D and D_{ave} in (1.7) and (1.12) respectively.

1.6
Effect of Perfusion and Low *b*-Value on ADC Estimation

The influence of blood flow and microcirculation on diffusion measurement warrants further discussion. The otherwise independent concepts of *perfusion* and *diffusion* have been inextricably linked since the landmark work by Denis Le Bihan where he defines intravoxel incoherent motion (IVIM) to include both thermally driven diffusion (ADC), as well as hyper diffusion-like motions of blood flow through randomly oriented capillaries (LE BIHAN et al. 1986, 1988, 2008). Le Bihan theorized that signal attenuation due to perfusion is most apparent at relatively low *b*-values (approximately $b \leq 100\,\text{s/mm}^2$) and relates to the fraction of perfusion signal, whereas slower true diffusion signal attenuation dominates at higher *b*-values. Therefore, an experiment pairing two low *b*-values to contrast with one high *b*-value could potentially isolate diffusion and perfusion contributions. However, perfusion should not be considered as a true diffusion process nor does *fraction of perfusion signal* even dimensionally relate to diffusion or traditional perfusion measures. Nevertheless, the two phenomena are intertwined in the low *b*-value regime.

In the context of diffusion studies, it is usually desirable to eliminate perfusion signal which we consider a contaminant in ADC estimation. As an approximation, we consider the fraction of water signal from the vascular space does not exchange with extravascular water over the measurement timescale ($\approx$TE), thus signal can be modelled as a composite of two distinct compartments (LE BIHAN et al. 1988)

$$S(b) = (1 - f_v) e^{-b \, \text{ADC}} + f_v \Phi_v(b), \qquad (1.15)$$

where f_v is the fractional volume of flowing spins and $\Phi_v(b)$ reflects the attenuation of perfusion signal due to flow dephasing in randomly oriented capillaries. Figure 1.2a illustrates a simulation of signal loss based on (1.14) and (1.15) for fractional perfusion volumes

of 0, 5, 10 and 20%. The remaining volume has an assigned ADC = 1×10^{-3} mm^2/s representative of tissue. Figure 1.2b indicates the impact of perfusion and choice of low b-value on measured ADC. That is, (1.7) was applied to calculate ADC using a fixed high b-value = 1,000 s/mm^2 and the low b-value varied from 0 to 999. As expected, ADC overestimation increases with greater perfusion fraction and is worst when $b = 0$ is used in the two-point ADC calculation. Perfusion error on ADC is reduced by use of moderately low b-values ($b = 100$–200 s/mm^2) that preferentially attenuate flow relative to other tissues. While the perfusion error further decreases as the low b-value is increased, it must be balanced with maintenance of

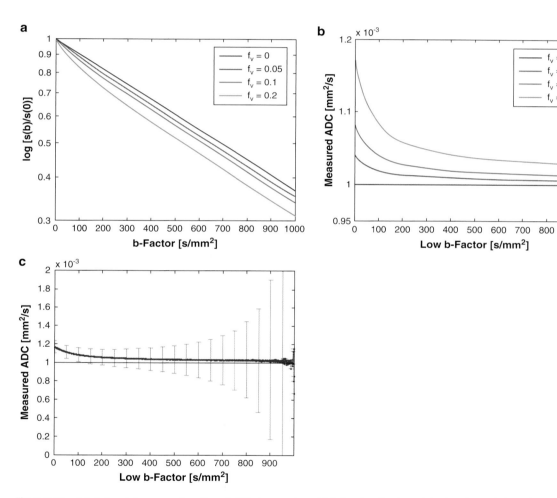

Fig. 1.2. Simulated signal decay as a function of diffusion sensitivity (i.e. b-value) and perfusion fraction (f_v). (**a**) Perfusion-induced deviation from mono-exponential decay increases with perfusion fraction and is most apparent in the low b-value regime. (**b**) Measured ADC via (1.7) as a function of perfusion fraction and choice of low b-value from 0 through 999 s/mm^2 with the high b-value fixed at 1,000 s/mm^2. Deviation of measured ADC from true ADC (equal to 1×10^{-3} mm^2/s in this simulation) increases for decreasing low b-value. (**c**) Plot of perfusion-induced bias error and noise-induced random error shown as *error bars*. While bias error decreases using a higher low b-value, random error increases due to reduced diffusion contrast-to-noise

sufficient diffusion contrast-to-noise between low and high b measurements. To illustrate this trade-off, Fig. 1.2c includes the effect of noise for a fractional perfusion volume $f_v = 0.2$ and a signal-to-noise (SNR) = 50. The error bars indicating random error due to noise clearly increases as the low b-value approaches the high b-value (held fixed at 1,000 s/mm²) due to reduced diffusion contrast. While a non-zero low b-value is preferred for improved ADC estimation, it is still recommended to also acquire an additional $b = 0$ image since it does not have to be repeated for three orthogonal directions, thus it is fast, and $b = 0$ offers consistency with most prior studies.

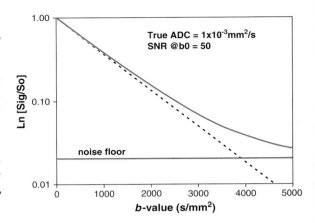

Fig. 1.3. Simulated signal (*blue line*) that deviates from true mono-exponential decay (*dashed line*) as signal approaches noise-floor (*red line*) at high b-values

Effect of SNR and High b-Value on ADC Estimation

Aside from undesired perfusion effects, the formalism above implies tissue diffusion is a simple mono-exponential decay with b-value. However, as has been demonstrated in multiple studies, diffusion in tissue truly is non-mono-exponential; moreover this multi-exponential behaviour is unrelated to perfusion arte-fact. Rather high b-values ($b \geq 3,000$ s/mm²) are required to elicit multi-exponential decay features from tissue (BURDETTE et al. 2001; DELANO et al. 2002). According to (1.6), b-value has a [time]³ dependence, thus a moderate increase in TE allows one to greatly increase b-value. Even $b = 10,000$ s/mm² can be readily achieved on clinical systems. Unfortunately, the signal loss due to diffusion at high b-value becomes a limiting factor in these studies. Baseline SNR and true diffusion determine how quickly signal drops to the noise-floor as b-value is increased. An unfortunate result is that signal decay will appear to exhibit multi-exponential features as it approaches the noise-floor – thus it may be confused with *true* tissue-related multi-exponential behaviour (DIETRICH et al. 2001). For illustration we again turn to simulations where we have control to define tissue as mono-exponential with no perfusion component. In this way, any apparent multi-exponential features must be artefactual in origin.

Figure 1.3 graphically illustrates false multi-exponential decay for simulated SNR = 50 (at $b = 0$) and a true tissue ADC = 1×10^{-3} mm²/s. That is, as the true signal decays below the noise-floor, the observed signal plus noise is buoyed by noise and appears to decay at a slower rate. For this example, signal decay in the $b = 0{\rightarrow}1,000$ s/mm² range appears mono-exponen-

tial but at higher b-values (i.e. $b > 2,000$ s/ mm²) noise dominates and the curve no longer appears mono-exponential (DIETRICH et al. 2001).

In most in vivo studies b-values are sparsely sampled so the risk of noise does not necessarily lead to mis-characterization of multi-exponential decay constituents. Instead, noise tends to lead to quantitative errors in ADC estimation. A common approach is to presume mono-exponential behaviour, acquire one low and one high b-value and estimate ADC via (1.7). Assuming this is the case, the regime where noise biases ADC estimation depends on baseline SNR, true diffusion coefficient and the chosen high b-value. Figure 1.4 summarizes results of Monte Carlo simulations where again for simplicity truth is defined as mono-exponential diffusion with no perfusion contribution. Baseline SNR = 25 was selected as it is representative of some body DW-MRI protocols. Top frames are measured ADC vs. true diffusion, and lower frames expand on random and bias error as a function of true diffusion value. Here random error is defined as the standard deviation of measured ADC and is illustrated by error bars, whereas bias error is shown as distance from the horizontal line. ADC estimations via three b-value pairs were simulated: $b = 0$ & 500; $b = 0$ & 1,000; and $b = 0$ & 2,000 s/mm² for left, middle and right columns respectively. At the expense of increased random error at low diffusion values, the modest b-value pair 0 & 500 s/mm² avoids significant bias over the relevant tissue ADC range (0.3$\rightarrow$3.0 $\times 10^{-3}$ mm²/s). Bias error begins to appear using pair $b = 0$ & 1,000 s/ mm² and increases for $b = 0$ & 2,000 s/ mm². It should be noted that the magnitude of these errors and b-value ranges are only applicable to the

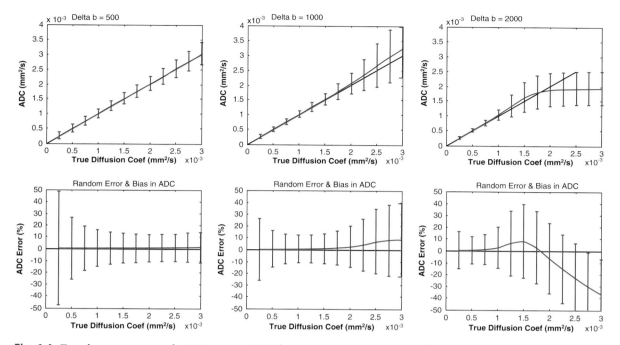

Fig. 1.4. *Top* plots are measured ADC vs. true ADC for a simulated baseline SNR = 25 (at b = 0) and choice of three b-value pairs: b = 0 & 500 *left* column; b = 0 & 1,000 *middle* column; b = 0 & 2,000 *right* column. *Bottom* plots expand on bias error (deviation from horizontal line) and random error *(error bars)*. Bias error increases at high b-value and/or high ADC where noise can dominate high b-value measurements. There is a transient overestimation in ADC that switches to large underestimate error at very high b-value extremes

conditions used in this simulation – results will vary for different baseline SNR values. In general, the observed bias is a direct result of noise becoming a significant component of the high b-value measurement which is naturally more probable as true diffusion increases and/or a greater high b-value is used. At the very high-b extreme, measured ADC is systematically lower than the true diffusion. Therefore, the proper choice of body DW-MRI b-values depends on baseline SNR and target tissue diffusion properties (XING et al. 1997; DIETRICH et al. 2001). For a body DW-MRI protocol that is limited to SNR $\approx$ 25, b-values 0$\rightarrow$500 s/mm² are a reasonable choice to avoid bias. Alternatively if one is not concerned with accuracy in the high ADC range (e.g. >2 × 10⁻³ mm²/s), then a b-value range b = 0$\rightarrow$1,000 s/mm² is not unreasonable. According to Xing, a reasonable guide for protocol design is to have ADC × $(b_2 - b_1)$ $\approx$ 1.1 (XING et al. 1997). Any factor that improves baseline SNR should be incorporated to reduce random error and allow greater low-b to high-b spread thus enhancing DW-MRI contrast and ADC estimate accuracy. For example, signal averaging and surface coils are commonly employed in clinical DW-MRI to enhance SNR as will be discussed in later chapters.

Simulations are useful to isolate impact of perfusion at low b-values from noise-related error at high b-values since these effects are independently controlled by the programmer (XING et al. 1997; DIETRICH et al. 2001). Simulation also provides guidance to design DW-MRI protocols for accurate ADC quantification (XING et al. 1997). To summarize simulation results, perfusion tends to inflate ADC estimates when the low b-value is too low to eliminate flow signal, whereas a high b-value that is too high for the available SNR of the high-b image tends to cause underestimation of ADC as the slope of log(signal) vs. b-value flattens when approaching the noise-floor.

In DW-MRI of real tissue, one cannot easily isolate or control the various signal modifiers, but their presence is perhaps more recognizable by understanding the basic principles involved. Consider, for example, diffusion-weighted images through normal kidneys shown in Fig. 1.5 for b-values: 0, 50, 100, 200, 500, 750, 1,000 and 2,000 s/mm². The noise-floor was estimated from mean plus two standard deviations from a non-signal background region and is shown as the horizontal dashed line. The logarithm of signal vs. b-value for a small region of interest in kidney cortex clearly is not mono-exponential over the full b-value range.

Fig. 1.5. Measured signal
decay in kidney cortex
as a function of *b*-value
in a normal volunteer.
Diffusion-weighted images
acquired at different
b-values are shown on the
right. Table inset shows
calculated ADC based on
selecting a subset of
b-values for the calculation. Perfusion contamination is increased by inclusion of *b*-values too low
and noise contamination
is increased by use of *b*-
values too high. The *solid
line* is a fit of intermediate
b-values = 100, 200, 500,
and 750 s/mm²

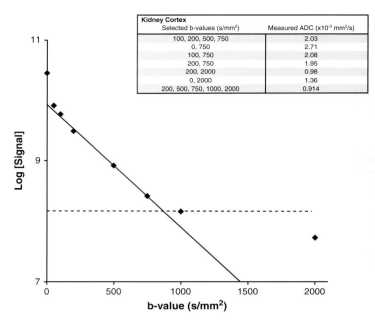

Kidney Cortex	
Selected b-values (s/mm²)	Measured ADC (x10⁻³ mm²/s)
100, 200, 500, 750	2.03
0, 750	2.71
100, 750	2.08
200, 750	1.95
200, 2000	0.98
0, 2000	1.36
200, 500, 750, 1000, 2000	0.914

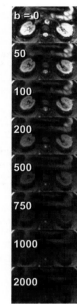

Based on arguments above, the steep slope of log(signal) over low *b*-value range ($b = 0 \rightarrow 100$ s/mm²) is partially driven by perfusion blood flow. At high *b*-values ($b = 1{,}000 \rightarrow 2{,}000$ s/mm²) the kidney signal is close to, if not below the noise-floor. In this regime, slope of log(signal) vs. *b*-value is reduced, thus ADC is being underestimated by including *b*-values greater than 1,000 s/mm². The inset table lists measured ADC values for this kidney based on which *b*-values are included in the log slope estimates. Based on arguments presented above, a reasonably accurate estimate of ADC of kidney cortex is derived from the *b*-value range $b = 100 \rightarrow 750$ s/mm². Kidney cortex has a relatively high ADC $\approx 2 \times 10^{-3}$ mm²/s even after suppression of perfusion contamination. Figures 1.6 and 1.7 follow the same format as Fig. 1.5, but focus on lower ADC tissues of liver and spleen respectively. Liver exhibits relatively low SNR and it is questionable if $b = 750$ is advisable for this protocol. On the other hand, spleen has a relatively high SNR and can tolerate a greater high *b*-value range. The *b*-value list in Figs. 1.5–1.7 is longer than normally performed for DWI of the body. Moreover, retrospective ad hoc selection of *b*-values to avoid perfusion and/or low SNR effects as well as ROI-based measurement of ADC values are not recommended procedures. They were performed here to graphically illustrate fundamental limitations on ADC quantification in the body when perfusion and SNR limits need to be considered by selection of appropriate *b*-values. In practice it is more common to acquire only two or three

b-values along three orthogonal axes with adequate signal averaging to quantify ADC in target organs/tissues in a reasonably short image acquisition time.

1.8
Multi-Exponential Diffusion in Tissues

As briefly mentioned above, tissue actually does exhibit true multi-exponential diffusion decay with *b*-value that is unrelated to false multi-exponential appearance due to perfusion and/or noise (Norris et al. 1995; Niendorf et al. 1996; Pfeuffer et al. 1999; Clark et al. 2000; Mulkern et al. 2000; Grant et al. 2001; Basser et al. 2002; Le Bihan 2007). Reliable demonstration of true multi-exponential decay features requires a very wide *b*-value range (*b*: 0 through ≥3,000 s/mm²). Given the relatively modest SNR in body DW-MRI and significant time penalty to acquire additional *b*-values with signal averaging, multi-exponential diffusion analyses are not common in DW-MRI of the abdomen. Nevertheless, it is worthwhile to summarize methods that address multi-exponential properties. To date most multi-exponential diffusion studies have been performed on the brain which offers several advantages: minimal cardiac/respiratory motion; high SNR due to long T2, favorable geometry and advanced high-channel array coils; and fat suppression is less problematic in the brain.

Fig. 1.6. Measured signal decay in liver as a function of *b*-value in a normal volunteer. Diffusion-weighted images acquired at different *b*-values are shown on the *right*. Table inset shows calculated ADC based on selecting a subset of *b*-values for the calculation. Perfusion contamination is increased by inclusion of *b*-values too low and noise contamination is increased by use of *b*-values too high. Liver has a moderate ADC but has lower baseline SNR, thus noise limitation occurs at lower *b*-values ($b \approx 750$–1,000 s/mm²). The *solid line* is a fit of intermediate *b*-values = 100, 200, 500, and 750 s/mm²

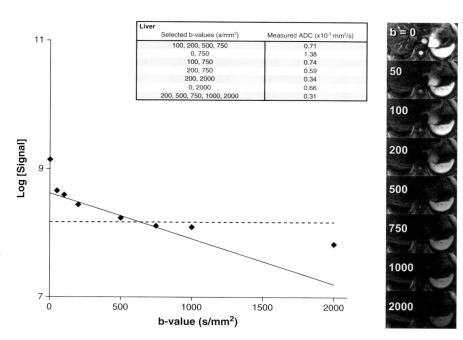

Liver	
Selected b-values (s/mm²)	Measured ADC (x10⁻³ mm²/s)
100, 200, 500, 750	0.71
0, 750	1.38
100, 750	0.74
200, 750	0.59
200, 2000	0.34
0, 2000	0.66
200, 500, 750, 1000, 2000	0.31

Fig. 1.7. Measured signal decay in spleen as a function of *b*-value in a normal volunteer. Diffusion-weighted images acquired at different *b*-values are shown on the *right*. Table inset shows calculated ADC based on selecting a subset of *b*-values for the calculation. Perfusion contamination is increased by inclusion of *b*-values too low and noise contamination is increased by use of *b*-values too high. Spleen has a moderate ADC and has a relatively high baseline SNR, thus noise limitation occurs at higher *b*-value. The *solid line* is a fit of intermediate *b*-values = 100, 200, 500, and 750 s/mm²

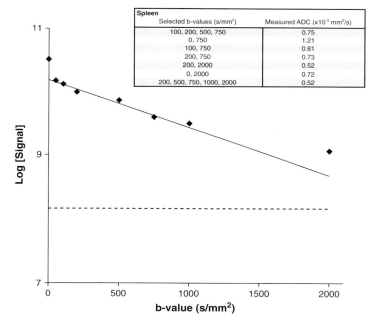
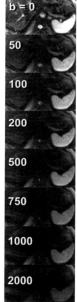

Spleen	
Selected b-values (s/mm²)	Measured ADC (x10⁻³ mm²/s)
100, 200, 500, 750	0.75
0, 750	1.21
100, 750	0.81
200, 750	0.73
200, 2000	0.52
0, 2000	0.72
200, 500, 750, 1000, 2000	0.52

The simplest extension of (1.7) is to allow for admixture of two diffusion pools. Models may allow for exchange of water between these pools depending on the timescale of measurement relative to exchange rate (CLARK et al. 2000; BASSER et al. 2002; LEE et al. 2003). For simplicity, consider non-exchanging pools where the majority of measurable signal originates from compartment A, characterized by diffusion coefficient D_A and the minority of signal from compartment B having diffusion coefficient D_B. The biexponential version of (1.7) is

$$S(b) = S_o [f \ e^{-bD_A} + (1-f)e^{-bD_B}] \qquad (1.16)$$

where f denotes the fractional size of the A compartment ($f \geq 0.5$). While this bi-exponential model

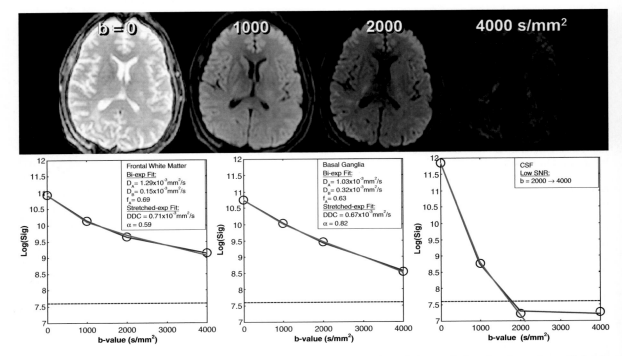

Fig. 1.8. Demonstration of true multi-exponential diffusion behaviour in brain observed over a wide *b*-value range (0 through 4,000s/mm²). Non-mono-exponential features are quantified via bi-exponential fit (*blue line*) and stretched exponential (*red line*) models. Unlike CSF, water mobility in brain tissues (white matter and basal ganglia illustrated here) is moderately low such that signal remains sufficiently above the noise-floor even at *b* = 4,000s/mm². While simple mathematical functions fit the data reasonably well, biophysical interpretation of models for water mobility in tissue require additional exchange between diffusion pools and/or other factors to account for observations

allows for coexistence of only one additional diffusion coefficient (or ADC), it introduces two additional fit parameters, *f* and D_B. In the presence of exchange between compartments, the fractional volumes and diffusion coefficients become *effective* values that incorporate other model parameters (LEE et al. 2003), although the bi-exponential functional form is still used for data fitting.

An alternative mathematical model has been introduced to fit non-mono-exponential diffusion data and is referred to as *stretched exponentials* (BENNETT et al. 2003, 2006) given by

$$S(b) = S_o \, e^{-[b\,\mathrm{DDC}]^{\alpha}} \qquad (1.17)$$

where DDC represents a *distributed diffusion coefficient* and α provides an index of diffusion heterogeneity. Dimensionally, DDC is equivalent to *D* (or ADC) whereas α is dimensionless and is bounded between 0→1. By inspection it is clear an $\alpha = 1$ is equivalent to mono-exponential decay. An α less than 1 signifies a mixture of exponentials with increasing intra-voxel diffusion heterogeneity as α decreases. A desirable

property of stretched exponentials is that the model introduces only one additional fit parameter over the mono-exponential model and yet is able to empirically fit a wide range of curve shapes.

Figure 1.8 illustrates DW-MRI of the brain for *b*-values = 0, 1,000, 2,000 and 4,000 s/mm² where again the noise-floor (estimated as mean pixel intensity plus 2× standard deviation in non-signal background) is illustrated as a horizontal dashed line. Logarithm signal decay curves are shown for representative grey matter, white matter and CSF regions avoiding blood vessels. Fitting the data by a least-squares-difference algorithm to the models in (1.16) and (1.17) are shown in blue and red lines respectively. Note bi-exponential and stretched exponential models fit the data reasonably well with the exception of CSF data. Despite its high baseline SNR, CSF has a high diffusion coefficient (CSF ADC ≈ 3 × 10⁻³ mm²/s) and thus falls into the noise-floor for *b* > 2,000 s/mm². Since two of four data points are dominated by noise, CSF is not reliably fit by either model.

At a minimum, bi-exponential and stretched-exponential models offer a practical means for data reduction. However, biophysical insight and interpretation of model parameters is less straightforward. For example, an early simple interpretation of bi-exponential compartments was for the majority compartment A to represent intracellular water presumably in a lower mobility environment relative to compartment B representing more mobile extracellular water. Unfortunately, as indicated by bi-exponential fits for white matter and basal ganglia in Fig. 1.8, the majority compartment has the higher diffusion coefficient. This unexpected finding is consistent with more detailed studies on brain, ischaemic brain and packed cell systems which clearly indicates that the simple interpretation of two independent compartments fail to reconcile known properties of cells with MR diffusion observations (LATOUR et al. 1994; CLARK et al. 2000; MULKERN et al. 2000). As a result, more elaborate models that add more compartments or allow compartment exchange are required (LEE et al. 2003). Unfortunately, these introduce more parameters and/or assumptions. Moreover, to test and apply these models a large number of measurements (b-values and/or diffusion intervals) are required which further limits their clinical utilization.

The stretched-exponential model is perhaps less intuitive, but does offer some biophysical interpretation. As outlined by Bennett, the stretched-exponential makes no assumption regarding the number of proton pools contributing to the signal, and thus may be more suitable for hierarchical complexities of tissue/cell structures (BENNETT et al. 2003, 2006). The DDC closely relates to a diffusion coefficient in that it quantifies signal decay with b-value, although the functional form of (1.17) suggests a distribution of diffusion coefficients each weighted by their fractional contribution to the net signal. Interpretation of the α index is simply that it defines the deviation away from mono-exponential decay. An $\alpha = 1$ equates to mono-exponential decay and an α approaching 0 is highly non-mono-exponential, suggesting a heterogeneous distribution of diffusion values – thus α is referred to as the heterogeneity index. Please note, however, that this heterogeneity refers to *intravoxel heterogeneity* and not heterogeneity across voxels as is usually the case.

1.9

Conclusion

Diffusion provides a unique probe into water interaction with cellular, subcellular and macromolecular entities that impede otherwise free water movement. While diffusion-weighted MR imaging is sensitive to these properties, it can only partially elucidate the level of complexity in tissue. Moreover, confounding factors affecting in vivo diffusion quantification include blood flow/perfusion, bulk tissue motion in the presence of diffusion-sensitization pulses and overall signal-to-noise. Despite these limitations, successful clinical protocols have been developed and are in widespread clinical use for many applications in the body including enhanced disease detection, diagnosis and treatment response assessment as is discussed in detail in subsequent chapters.

References

Alexander AL, Hasan K, Kindlmann G et al (2000) A geometric analysis of diffusion tensor measurements of the human brain. Magn Reson Med 44: 283–291

Basser PJ, Jones DK (2002) Diffusion-tensor MRI: theory, experimental design and data analysis – a technical review. NMR Biomed 15: 456–467

Basser PJ, Pierpaoli C (1998) A simplified method to measure the diffusion tensor from seven MR images. Magn Reson Med 39: 928–934

Beaulieu C (2002) The basis of anisotropic water diffusion in the nervous system – a technical review. NMR Biomed 15: 435–455

Bennett KM, Hyde JS, Schmainda KM (2006) Water diffusion heterogeneity index in the human brain is insensitive to the orientation of applied magnetic field gradients. Magn Reson Med 56: 235–239

Bennett KM, Schmainda KM, Bennett RT et al (2003) Characterization of continuously distributed cortical water diffusion rates with a stretched-exponential model. Magn Reson Med 50: 727–734

Burdette JH, Durden DD, Elster AD et al (2001) High b-value diffusion-weighted MRI of normal brain. J Comput Assist Tomogr 25: 515–519

Chenevert TL, Brunberg JA, Pipe JG (1990) Anisotropic diffusion in human white matter: demonstration with MR techniques in vivo. Radiology 177: 401–405

Chenevert TL, Pipe JG (1991) Effect of bulk tissue motion on quantitative perfusion and diffusion magnetic resonance imaging. Magn Reson Med 19: 261–265

Clark CA, Hedehus M, Moseley ME (2001) Diffusion time dependence of the apparent diffusion tensor in healthy human brain and white matter disease. Magn Reson Med 45: 1126–1129

Clark CA, Le Bihan D (2000) Water diffusion compartmentation and anisotropy at high b values in the human brain. Magn Reson Med 44: 852–859

Crank J (1975) The mathematics of diffusion. Oxford University Press, New York

DeLano MC, Cao Y (2002) High b-value diffusion imaging. Neuroimaging Clin N Am 12: 21–34

Dietrich O, Heiland S, Sartor K (2001) Noise correction for the exact determination of apparent diffusion coefficients at low SNR. Magn Reson Med 45: 448–453

Ennis DB, Kindlmann G (2006) Orthogonal tensor invariants and the analysis of diffusion tensor magnetic resonance images. Magn Reson Med 55: 136–146

Enzmann DR, Pelc NJ (1992) Brain motion: measurement with phase-contrast MR imaging. Radiology 185: 653–660

Fukuda Y, Ohashi I, Hanafusa K et al (2000) Anisotropic diffusion in kidney: apparent diffusion coefficient measurements for clinical use. J Magn Reson Imaging 11: 156–160

Gellermann J, Wlodarczyk W, Feussner A et al (2005) Methods and potentials of magnetic resonance imaging for monitoring radiofrequency hyperthermia in a hybrid system. Int J Hyperthermia 21: 497–513

Grant SC, Buckley DL, Gibbs S et al (2001) MR microscopy of multicomponent diffusion in single neurons. Magn Reson Med 46: 1107–1112

Gurses B, Kabakci N, Kovanlikaya A et al (2008) Diffusion tensor imaging of the normal prostate at 3 Tesla. Eur Radiol 18: 716–721

Haacke EM, Brown RW, Thompson MR et al (1999) Magnetic resonance imaging: physical principles and sequence design. John Wiley, Chichester

Hagmann P, Jonasson L, Maeder P et al (2006) Understanding diffusion MR imaging techniques: from scalar diffusion-weighted imaging to diffusion tensor imaging and beyond. Radiographics 26(Suppl 1): S205–S223

Hasan KM, Basser PJ, Parker DL et al (2001) Analytical computation of the eigenvalues and eigenvectors in DT-MRI. J Magn Reson 152: 41–47

Karampinos DC, King KF, Sutton BP et al (2007) In vivo study of cross-sectional skeletal muscle fiber asymmetry with diffusion-weighted MRI. Conf Proc IEEE Eng Med Biol Soc 2007: 327–330

Kauppinen RA (2002) Monitoring cytotoxic tumour treatment response by diffusion magnetic resonance imaging and proton spectroscopy. NMR Biomed 15: 6–17

Kinsey ST, Locke BR, Penke B et al (1999) Diffusional anisotropy is induced by subcellular barriers in skeletal muscle. NMR Biomed 12: 1–7

Latour LL, Svoboda K, Mitra PP et al (1994) Time-dependent diffusion of water in a biological model system. Proc Natl Acad Sci U S A 91: 1229–1233

Le Bihan D (2007) The 'wet mind': water and functional neuroimaging. Phys Med Biol 52: R57–R90

Le Bihan D (2008) Intravoxel incoherent motion perfusion MR imaging: a wake-up call. Radiology 249: 748–752

Le Bihan D, Breton E, Lallemand D et al (1986) MR imaging of intravoxel incoherent motions: application to diffusion and perfusion in neurologic disorders. Radiology 161: 401–407

Le Bihan D, Breton E, Lallemand D et al (1988) Separation of diffusion and perfusion in intravoxel incoherent motion MR imaging. Radiology 168: 497–505

Le Bihan D, Delannoy J, Levin RL (1989) Temperature mapping with MR imaging of molecular diffusion: application to hyperthermia. Radiology 171: 853–857

Le Bihan D, Mangin JF, Poupon C et al (2001) Diffusion tensor imaging: concepts and applications. J Magn Reson Imaging 13: 534–546

Lee JH, Springer CS Jr (2003) Effects of equilibrium exchange on diffusion-weighted NMR signals: the diffusigraphic "shutter-speed". Magn Reson Med 49: 450–458

Manenti G, Carlani M, Mancino S et al (2007) Diffusion tensor magnetic resonance imaging of prostate cancer. Invest Radiol 42: 412–419

Mattiello J, Basser PJ, Le Bihan D (1997) The b matrix in diffusion tensor echo-planar imaging. Magn Reson Med 37: 292–300

Moseley M (2002) Diffusion tensor imaging and aging – a review. NMR Biomed 15: 553–560

Moseley ME, Kucharczyk J, Asgari HS et al (1991) Anisotropy in diffusion-weighted MRI. Magn Reson Med 19: 321–326

Mulkern RV, Zengingonul HP, Robertson RL et al (2000) Multicomponent apparent diffusion coefficients in human brain: relationship to spin-lattice relaxation. Magn Reson Med 44: 292–300

Niendorf T, Dijkhuizen RM, Norris DG et al (1996) Biexponential diffusion attenuation in various states of brain tissue: implications for diffusion-weighted imaging. Magn Reson Med 36: 847–857

Niendorf T, Norris DG, Leibfritz D (1994) Detection of apparent restricted diffusion in healthy rat brain at short diffusion times. Magn Reson Med 32: 672–677

Norris DG (2001a) The effects of microscopic tissue parameters on the diffusion weighted magnetic resonance imaging experiment. NMR Biomed 14: 77–93

Norris DG (2001b) Implications of bulk motion for diffusion-weighted imaging experiments: effects, mechanisms, and solutions. J Magn Reson Imaging 13: 486–495

Norris DG, Niendorf T (1995) Interpretation of DW-NMR data: dependence on experimental conditions. NMR Biomed 8: 280–288

Notohamiprodjo M, Glaser C, Herrmann KA et al (2008) Diffusion tensor imaging of the kidney with parallel imaging: initial clinical experience. Invest Radiol 43: 677–685

Pfeuffer J, Provencher SW, Gruetter R (1999) Water diffusion in rat brain in vivo as detected at very large b values is multicompartmental. MAGMA 8: 98–108

Pipe JG, Farthing V, Forbes KP (2002) Multishot diffusion-weighted FSE using PROPELLER MRI. Magn Reson Med 47: 42–52

Poncelet BP, Wedeen V, Weisskoff RM et al (1992) Brain parenchyma motion: measurement with cine echo-planar MR imaging. Radiology 185: 645–651

Ries M, Jones RA, Basseau F et al (2001) Diffusion tensor MRI of the human kidney. J Magn Reson Imaging 14: 42–49

Rohmer D, Sitek A, Gullberg GT (2007) Reconstruction and visualization of fiber and laminar structure in the normal human heart from ex vivo diffusion tensor magnetic resonance imaging (DTMRI) data. Invest Radiol 42: 777–789

Sinha S, Sinha U (2004) In vivo diffusion tensor imaging of the human prostate. Magn Reson Med 52: 530–537

Sinha S, Sinha U, Edgerton VR (2006) In vivo diffusion tensor imaging of the human calf muscle. J Magn Reson Imaging 24: 182–190

Stejskal EO, Tanner JE (1965) Spin diffusion measurements: spin echoes in the presence of a time-dependent field gradient. J Chem Phys 42: 288–292

Szafer A, Zhong J, Gore JC (1995) Theoretical model for water diffusion in tissues. Magn Reson Med 33: 697–712

Torrey HC (1956) Bloch equations with diffusion terms. Phys Rev 104: 563–565

Turner R, Le Bihan D, Chesnick AS (1991) Echo-planar imaging of diffusion and perfusion. Magn Reson Med 19: 247–253

Westin CF, Maier SE, Mamata H et al (2002) Processing and visualization for diffusion tensor MRI. Med Image Anal 6: 93–108

Wright AC, Bataille H, Ong HH et al (2007) Construction and calibration of a 50 T/m z-gradient coil for quantitative diffusion microimaging. J Magn Reson 186: 17–25

Xing D, Papadakis NG, Huang CL et al (1997) Optimised diffusion-weighting for measurement of apparent diffusion coefficient (ADC) in human brain. Magn Reson Imaging 15: 771–784

Techniques and Optimization

2

David J. Collins and Matthew Blackledge

SUMMARY

In this chapter, we discuss the factors that affect image quality of DW-MRI and practical methods to improve the quality of DW-MR images obtained from clinical scanners. We demonstrate how simple phantoms may be used to improve image quality so that high-quality images can be attained consistently. We review the relative merits of fat-suppression schemes and how these may be applied to different clinical applications. We discuss the optimization of b-values and the number of b-values required for clinical imaging and further illustrate the range of considerations required for these choices. We survey the different data acquisition methods using breath-holding, physiological gating or free breathing, and how the choice of data acquisition method may relate to a particular scanning application. Finally, we provide recommendations to enable the reader to develop their own practical diffusion-weighted imaging protocols in the body.

David J. Collins, MInstP
Matthew Blackledge, MSc
CR UK – EPSARC Cancer Imaging Centre, Institute of Cancer Research & Royal Marsden Hospital, Downs Road, Sutton SM2 5PT, UK

2.1

Introduction

Over the past decade, DW-MRI has been a great success in neurological imaging, particularly for the assessment of acute cerebral vascular events (Bammer et al. 2001; Marks et al. 2008) and in mapping the anatomical cerebral pathways using DTI (Chen et al. 2001; Bammer et al. 2002). DW-MRI has become practical in extracranial applications following the introduction of parallel imaging techniques in the late 1990s (PRUESSMANN et al. 1999; BLAIMER et al. 2004; LARKMAN et al. 2007) and the continued improvements in MR hardware. The use of parallel imaging in combination with diffusion-weighted single-shot echo-planar imaging (EPI) has overcome many of the challenges that have limited its earlier implementation in the body. Although using EPI DW-MRI acquisition and enhanced hardware advances have enabled high-quality DW-MR images in the body to be acquired within a reasonable time frame, a number of challenges still remain.

As is well known, EPI is highly sensitive to static magnetic field inhomogeneity, chemical shift artefacts and eddy currents resulting from the application of the diffusion encoding gradients (LE BIHAN et al. 2006). Physiological motions within the body are an additional challenge and the number and range of diffusion weightings (*b*-values) used within a measurement also require consideration for DW-MRI in the body, which could be tailored for disease evaluation at specific anatomical sites. Methods to overcome, or at least reduce, the impact of a range of artefacts in DW-MRI (e.g. geometric distortion, chemical shift, N/2 ghosting, susceptibility artefacts, G-noise) are required to ensure consistent high-quality images. Many post-processing methods for correcting and eliminating DW-MRI artefacts have been developed for neurological applications (LE BIHAN et al. 2006). However, many of these techniques have failed to deal with the challenges in body DW-MRI.

In this chapter, we discuss the factors that affect the image quality of echo-planar DW-MRI acquisitions. An imaging optimization strategy that can be conducted at any institution to optimize the MR data acquisition to an acceptable level of image artefact and image signal-to-noise is presented. As the process of imaging optimization can be quite complex, it is recommended that this should be done in collaboration with an experienced physicist or vendor application specialist. Clearly, improvements in image quality can also be achieved through post-processing of the DW-MRI data (BODAMMER et al. 2004). However, in clinical practice, DW-MR images enter the radiological workflow immediately after acquisition and therefore acquisition schemes should be as robust as possible. Image post-processing can be very useful but these techniques are largely being developed and used on a research basis. However, such developments may be integrated onto future image-viewing platforms for wider access.

Imaging phantoms are useful devices that can help to test and improve the image quality from DW-MRI

acquisition protocols on clinical MR scanners and we will describe how these could be applied for this purpose. The key factors that affect image signal-to-noise and image artefacts using single-shot echo-planar DW-MRI acquisitions, are discussed alongside how these may be optimized. Breath-hold, free-breathing and physiologically gated DW-MR imaging techniques in the body are reviewed, highlighting the advantages and disadvantages of each method.

2.2
Factors that Affect Image Quality Using EPI DW-MRI Acquisition

There are many factors that affect image quality in an EPI DW-MRI image acquisition scheme. These can be divided into factors that influence image signal-to-noise and artefacts.

2.2.1
Image Signal-to-Noise (SNR)

DW-MR images are inherently noisy because of the EPI technique and range of signal attenuating gradients used for image acquisition, and hence the image signal-to-noise should be optimized. The following factors can be adjusted to improve image signal-to-noise: matrix size (smaller), echo-time (shorter), number of signal average (higher), section thickness (increase), receiver bandwidth (optimized), parallel imaging (optimized) and choice of fat-suppression scheme.

2.2.2
Image Artefacts

These include motion, chemical shift artefacts, eddy currents effects, N/2 ghosting, susceptibility artefacts and G-noise. Motion can cause image blurring, spin dephasing and signal loss on DW-MRI. Chemical shift artefact can result from the misregistration of the fat and water signal when the protons imaged in the same voxel result in a "banding" artefact. Eddy currents (residual gradient fields) are formed in the presence of a changing magnetic field, i.e. when gradients are rapidly turned on and off as in EPI. This results in geometric distortion and misaligned images with the appearance of "shearing", "translational" and "scaling" (magnification) artefacts. N/2 ghosting artefact results from phase errors due to a phase difference between each echo acquisition during readout, and is seen as a repeated image "ghost" throughout the image in the phase-encode direction. Susceptibility artefact occurs due to $T2'$ relaxation as a result of inhomogeneities in the main magnetic field, which is accentuated in EPI because of the small bandwidth (BW) per pixel. Last but not least, G-noise results from the use of parallel imaging, which results from noise already inherent in the data being amplified during parallel imaging reconstruction.

Bulk Diffusion Phantoms

Appropriate phantoms are useful for DW-MRI optimization as they enable quantitative assessment of artefacts and distortions. Phantoms are also being widely applied for evaluating the accuracy of the diffusion encoding b-factor on clinical and research MR scanners.

A range of materials including water, alkanes, sucrose and copper sulphate solutions, are suitable for use as diffusion phantoms on clinical MR systems (TOFTS et al. 2000; PADHANI et al. 2009). At our institution, we have made extensive use of different phantoms containing polydimethylsiloxane (PDMS), ice water and sucrose solutions to evaluate the performance of MR systems.

PDMS is a viscoelastic material that can be considered non-diffusing because of its high molecular weight and viscosity (PRICE 1998). This enables DW-MRI protocols to be evaluated using a phantom containing PDMS in a quantitative manner without having to account for the effects of diffusion. Water is non-toxic and readily available but its diffusion properties are temperature-dependent, its diffusion rates being higher than in tissues at body temperature and it also has a longer relaxation time compared with tissues. One way of minimizing variations is to use ice water that is held at a constant temperature of about 0°C such that the diffusion measurement data are constant (insensitive to the ambient temperatures in the scanner) over repeat measurements (PADHANI et al. 2009). In addition, the diffusivity of water at 0° is about $1.12 \times 10^{-3}\,mm^2/s$, which is in the range found in human tissues. For these reasons, a phantom made out of ice water is highly suitable for quality assurance and b-value calibrations. Another material that can be used to measure diffusivity is sucrose, which is more viscous than water. Sucrose phantoms are highly stable and can be manufactured, depending on their solution concentration, to obtain a wide range of diffusivities and are thus also suitable for quality-assurance procedures. Sucrose phantoms are usually scanned at room temperature. However, sucrose phantoms are temperature-sensitive and the results may thus differ if the ambient room temperature varies between measurements.

2.3.1
Optimizing Image Quality Using a Phantom

EPI data acquisitions are highly sensitive to static field inhomogeneity, causing geometric distortions in the phase-encoding direction. These distortions are proportional to the ratio of the field of view and the image acquisition receiver BW. This relationship would suggest that the DW-MR images should be acquired with the minimum field of view and the highest BW possible. However, in practice it is found that increasing the imaging BW (reducing the inter-echo spacing of the EPI readout) introduces and increases an artefact known as N/2 ghosting (formally Nyquist ghosting), as demonstrated in Fig. 2.1. N/2 ghosts arise from a number of factors including gradient switching timing errors, residual eddy currents which are b-value-dependent (increases with b-values) and non-linearity in the low pass filters. These factors are highly scanner-dependent and hence need to be individualized for each scanner and acquisition protocol used, as factors such as imaging field of view, the choice of b-values and the receiver BW all contribute to the magnitude of both the geometric distortion and N/2 ghosting.

In practice the magnitude of these effects can be quantified using a suitable phantom. PDMS is well suited for these evaluations as subtraction images obtained from a number of images obtained with and without diffusion weighting can be used to establish the magnitude of N/2 ghosts and eddy current induced geometric distortions over a range of different experimental conditions including alterations in the receiver BWs (Fig. 2.1). One possible optimization strategy would be to establish a balance between the magnitude of N/2 ghosting and the geometric distortions. To do this, a number of measurements are performed with a fixed b-value (typically the largest b-value employed in the measurement protocol) on the PDMS phantom with varying BWs, whilst measuring the magnitude of the distortions by recording

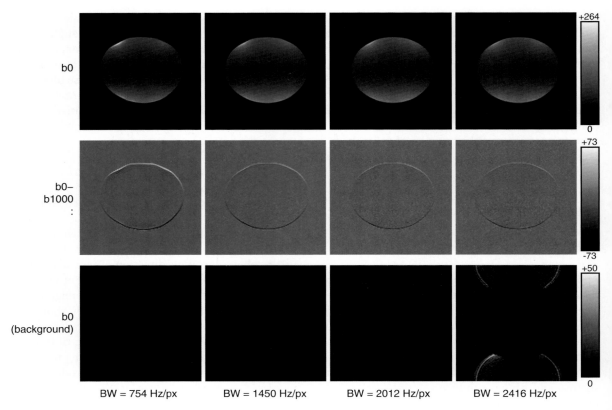

Fig. 2.1. *Top*: $b = 0 \, \text{s/mm}^2$ ($b0$) images of a polydimethylsiloxane (PDMS) phantom taken at different readout bandwidths (BWs) (displayed at bottom in Hertz per pixel, Hz/px) using a Stejskal–Tanner DW-MRI pulse sequence. *Middle*: Difference of $b0$ and $b = 1000 \, \text{s/mm}^2$ ($b1, 000$) images at the respective BWs. *Bottom*: Background $b0$ images of the phantom. It is clear from the difference images that distortions due to eddy currents at high b-values are reduced at higher BWs but N/2 ghosting on the background images also increases as BW increases

displacements in the difference images of the phantom. Figure 2.1 illustrates that as the BW is increased, the magnitude of the displacements observed on the subtraction images is reduced. Measurements in a fixed region of interest outside of the phantom can be used to measure the magnitude of the N/2 ghosting. In general, a readout BW value can be determined, which reduces the magnitude of the distortion to an acceptable level of ±1 px with a ghosting magnitude of less than 10%. If this cannot be achieved, it may be necessary to reduce the magnitude of the b-value until this is attained. This process can be repeated by independently applying the b-factor in all three orthogonal magnet axes, to determine whether there is any directional dependency in the gradient performance. It is not uncommon for one gradient direction to perform less well compared to the other encoding directions, and this axis may thus limit the maximum b-factors that can be employed in an imaging

protocol using orthogonal diffusion gradient encoding. A similar optimization process can be performed for other diffusion gradient encoding methods (e.g. tetrahedral encoding or three-scan trace approach), parallel imaging factors or the types of parallel imaging applied (Fig. 2.2).

A major advantage of applying parallel imaging to single-shot DW-MRI is the reduction in the echo-train length of the EPI readout. This in turn reduces the number of phase encoding steps which brings substantial benefits to the DW-MRI measurement as it reduces the magnitude of ghosting in the phase encoding direction and enables a reduction in the minimum echo-time achievable by the measurement. This, in turn, helps to maintain image quality and image signal-to-noise. The advantages of applying parallel imaging (e.g. using GeneRalized Autocalibrating Partially Parallel Acquisitions or GRAPPA) are shown in Fig. 2.2. We have evaluated a number of parallel

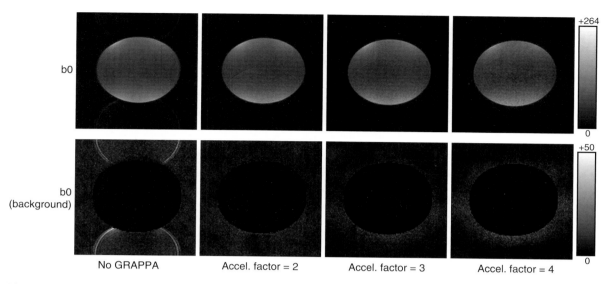

b0

b0
(background)

No GRAPPA   Accel. factor = 2   Accel. factor = 3   Accel. factor = 4

Fig. 2.2. *Top*: $b = 0\,\text{s/mm}^2$ (*b0*) images of a PDMS phantom acquired using a readout BW of 2,416 Hz/pixel and utilizing parallel imaging technique known as generalized autocalibrating partially parallel acquisitions (GRAPPA) at various acceleration factors. *Bottom*: Background *b0* images of the phantom. It can be seen that using GRAPPA reduces the magnitude of N/2 ghosting observed on the background image. There does not seem to be any additional advantage in this case of using acceleration factors greater than 2 and it can be seen that the signal-to-noise and noise heterogeneity worsen when acceleration factors of 3 or 4 are used

imaging techniques (Sensivity Encoding SENSE, mSENSE and GRAPPA) employed in DW-MRI and all methods have demonstrated improvements in the DW-MR image quality.

In clinical studies, it is usually advantageous to apply reduced phased encoding steps in the direction requiring the least volume coverage. For example, in axial acquisition of the body, this would be in the anterior–posterior (AP) direction. In general, a successful strategy to high-quality DW-MRI using EPI technique is to reduce both the echo-time and the number of phase-encoding steps to the minimum for the clinical studies. However, it must also be remembered that parallel imaging itself does reduce the signal-to-noise by a factor proportional to √(parallel imaging acceleration factor) and also changes the distribution of both noise and ghosting artefacts within the image. However, as the application of parallel imaging allows shortening of the echo-time and echo-train length, these help to improve the overall image quality. Nevertheless, a poor choice of imaging field of view and parallel imaging acceleration factor can result in additional noise and artefacts within the image. Detailed discussions of the various implementations of parallel imaging are beyond the scope of this chapter although the interested reader is directed to an excellent review by Blaimer et al. 2004. It is important

to mention that when applying parallel imaging techniques (e.g. GRAPPA) that allow the user to specify the number of reference scan lines, this should be checked to establish that sufficient reference lines are specified to minimize image ghosting.

A number of measurement-specific methods have been developed to reduce the effect of eddy-current-induced distortions, the most effective of which have been the following: (a) simultaneous application of diffusion encoding gradients in more than one direction, implemented on clinical scanners as tetrahedral encoding or three-scan trace approaches and (b) the use of the twice refocused spin-echo with diffusion weighting (Alexander et al. 1997; Koch et al. 2000; Reese et al. 2003).

The application of simultaneous diffusion-weighted encoding gradients results in a reduction in both the magnitude and rate of change of diffusion encoding gradients as the vector sum of the applied gradients creates the required *b*-value. This can significantly improve image quality by reducing the magnitude of eddy currents. An additional benefit of using a simultaneous gradient application scheme is the ability to reduce the measurement echo-time to a minimum. The minimum echo-time achievable at clinical DW-MRI may be proportional to the magnitude of the diffusion-weighting *b*-value applied, as most gradient

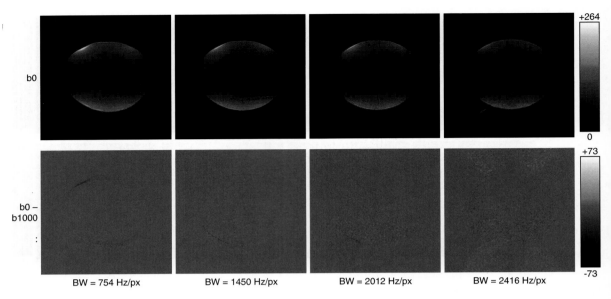

Fig. 2.3. *Top*: $b = 0\,s/mm^2$ (b0) images of a PDMS phantom taken at different readout BWs acquired using the double spin-echo (DSE) DW-MRI pulse sequence. *Bottom*: Difference of b0 and $b = 1,000\,s/mm^2$ (b1,000) images at the respective BWs (displayed at *bottom* in Hertz per pixel, Hz/px).

There is a clear improvement in the eddy current distortion across all BWs compared to the Stejskal–Tanner DW-MRI pulse sequence (Fig. 2.1) as observed from the difference images. However, the effects of N/2 ghosting are worse using higher BW = 2,416 Hz/px

systems operate at the maximum possible slew rate. Thus, an increase in *b*-values may necessitate increasing either the duration of the applied gradient or the time delay between diffusion encoding gradients; both of these will lead to longer echo times (KINGSLEY 2006). A reduction in the echo-time at DW-MRI can be highly advantageous in tissues with short T2 relaxation times such as the liver by maintaining good image signal-to-noise.

The twice-refocused spin-echo technique is very effective in cancelling the effects of eddy currents (Figs. 2.3 and 2.4). Briefly, the diffusion encoding gradients normally employed in a standard Stejskal–Tanner DW-MRI measurement scheme are split by the introduction of a 180° refocusing pulse. In the twice-refocused spin echo implementation, the diffusion encoding gradients are applied in reverse polarity around each RF pulse thereby cancelling the eddy currents which are set up by the diffusion encoding gradients applied in the opposite direction. The net result of the application of these four diffusion-encoding gradients is substantial reduction of eddy currents during the EPI readout (ALEXANDER et al. 1997; KOCH et al. 2000; REESE et al. 2003). The twice-refocused spin-echo method can be combined with the three-scan trace or tetrahedral diffusion-

weighted encoding scheme to further reduce the effects of eddy currents in the measurement. By using such a combination of approaches, diffusion-weighting factors employing *b*-values $>1,000\,s/mm^2$ can be applied over relatively large field of view for DW-MRI studies with minimal geometric distortion. In our experience, a maximum pixel displacement of 2 mm or less can be achieved when imaging is performed using a relatively large field of view (400 mm) with a well-optimized imaging protocol.

As the information gained from phantom studies can be very helpful towards the understanding and optimization of a DW-MRI technique, we have found it advantageous to initially test new imaging protocols on phantoms prior to volunteer or patient studies.

2.4

Optimizing Image Quality on Volunteer or Patient Studies

Phantom studies are useful to check diffusion gradient performance on MR scanners and to quantify image signal-to-noise, image ghosting and geometric

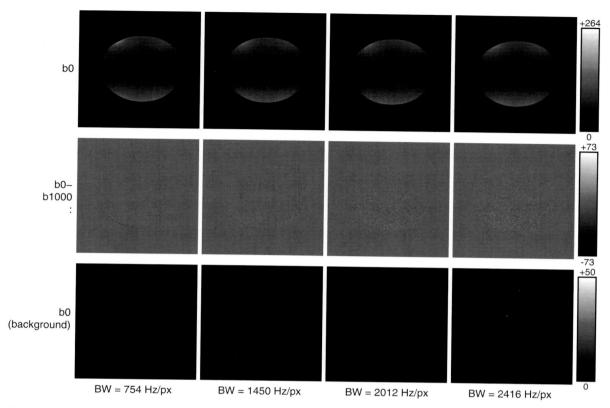

Fig. 2.4. Top: $b = 0 \, \text{s/mm}^2$ ($b0$) images of a PDMS phantom acquired using both DSE and parallel imaging GRAPPA at acceleration factor 2. *Middle*: Difference of $b0$ and $b = 1,000 \, \text{s/mm}^2$ ($b1,000$) images. *Bottom*: Background $b0$ images of the phantom. Using both GRAPPA and DSE techniques, both N/2 ghosting and eddy current distortion artefacts have been reduced over the range of imaging BWs (displayed at *bottom* in Hertz per pixel, Hz/px)

distortion. However, there are other factors that come into play that have a major effect on the quality of DW-MRI studies that cannot be adequately or reliably addressed using a phantom. For these, volunteer and/or patient studies are required.

2.4.1
Fat Suppression

Eliminating signals from the methylene resonances in fat is an essential requirement in DW-MRI body applications. Fat signals produce significant artefacts in EPI in general but can be particularly pronounced in EPI DW-MRI as a result of a lower rate of signal attenuation in fat on DW-MR imaging compared to other tissues. Signal arising from protons associated with fat typically has a resonant frequency difference of 220 Hz from protons associated with water at 1.5 T and significantly lower diffusion rates than tissue

water. Water and fat signals arising from the same pixel location will appear within the same pixel provided that the pixel BW is greater than the fat–water chemical shift of 220 Hz. In EPI DW-MRI experiments, the BW per pixel in the phase-encoding direction is substantially less than the chemical shift difference of fat and water: the typical pixel BWs for single-shot EPI are 10–30 Hz in the phase-encoding direction. As a result, unsuppressed fat signals in EPI DW-MRI appear as high signal intensity ghosting through the image. Ghosting artefacts arising from fat–water chemical shift can be displaced by 10–15 pixels from their source location. The typical pixel dimensions for DW-MRI in the body are 2–4 mm, and the chemical shift ghosting artefact observed can therefore be distant from the source of the artefact by distances ranging from 2 to 6 cm. These chemical shift artefacts can propagate further ghosting artefacts as a result of N/2 induced ghosting. It is therefore of great importance to evaluate and optimize the performance of fat suppression techniques for DW-MRI applications in the body.

It is a great credit to the equipment designers and vendors that modern clinical MR machines are able to suppress fat signals very effectively over very large fields of view. Nevertheless, it is still essential that the quality of fat suppression is checked and optimized on a per-protocol and per-scanner basis. The choice of fat suppression technique used in part depends on the ability of the scanner to optimize the B0 field homogeneity over relatively large fields of view. This in turn, is influenced by the magnitude of the static field strength, the presence or absence of adjustable higher-order shimming currents and the shimming technique employed. Other factors that are important include the BW of the fat suppression pulses, as well as the accuracy and efficiency of the inversion pulses. Fat suppression techniques that are routinely employed on clinical scanners include water only excitation, chemical fat suppression (frequency selective fat excitation and magnetization spoiling), STIR (short-tau inversion recovery) and SPAIR (spectral selection attenuated inversion recovery). STIR and SPAIR are inversion-recovery-based techniques.

In our experience, the SPAIR method works well in nearly all circumstances across different vendors' platforms except when the field of view is very large (>25 cm in major magnet axis) or when there is a significant transition in the normal anatomy (e.g. at the interphase of the shoulders/neck and pelvis/legs). In these cases, conventional inversion recovery fat suppression techniques are recommended, and may be preferred in whole-body DW-MRI examinations. For whole-body DW-MRI, a further advantage of using the inversion recovery techniques is that imaging of multiple image stations can be conducted at the same resonant frequency (Li et al. 2007) following initial station specific shimming, which helps to overcome station-to-station misregistrations that frequently occur in whole-body DW-MRI. A 20–30 Hz difference of the water resonance following shimming at each imaging station for whole-body DW-MRI can result in a geometric shift of at least one or two pixels in the phase-encoding direction. Resonant frequency shifts of 1–2 ppm following shimming are not uncommon particularly in the head and neck region. However, the disadvantages of using inversion recovery prepared DW-MRI protocols are the increased measurement time, altered T1 contrast on the b0 image and reduced signal-to-noise as the full longitudinal magnetization is no longer available.

2.4.2
Single-Shot Acquisition vs. Multiple Signals Averaging

Clearly, a major problem with imaging in the body is physiological motion. The major advantage of single-shot DW-MRI is that the image data is acquired within 60–100 ms, thereby effectively freezing motion in any given image. The challenge to performing DW-MRI in the body is to acquire DW-MR images of different b-values sufficient for ADC quantification from the same image location within a single measurement time. There are three acquisition methods that are in use to address this challenge.

The first is to acquire all the DW-MRI data required for an ADC calculation in a breath-hold using a single-shot EPI technique. Clearly this limits the number of b-values and/or the number of signal averages that can be accommodated in a breath-hold for ADC calculation and the anatomical coverage that can be achieved. A significant limitation is that the DW-MRI data are inherently noisy and the signal-to-noise is reduced exponentially with increasing b-values. Breath-hold data are therefore signal-to-noise-limited and the ADC estimates will have larger uncertainty.

The second method is to acquire DW-MRI data with multiple averaging with some form of physiological triggering. For respiratory motion, a navigator is typically used at the diaphragm, and this may be combined with cardiac triggering. The two main problems with this approach are poor measurement efficiency and that the navigator does not entirely eliminate motion-induced artefacts as it normally has an acceptance window of the order of the slice thickness. In addition, the liver is an elastic organ and will not necessarily deform in a consistent manner during the course of the DW-MRI measurement. Despite these issues, navigator-controlled DW-MRI with multiple averaging is an effective and robust technique when well-implemented.

The final option is to acquire DW-MRI data in free-breathing with multiple b-values and averages. The advantage of this approach is the high efficiency of data acquisition and increased coverage that can be achieved in a similar imaging time compared with DW-MRI measurements with physiological gating. DW-MR images are averaged in image space where only the magnitude of the image data is used. Motions occurring during imaging results in a phase shift in the complex image data and by discarding the phase information during averaging, the effects of motion on the resultant image are reduced. The important question is how much averaged data is required to obtain an ADC estimate with comparable accuracy and repeatability as a breath-hold study. Based on our observations, a factor of six provides similar ADC estimates with improved repeatability over breath-hold studies. Suggested clinical DW-MRI protocols are presented in Table 2.1.

2.5
Optimization Strategies for the Selection of *b*-Values

While DW-MRI is being applied in the body to evaluate non-oncological and oncological conditions, it is the oncological application of the technique that is being widely investigated. In particular, there is growing interest in the development of DW-MRI as a potential biomarker for the assessment of tumour response to treatment.

When developing DW-MRI protocols for evaluating cancers, it is important to consider the choice of *b*-values so that the resulting images provide the most accurate information. The optimization processes depend in part on whether DW-MRI is used as a qualitative tool to provide image contrast between diseased and normal tissue, or the technique is applied primarily to quantify the diffusivity of the tissue by means of calculating the ADC. Hence, we will discuss *b*-value optimization along two lines: *quantitative* (ADC maps) and *qualitative* (anatomical diffusion-weighted images). This section briefly outlines the optimization strategies that may be applied in each case, taking into account the fundamental considerations. We will also illustrate these with clinical examples.

In all cases, a clear knowledge of the relationship between image signal intensity and *b*-value (STEJSKAL et al. 1965) is essential:

$$S(b) = S(0)e^{-bD}. \qquad (2.1)$$

When DW-MRI is performed at a particular *b*-value, the relation of the measured signal intensity $S(b)$ with other parameters is as shown in the equation where D is the apparent diffusion coefficient of the tissue (mm^2/s) and b is the *b*-value (s/mm^2). $S(0)$ is the signal intensity of the tissue when $b = 0\,s/mm^2$. The equation has two unknown quantities, namely D and $S(0)$, such that at least two DW-MRI measurements using different *b*-values will be required to estimate D.

2.5.1
Quantitative Data

Statistical noise is an inherent characteristic in all MR images and efforts should be made to reduce its presence as far as possible. In the calculation of ADC maps, image noise causes errors in the ADC estimates and so it is important to choose *b*-values which will minimize the effects of noise. A simple approach is to use error propagation to derive an expression for the standard deviation in ADC calculations from N independent *b*-values (BITO et al. 1995);

$$\sigma_D = \frac{D_0}{SNR_0} \times \sqrt{\frac{\sum_n (b_n N - \sum_n b_n)^2 e^{2b_n D_0}}{N \sum_n b_n^2 - (\sum_n b_n)^2}}. \qquad (2.2)$$

Here, D_0 represents the true ADC of the tissue and SNR_0 is the signal-to-noise ratio of a *single* $b = 0\,s/mm^2$ image. Minimization of this function with respect to b_n then provides the optimum set of *b*-values. It may be shown (BITO et al. 1995) that for the case of a single D_0, the ideal sequence consists of n image acquisitions at $b = 0$ and m acquisitions at some other *b*-value which may be found by numerically solving;

$$e^{2bD_0}(bD_0 - 1) = \frac{m}{n}(m + n = N). \qquad (2.3)$$

Furthermore, if the function is optimized with respect to m/n then;

$$\frac{m}{n} \approx 3 \quad \text{and} \quad bD_0 \approx 1.25. \qquad (2.4)$$

An important consideration is that prior knowledge of the D_0 values is required in all calculations. Such information could be obtained from previous reports or if direct measurement is needed then a range of *b*-values (e.g. $0-1,000\,s/mm^2$) should be used so that at least one is near optimum. When a distribution of D_0 is encountered, the mean value should provide a reasonable approximation.

To demonstrate the processes involved in this optimization scheme consider the test case shown in Fig. 2.5. A patient with liver metastases from colorectal cancer has been scanned using six *b*-values from 0 to $750\,s/mm^2$ and regions of interest have been hand-drawn around four index lesions, each measuring $>2\,cm$ in diameter, on the b-$750\,s/mm^2$ images. Using all of the *b*-values, the ADC map was generated

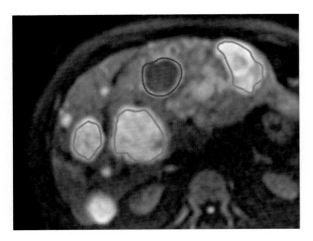

Fig. 2.5. A $b = 750 \, \text{s/mm}^2$ image of a patient with multiple colorectal metastases in the liver. Regions of interest have been drawn around four index lesions with a largest diameter greater than 2 cm. Note the dark central signal intensity of the lesion with a *red outline* due to central necrosis. This lesion returned a high ADC (not shown) and thus can bias the calculation of the optimum b-value for imaging

and voxel-wise ADC values from all ROIs were exported for analysis in a statistics software package. The mean ADC value from all voxel ADC values was calculated to be $1.54 \times 10^{-3} \, \text{mm}^2/\text{s}$ suggesting that the optimum single b-value for use in this study was:

$$b = \frac{1.25}{D_0} \Rightarrow b = 814 \, \text{s/mm}^2$$

In practice, however, it would be rare for a scanner to achieve any arbitrary b-value and so this value should be rounded to the nearest whole value possible. As an example we would say that b-values of 800 or 850 s/mm^2 would be optimal in this test case. It is noticed in Fig. 2.1 that one of the lesions (outlined in red) is necrotic and has a higher ADC than the others. The implications of this are that the mean ADC is increased when including the necrotic tumour and so the optimum b-value calculated may be too low for the other non-necrotic metastases (which have a mean ADC in this example of $1.25 \times 10^{-3} \, \text{mm}^2/\text{s}$). It may be worthwhile considering whether a tailored optimization to a specific tissue is needed or whether a slightly less optimized but global solution is preferred as has been presented here.

Once the optimization calculations are complete, tests can be conducted to check that the optimum b-value has been approximated. A useful approach is to plot frequency histograms of the voxel ADC data calculated using the $b = 0 \, \text{s/mm}^2$ image and each individual b-value in the imaging range, as well as all b-values within the imaging range. It is important to normalize the histograms from each ROI (i.e. divide by the number of voxels) before consolidating them into a single population histogram. The plots in our example are as shown in Fig. 2.6. From these data it is clear that as the optimum b-value is approached ($\sim 900 \, \text{s/mm}^2$) the ADC histogram more closely resembles the ADC profile with the narrowest distribution obtained using all b-values in the range between 0 and $750 \, \text{s/mm}^2$ suggesting an improvement in the accuracy of ADC measurement.

In some circumstances it may be necessary to consider including T2 dependence into the optimization (Jones et al. 1999) and also the form of the noise distribution in the optimization calculations (Saritas et al. 2007). The mathematics governing these methods is beyond the scope of this chapter but may need to be taken into account when the tissue T2 values are short (roughly <60 ms) (Saritas et al. 2008) or the SNR_0 is low (roughly <6) (Gudbjartsson et al. 1995). It should also be mentioned that parallel imaging, which is now routinely applied in diffusion imaging to improve spatial integrity, introduces a problem in the above discussion as SNR_0 is no longer homogeneous throughout the image. However, signal-to-noise estimation based on the ratio between mean lesion signal and the standard deviation of pixel values within a region of interest drawn over a large background area may be adopted when parallel imaging is employed.

2.5.2
Qualitative Data

The acquisition of high b-value images in the body is now possible due to the advances in gradient technology and the development of strategies to improve imaging artefacts. DW-MRI in the body, using b-values as high as $1{,}000 \, \text{s/mm}^2$ is now being applied to provide contrast between lesions and background tissue for tumour localization (Kwee et al. 2008). However, at these high values the signal-to-noise ratio decreases exponentially and it is thus important to find optimum b-values that provide a compromise between tissue contrast and signal-to-noise.

A relationship has been described for finding the b-value which maximizes the contrast between two homogeneous tissues with apparent diffusion coefficients of D_1 and D_2 at $b = 0 \, \text{s/mm}^2$. The definition of

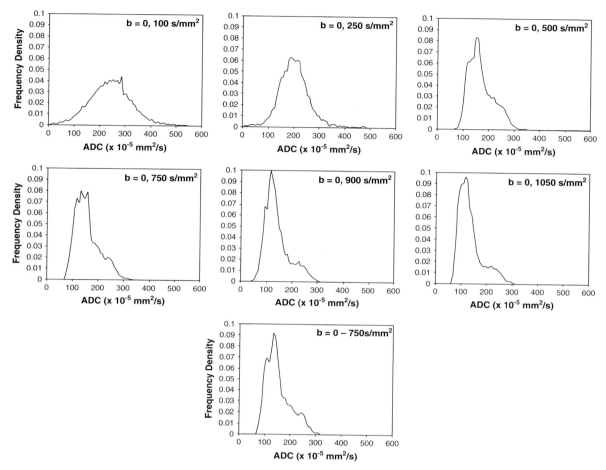

Fig. 2.6. Frequency density histograms of ADC values calculated for the four tumour volumes shown in Fig. 2.5 using b = 0 s/mm² and each of the other b-values (b = 100, 250, 500, 750, 900 and 1,050 s/mm²). The distribution is narrowest and most closely resembles the ADC histograms calculated using all b-values (*bottom*) at the b-value of 900 s/mm² indicating the least error ADC in calculations

contrast that can be applied is known as the Michelson contrast and is defined as:

$$C_{1,2} = \frac{L_1 - L_2}{L_{max} + L_{min}} \qquad (2.5)$$

where L_{max} and L_{min} repesent the maximum and minimum "lightness" in the image respectively as perceived by the observer. We will assume that the minimum lightness of the image is black ($L_{min} = 0$), the image contrast is stretched such that L_{max} is as high as can be for a given viewing monitor and that there is a linear relationship between the lightness of tissue i and signal intensity as defined by (2.1);

$$L_i(b) = k\, S_i(0) e^{-b D_i} \quad k = \text{constant} \qquad (2.6)$$

The Michelson contrast may then be written as:

$$C_{1,2} = \frac{k\, S_1(0) e^{-b D_1} - k\, S_2(0) e^{-b D_2}}{L_{max}} \qquad (2.7)$$

The standard approach is then to assume that L_{max} remains constant in all images (i.e. it is independent of b-value) and that the maximization of the contrast is achieved by differentiation with respect to "b" and equating to 0:

$$b_{opt} = \frac{\ln(D_1 / D_2) + \ln(S_1(0)/S_2(0))}{D_1 - D_2} \qquad (2.8)$$

If $S_1(0)$ is approximately equal to $S_2(0)$ then we have (KINGSLEY 2006)

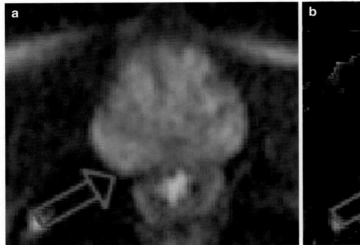
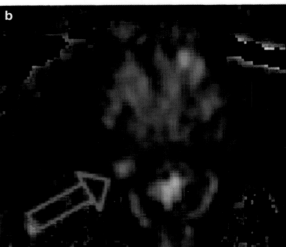

Fig. 2.7. (a) An acquired $b = 1,000\,s/mm^2$ image of the prostate. It is very difficult to distinguish the focus of prostate carcinoma (*red arrow*) from healthy tissue on this b-value image due to the high signal intensity of the normal peripheral zone. (b) A computed $b = 2,000\,s/mm^2$ image of the same region shows clearly the focus of high signal intensity prostate cancer

$$b_{opt} = \frac{\ln D_1 - \ln D_2}{D_1 - D_2} \qquad (2.9)$$

which may be applied as a reasonable approximation in most circumstances.

As an example of this optimization procedure, the mean ADC for a region of background liver from the previous section was found to be $D_2 = 1.38 \times 10^{-3}\,mm^2/s$. Applying this to Equation 7 along with the ADC value for the liver metastases excluding necrotic regions ($D_1 = 1.25 \times 10^{-3}\,mm^2/s$), gives us $b_{opt} = 761\,s/mm^2$. Figure 2.5 shows an image acquired using $b = 750\,s/mm^2$ where the metastases are clearly visible against the background liver tissue. In this way, the choice of b-value can be optimized for the detection of tissue within a certain ADC value range.

We finish this section with some thoughts regarding the choice of whether to acquire data using b-values that optimize ADC accuracy or b-values that optimize image contrast. From a diagnostic point of view it is clearly advantageous to have superior contrast between diseased and healthy tissue. It may be argued, therefore, that the total scanning time should be used to acquire the maximum possible number of signal averages at a single optimized b-value to improve the signal-to-noise ratio. However, it is our belief that wherever possible, images should be acquired with the intent of calculating ADC values. The estimated ADC may then be substituted into the Stejskal–Tanner relationship enabling the computation of images at *any* desired b-value providing the clinician with an increased degree of freedom to adjust image contrast. Furthermore, the signal-to-noise ratio is improved this way as noise decreases with increasing b-value, and high b-value images which are difficult to achieve using commercial scanners due to large image distortions may be simulated with ease (BLACKLEDGE 2009). Figure 2.7 shows an example where extrapolating a computed image out to $b = 2,000\,s/mm^2$ revealed the presence of a cancer within the prostate that was not observed on the acquired $b = 1,000\,s/mm^2$ image. The use of computed b-value images will be a welcomed development in the future.

2.6 Summary of Technique Optimization for DW-MRI in the Body

In summary, DW-MR imaging in the body can be optimized to improve image quality and minimize artefacts using phantoms and patient/volunteer studies. DW-MRI phantoms can provide quality assurance and also be used for sequence optimization. For sequence optimization, it is advantageous to reduce the phase-encoding field of view to the minimum required for a given measurement acquisition. The receiver BW should be adjusted to minimize geometric distortion and image ghosting. Parallel imaging should be applied to reduce the length of the EPI readout. Where possible, the lowest possible echo-time achievable for any given DW-MRI measurement protocol should be used. Where

Table 2.1. Examples of currently used imaging protocols for free-breathing, axial, single-shot DW-EPI with tetrahedral encoding

	Abdomen	Pelvis LFOV	Pelvis SFOV
Field of View (mm)	380	380	220-280
RFOV	80	80	80
No of Slices	26-33	40-48	18
Slice Thickness (mm)	6-7	6	5
Slice Gap (mm)	10%	10%	10%
Matrix	104-112/256	104-112/256	112/256
Foldover Direction	AP	AP	AP
TE (ms)	66-70	66	66-70
TR (ms)	5000	5600-7400	2500-3100
PI factor	2	2	2
Fat Sat	SPAIR	IR/SPAIR	SPAIR
EPI Factor	59-104	59-104	75-112
Signal Averages	4-5	4	4-8
Bandwidth (Hz/Px)	1800	1800	1800
b – values (s/mm^2)	0,100,500,750	0,900	0,300,750
Acquisition time	4.5 minutes	2.5 minutes	3 minutes

available, simultaneous diffusion gradient application schemes or double spin-echo (DSE) acquisition techniques should be considered, to reduce eddy-current-induced geometric distortion.

The use of at least two b-values is recommended for DW-MRI measurements, the higher b-value could be optimized for image contrast or ADC accuracy as discussed in the chapter. Multiple b-values, which include lower (≤ 100 s/mm^2) and higher b-values (>100 s/mm^2) could be applied if ADC calculation is the primary purpose for the DW-MRI study, especially when fractionation of the ADC calculation (perfusion sensitive vs. perfusion insensitive) or bi-exponential fitting of the data is desired (see Chap. 1).

When performing DW-MRI in the body, multiple averaging techniques provide better signal-to-noise. Navigator-triggered acquisitions can be applied in the thorax or upper abdomen. If physiological triggering is not possible or practical, multiple signal averaging with multiple b-values in shallow free-breathing are also robust. Breath-hold DW-MRI studies, although quick to perform, have lower signal-to-noise and offer limited coverage in terms of range of b-values employed and the volume of coverage.

When applying fat-suppression schemes, SPAIR is the fat saturation method of choice over small fields of view (less than 20 cm in the magnet z-orientation). The use of STIR for fat suppression is usually applied over larger fields of view such as in whole-body imaging (DWIBS). STIR fat suppression is also preferred in head and neck region and in the upper thorax.

References

Alexander AL, Tsuruda JS, Parker DL (1997) Elimination of eddy current artifacts in diffusion-weighted echo-planar images: the use of bipolar gradients. Magn Reson Med 38:1016–1021

Bammer R, Auer M, Keeling SL et al (2002) Diffusion tensor imaging using single-shot SENSE-EPI. Magn Reson Med 48:128–136

Bammer R, Keeling SL, Augustin M et al (2001) Improved diffusion-weighted single-shot echo-planar imaging (EPI) in stroke using sensitivity encoding (SENSE). Magn Reson Med 46:548–554

Bito Y, Hirata S, Yamamoto E (1995) Optimum gradient factors for apparent diffusion coefficient measurements. Proc Intl Soc Mag Reson Med 913

Blackledge M, Wilton B, et al (2009). "Computed Diffusion Weighted Imaging (cDWI) for Improving Imaging Contrast." Proc. Intl. Soc. Mag. Reson. Med.: 4005.

Blaimer M, Breuer F, Mueller M et al (2004) SMASH, SENSE, PILS, GRAPPA: how to choose the optimal method. Top Magn Reson Imaging 15:223–236

Bodammer N, Kaufmann J, Kanowski M et al (2004) Eddy current correction in diffusion-weighted imaging using pairs of images acquired with opposite diffusion gradient polarity. Magn Reson Med 51:188–193

Chen ZG, Li TQ, Hindmarsh T (2001) Diffusion tensor trace mapping in normal adult brain using single-shot EPI technique. A methodological study of the aging brain. Acta Radiol 42:447–458

Gudbjartsson H, Patz S (1995) The Rician distribution of noisy MRI data. Reson Med 34:910–914

Jones DK, Horsfield MA, Simmons A (1999) Optimal strategies for measuring diffusion in anisotropic systems by magnetic resonance imaging. Magn Reson Med 42:515–525

Kingsley PB (2006a) Introduction to diffusion tensor imaging mathematics: part II. Anisotropy, diffusion-weighting factors, and gradient encoding schemes. Concepts Magn Reson A 28A:123–254.

Kingsley PB (2006b) Introduction to diffusion tensor imaging mathematics: part III. Tensor calculation, noise, simulations, and optimization. Concepts Magn Reson A 28A:155–179

Koch M, Norris DG (2000) An assessment of eddy current sensitivity and correction in single-shot diffusion-weighted imaging. Phys Med Biol 45:3821–3832

Kwee TC, Takahara T, Ochiai R et al (2008) Diffusion-weighted whole-body imaging with background body signal suppression (DW-MRIBS): features and potential applications in oncology. Eur Radiol 18:1937–1952

Larkman DJ, Nunes RG (2007) Parallel magnetic resonance imaging. Phys Med Biol 52:R15–R55

Le Bihan D, Poupon C, Amadon A et al (2006) Artifacts and pitfalls in diffusion MRI. J Magn Reson Imaging. 24:478–488

Li S, Sun F, Jin ZY et al (2007) Whole-body diffusion-weighted imaging: technical improvement and preliminary results. J Magn Reson Imaging 26:1139–1144

Marks MP, Olivot JM, Kemp S et al (2008) Patients with acute stroke treated with intravenous tPA 3–6 hours after stroke onset: correlations between MR angiography findings and perfusion- and diffusion-weighted imaging in the DEFUSE study. Radiology 249:614–623

Padhani AR, Liu G, Mu-Koh D et al (2009) Diffusion-weighted magnetic resonance imaging as a cancer biomarker: consensus and recommendations. Neoplasia 11:102–125

Price WS (1998) Pulsed-field gradient NMR as a tool for studying translational diffusion. Part II: experimental aspects. Concepts Magn Reson 10:197–237

Pruessmann KP, Weiger M, Scheidegger MB et al (1999) SENSE: sensitivity encoding for fast MRI. Magn Reson Med 42:952–962

Reese TG, Heid O, Weisskoff RM et al (2003) Reduction of eddy-current-induced distortion in diffusion MRI using a twice-refocused spin echo. Magn Reson Med 49:177–182

Saritas EU, Lee JH, Nishimura DG (2007) Optimum b-value vs. SNR for apparent diffusion coefficient measurements. Proc Intl Soc Mag Reson Med 1508

Saritas EU, Lee JH, Nishimura DG (2008) Effects of T2-weighting on optimum b-value vs. SNR for ADC measurements. Proc Intl Soc Mag Reson Med 1798

Stejskal EO, Tanner JE (1965) Spin diffusion measurements: spin echoes in the presence of a time-dependent field gradient. J Chem Phys 42:288–292

Tofts PS, Lloyd D, Clark CA et al (2000) Test liquids for quantitative MRI measurements of self-diffusion coefficient in vivo. Magn Reson Med 43:368–374

Qualitative and Quantitative Analyses:
Image Evaluation and Interpretation

Dow-Mu Koh

3

CONTENTS

SUMMARY

DW-MR images and their corresponding apparent diffusion coefficient (ADC) maps provide unique information that reflects tissue cellularity and organization. The *b*-value images and ADC maps can be assessed qualitatively, and by comparing the varying signal intensities and appearances of tissues on these images, it is possible to characterize tissues and diseases. However, the ADC maps can also provide quantitative measurements of tissue water diffusivity, which can be used not only for disease assessment, but also for the evaluation of disease response to treatment. In order to achieve optimal image interpretation, the DW-MR images and ADC maps should be displayed with conventional morphologic images to enable the best assessment to be made. A pragmatic approach to utilizing DW-MR images and ADC maps for disease assessment is discussed in this chapter.

3.1

Introduction

Image interpretation of DW-MRI studies has a steep learning curve, and requires the radiologist to understand how and why the images are to be reviewed. There are some differences in the way one may look at DW-MR images compared with conventional morphological MR images. Firstly, whilst most conventional morphological MR images are only assessed visually, interpretation of DW-MR images can be performed qualitatively by visual assessment whilst quantitative assessment can be performed by analysing the apparent diffusion coefficient (ADC) maps.

Dow-Mu Koh, MD, MRCP, FRCR
Department of Diagnostic Radiology, Royal Marsden Hospital, Downs Road, Sutton, Surrey SM2 5PT, UK

Secondly, because disease assessment is based on differential signal attenuation with increasing *b*-values on DW-MRI between tissues, it is often helpful to display images acquired using different *b*-values side-by-side to facilitate this evaluation. Thirdly, when applying DW-MRI for disease characterization, the quantitative ADC maps calculated from the DW-MR images should be interpreted in conjunction with the *b*-value images to avoid misinterpretation. Last, but not the least, using multi-planar reformats or fusion imaging with conventional morphological images can aid disease localization and assessment (Koh et al. 2008).

In this chapter, we will discuss how to qualitatively assess DW-MR images and the limitations of interpreting just the *b*-value images alone. The basic concepts of tissue characterization and disease interpretation using *b*-value images and ADC maps will be outlined. The advantages of combining morphological images, DW-MR images obtained at different *b*-values and the ADC maps to optimize disease assessment will be emphasized. The potential applications of using ADC maps for quantitative evaluation, especially for disease characterization and for the assessment of tumour response to treatment will be reviewed. We will also survey the different methods of image displays to optimize radiological assessment and image interpretation.

3.2
Qualitative Assessment of DW-MR Images

3.2.1
DW-MR Images Acquired Using Different *b*-Values

When performing DW-MRI, there is differential signal attenuation with increasing *b*-values (diffusion weighting) between tissues, which is related to tissue cellularity, the tortuosity of the extracellular space and the integrity of the cell membranes (Koh et al. 2007; Thoeny et al. 2007; Patterson et al. 2008). Generally, with increasing *b*-values, there is less signal attenuation from cellular tissues (e.g. tumour tissue) compared with cystic structures. When diffusion-weighting is applied at DW-MRI, signal attenuation is also observed from protons with larger diffusion distances (i.e. mean displacement per unit time), such as from intravascular blood flow. Generally, with increasing

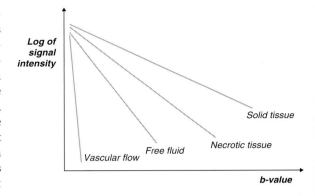

Fig. 3.1. Simplified schematic diagram showing the signal attenuation of different tissues with increasing *b*-values. Signal from vascular flow is rapidly attenuated with a small *b*-value. However, solid cellular tissues such as tumours show a lesser degree of signal attenuation at higher *b*-values compared with free fluids or necrotic tissues

diffusion weighting or *b*-values, there is a steeper gradient of signal attenuation from protons with greater diffusion distances compared with those from protons with smaller diffusion distances. As a corollary, cellular tumour tissues containing water protons with shorter diffusion distances will demonstrate greater preservation of the measured signal intensity at higher *b*-values (i.e. *b*-value >500 s/mm²). A simplified scheme which illustrates the differential signal attenuation of tissues with increasing *b*-values is shown in Fig. 3.1.

Based on this understanding, when DW-MR imaging is performed using two or more *b*-values, tissue characterization becomes possible based on the differences in the degree and rate of signal attenuation. By way of an example, when DW-MRI is performed on a large variegated metastasis in the liver, the necrotic central component of the tumour shows greater signal attenuation as the *b*-value increases, while the signal intensity from its cellular rim is relatively preserved (Fig. 3.2). Note also how the application of a low diffusion weighting (e.g. *b* = 50 s/mm²) results in nulling of the high signal intensity arising from intrahepatic vasculature.

As tumour tissues usually maintain their signal intensity on the higher *b*-value images due to restricted water diffusion, this imaging feature is harnessed to aid tumour detection using DW-MRI. DW-MRI performed using *b*-values of 800–1,000 s/mm² usually results in significant signal suppression of normal tissues or the background signal intensity, allowing foci

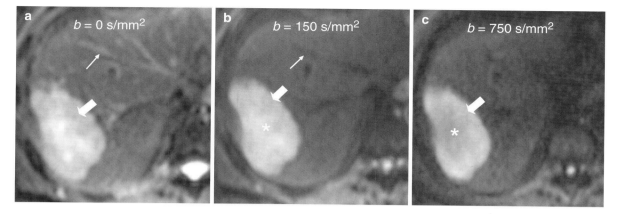

Fig. 3.2. Qualitative evaluation of DW-MR images. By performing DW-MRI using different *b*-values, tissue characterization is possible based on the differential signal attenuation between tissues. In this example of a man with a metastasis in the right lobe of the liver arising from colorectal cancer, DW-MRI was performed using 3 *b*-values (**a–c**) of 0, 150 and 750 s/mm^2. Note that the application of diffusion-weighting results in the nulling of signal arising from intrahepatic vasculature (*small arrows*). With increasing *b*-value or diffusion-weighting, note that the cellular tumour rim (*large arrows*) show relative preservation of signal intensity compared with the necrotic centre (*asterisk*)

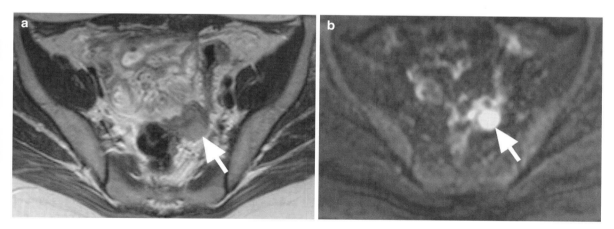

Fig. 3.3. Using high *b*-value DW-MR image to visualize areas of restricted diffusion. A 43-year-old man with sigmoid carcinoma. (**a**) Axial T2-weighted image through the mid-pelvis shows focal thickening of intermediate signal intensity in the sigmoid colon (*arrow*) consistent with a tumour. (**b**) On the high *b*-value ($b = 900$ s/mm^2) DW-MR image, the tumour appears as a very high signal intensity polypoidal focus (*arrow*) of restricted diffusion against the largely signal-suppressed background. Note that some high signal intensity persists in a few of the normal bowel loops

of high signal intensity impeded diffusion of tumours to be more readily identified. This has been the basis for using higher *b*-value images for tumour detection using the whole-body diffusion-weighted imaging with background suppression (DWIBS) technique. A similar rationale applies when high *b*-value images are used to aid the detection of primary tumours in patients with suspected prostate or gynaecological malignancies (Fig. 3.3).

3.2.1.1
T2 Shine-Through

One of the limitations of relying solely on the *b*-value images for disease assessment is the "T2 shine-through" effect. The T2 shine-through effect occurs because the measured signal intensity on the high *b*-value images depends not only on the water proton diffusivity but also on the intrinsic tissue

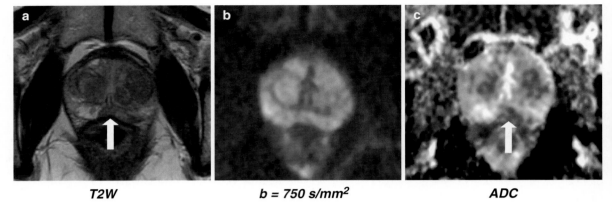

Fig. 3.4. Combining morphological DW-MRI b-value image and ADC map for image interpretation. (**a**) Axial T2-weighted, (**b**) $b = 750\,\mathrm{s/mm^2}$ DW-MR image and (**c**) ADC map in a 63-year-old man with pathological proven prostate cancer. The tumour is visualized as area of low signal intensity in the peripheral zone of the prostate gland (*arrow*) on the T2- weighted scan. On the b-value image, the tumour is poorly seen because of T2 shine-through from the normal peripheral zone. Note, however, that the tumour area returns low ADC value (*arrow*) on the ADC map in contrast to the high ADC from the normal peripheral gland exhibiting the T2 shine-through effect

T2-relaxation time. This is perhaps not surprising since the most commonly used DW-MRI echo-planar imaging acquisition scheme used for body imaging is adapted from a T2-weighted spin-echo sequence. As a result, a tissue may appear to exhibit high signal intensity on the higher b-value image (e.g. $>500\,\mathrm{s/mm^2}$), not because of the restricted mobility of the water protons, but because of the long intrinsic T2-relaxation time of the tissue. However, the mechanisms accounting for T2 shine-through is complex and may be contributed to by macromolecules that alter tissue diffusivity and relaxivity. The choice of b-value can also affect the perception of this phenomenon. In the range of b-values used for body imaging (e.g. up to $1,000\,\mathrm{s/mm^2}$) T2 shine-through effects can not only be observed in pathological tissues, but may also be observed in benign conditions such as cysts and glandular structures, and also in some normal anatomical regions such as the peripheral zone of the prostate gland (Fig. 3.4).

In order to avoid spurious interpretation of T2 shine-through effect on imaging as restricted diffusion, the high signal intensity observed on a high b-value image could be related to the native T2-weighted image (especially the long echo time acquisition) to have an appreciation of the native T2 relaxivity of the tissue. One simple method of overcoming T2 shine-through is by calculating the "exponential image" (Provenzale et al. 1999). This is produced by dividing the high b-value image by the $b = 0\,\mathrm{s/mm^2}$ image. An area with significant T2 shine-through will remain bright on the exponential image whereas areas of restricted diffusion will appear dark. However, the most common method to avoid misinterpretation of the presence and degree of T2 shine-through is to compare the high b-value image with the corresponding ADC map (Koh et al. 2007). A region with significant T2 shine-through will show high signal intensity on the high b-value image but also returns a high ADC value (Fig. 3.4).

3.2.1.2
Diffusion Anisotropy

Diffusion anisotropy refers to unequal diffusivity of the water protons, usually as a result of structural organization of tissues. Diffusion anisotropy can be observed at DW-MRI when the motion-probing gradients are applied in more than one direction (typically three or more). Many DW-MRI acquisition schemes used in clinical practice apply motion-probing gradients sequentially in three orthogonal directions of the MR gradient system: frequency select (x), phase select (y) and slice select. This results in three different directional DW-MR images for each b-value used.

An area of the body that demonstrates high diffusion anisotropy is in the brain, where the organization of the white matter fibres confers directionality to the water diffusion. For example, in the body of the corpus callosum, the neural tracts that connect the two cerebral hemispheres will show less restricted diffusion in the transverse orientation, compared to the anterior–posterior or foot–head directions.

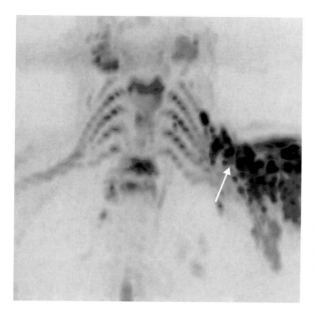

Fig. 3.5. The principle of diffusion anisotropy is harnessed for MR neurography. DW-MRI performed with the diffusion sensitizing gradient applied in a single direction (anterior-posterior) perpendicular to the travel of brachial plexus demonstrates the nerve roots, cords and trunks of the brachial plexus to advantage. On this inverted grey-scale coronal maximum intensity projection image of the neck acquired using $b = 900\,s/mm^2$, note the normal appearing nerves of the right brachial plexus. On the left, there is tumour infiltration of left brachial plexus (*arrows*) arising from breast carcinoma

The directionality of water diffusion can be harnessed by using a special diffusion-weighted imaging technique known as diffusion-tensor imaging (DTI), where the motion-probing gradient is applied in multiple directions (typically 12 or more) (BAMMER et al. 2002). DTI has been used in neurological imaging to reveal the complex organization of the white matter tracts in the brain. The application of DTI is currently being investigated in a number of sites in the body including the kidneys (FUKUDA et al. 2000; RIES et al. 2001) and the prostate gland (SINHA et al. 2004; MANENTI et al. 2007; GURSES et al. 2008; XU et al. 2009).

In oncology, diffusion anisotropy is usually not encountered because tumours typically grow in a random fashion. For this reason, the orthogonal motion probing gradients are usually applied simultaneously rather than sequentially to yield only the "trace" or "index" image. However, certain regions in the body do demonstrate structural organization that can be differentiated by their directional water diffusivity. For example, the prostate gland and uterus show varying degrees of diffusion anisotropy

due to the anatomical arrangement of the collecting ducts or muscular fibres. The directional unequal barrier to water motion is also being utilized in MR neurography, where the motion-probing gradient could be applied in a single direction perpendicular to the long axis of the nerves, to maximize neural visualization (Fig. 3.5).

There is growing awareness of the potential of utilizing the principles of diffusion anisotropy to improve disease detection and assessment both in oncological and non-oncological practices in the body. However, much of this work remains developmental, although there appears to be substantial promise in the technique (XU et al. 2009). It is likely that DW-MRI performed to harness differences in the anisotropic diffusion of tissues is likely to evolve over the next few years.

3.2.2
ADC Maps

Calculation of the ADC provides a means by which tissue water diffusivity can be quantified. The ADC map is easily generated on most modern-day MR scanners at a push of a button. On most MR systems, a mono-exponential fit is applied to the relationship between the logarithm of the measured signal intensity and the b-value for each voxel on the DW-MR images. The slope of the mono-exponential line fit represents the ADC. The calculated ADC for each voxel is usually displayed as a parametric map, which can be visually appraised. By drawing regions of interest (ROI) on the ADC map, the apparent water diffusivity of different tissues can be recorded. ADC is usually expressed in units of x $10^{-3}\,mm^2/s$.

The calculated ADC is unique amongst imaging techniques as it provides a quantitative measure of water diffusivity, which indirectly reflects tissue cellularity and tissue organization. The calculated ADC is independent of magnetic field strength, and helps to overcome the effects of T2 shine-through.

To the eye, the ADC maps usually appear rather noisy compared with the b-values DW-MR images. This is in part due to the propagation of noise from the native DW-MR images and poorly fitted pixels that arise from a variety of artefacts. Hence, interpretation of ADC maps on their own can be difficult; and the quality of the ADC map will be limited by the quality of the DW-MRI b-value images.

Areas of true restricted water diffusion will appear high signal intensity on the high b-value image but

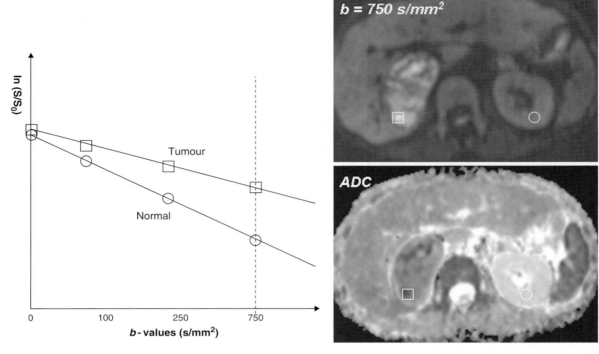

Fig. 3.6. Simplified schematic diagram showing relationship between the *b*-values and ADC. A 53-year-old man with right renal cell carcinoma. On the *b* = 750 s/mm² DW-MR image, the tumour (*box*) area shows higher signal intensity compared with the normal kidney (*circle*). Graph shows the relationship of the logarithm ratio of signal intensities vs. *b*-values, where S_0 is the signal intensity at $b = 0$ s/mm². Note the signal attenuation plots for the tumour (*box*) vs. normal renal tissue (*circle*). The slope of these plot lines represents the ADC for the individual tissues. Hence, although the tumour area returns higher signal intensity at $b = 750$ s/mm² compared with normal renal tissue (marked by *dotted line* on graph), the slope or gradient of the line is steeper for normal tissue than tumour. Hence, in this example, the renal tumour has a lower ADC compared with normal renal tissue. This difference can be readily appreciated on the ADC map

return a low ADC value. This apparent inverse "contrast" between the DW-MRI *b*-value images and the ADC map is worth remembering when interpreting images. It is easy to appreciate this by considering a tumour that shows little attenuation of its signal intensity at high *b*-value compared with normal tissue. The tumour therefore appears higher in signal intensity on the high *b*-value DW-MR image. However, because there is little signal attenuation, the slope or gradient of the line that describes the relation between the measured signal intensity and *b*-value will be shallow, thus returning a low ADC value (Fig. 3.6).

As discussed in Chap. 1, DW-MR imaging can be performed by omitting the lower (<100 s/mm²) *b*- values to derive a perfusion-insensitive ADC (Koh et al. 2007). If only low *b*-values are used for ADC calculations, then the resultant ADC value will be perfusion-sensitive (Thoeny et al. 2005a, b). Where a more sophisticated model is employed, such as by applying

the principles of intravoxel incoherent motion (IVIM) (Le Bihan et al. 1988), maps of the "True Diffusion (D)" and the perfusion fraction (f) may be derived by applying a bi-exponential data fitting. However, for accurate IVIM calculations, multiple *b*-values need to be acquired, which is usually not performed in clinical practice. There is also a need to quality assure that the DW-MRI performed using low *b*-values is accurate. IVIM analysis is also performed off-line, as current vendor softwares do not support this methodology. Thus, although the IVIM methodology may appear appealing, it is currently only used in a research setting in the body. For most clinical departments, the ADC calculated using two to three *b*-values appears to suffice on a practical basis.

The diffusion measurements and ADC calculations are usually made over a range of *b*-values ($b = 0$–1,000 s/mm²) and could include or exclude the lower *b*-values ($b = 0$–100 s/mm²). The lower

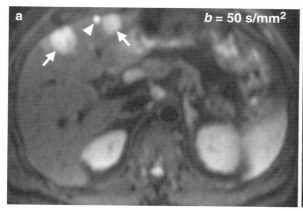
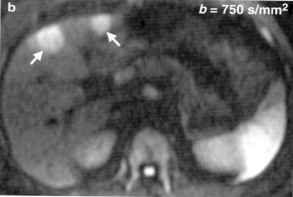

Fig. 3.7. Tissue characterization by comparing signal attenuation from tissues at different b-values. DW-MR images of the liver acquired using b-values of (**a**) 50 and (**b**) 750 s/mm^2 in a patient with colorectal cancer. On the low b-value (50 s/mm^2) image, the metastases (*arrows*) and cyst (*arrowhead*) all return high signal intensities. However, the signal intensity within the cyst is suppressed on the high b-value (750 s/mm^2) image, confirming its fluid content; whereas the metastases show persistent high signal intensity (*arrows*)

b-values are omitted if calculation of the perfusion-insensitive ADC is desired.

3.2.3
Principles of Image Interpretation Using DW-MRI and ADC Maps

The DW-MR images acquired at different b-values can be first visually surveyed to look for areas of differential signal attenuation, which aids disease and lesion characterization. For example, a simple hepatic cyst and a liver tumour will both return high signal intensity on the low b-value image. However, because of the higher water diffusivity within the cyst, the hepatic cyst will generally appear isointense to the hepatic parenchyma at higher b-values of >500 s/mm^2, whereas a solid tumour in the liver would maintain its high signal intensity (Fig. 3.7).

When surveying the high b-value images, the eye is trained to pick out foci of relatively high signal intensity against the low signal intensity background, which should be optimally suppressed. This is the basis of using DW-MRI as a tool to aid disease detection. The definition of a "high" b-value image is relative and may vary to some extent upon the organ or region of study. In the liver, because of the short T2-relaxation of the normal liver parenchyma, b-values between 500 and 800 s/mm^2 may be regarded as relatively high b-values. However, in pelvic or whole-body imaging (TAKAHARA et al. 2004), b-values

DW-MRI signal intensity (high b-value)	ADC	Interpretation
⬜	⬛	Cellular tissue, tumour
⬛	⬜	Cystic or necrotic tissue
⬜	⬜	T2 shine through
⬛	⬛	Artefacts, fat

Fig. 3.8. Summary of the common patterns of DW-MRI appearances on the high-b-value images and ADC maps, and their diagnostic interpretations. Boxes in *white* indicate high signal intensity/ADC values and boxes in *black* indicate low signal intensity/ADC values

of 1,000 s/mm^2 or higher are often employed for disease assessment.

When surveying high b-value images, it has to be borne in mind that there are a number of normal anatomical structures that show impeded water diffusion. The brain, salivary glands, normal lymph nodes, spleen, uterus, ovaries, testes, spinal cord and peripheral nerves all appear relatively bright at DW-MRI on the high b-value images (TAKAHARA et al. 2004). The normal bowel wall also demonstrates varying degrees of high signal intensity, which can be difficult to eliminate.

Figure 3.8 summarizes the common signal intensity patterns that may be encountered on qualitative visual assessment of the high b-value DW-MR images and their corresponding ADC maps. When a lesion returns high signal intensity on the DW-MR image but

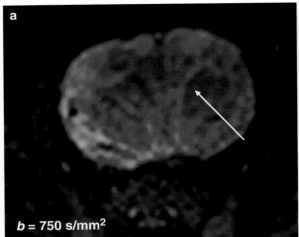

Fig. 3.9. Appearance of cystic ovarian tumour on high *b*-value DW-MR image and ADC map. (**a**) DW-MRI *b* = 750 s/mm² image showing signal suppression (low signal intensity) within the cystic locules of this ovarian cystadenocarcinoma. (**b**) The ADC map returns high ADC values in the cystic areas (*arrow*)

appears dark on the ADC map, the radiological interpretation is usually one of cellular tissue. However, not all cellular tissues are malignant, although solid neoplasm is within the differential diagnoses. It has to be remembered that abscesses are also cellular in nature, and would show a similar imaging appearance to tumours at DW-MRI. Thus, DW-MRI *b*-value images should always be interpreted with the relevant accompanying clinical details. Fibrotic tissues can show low signal intensity on the DW-MR images and return intermediate to low ADCs. However, the full range of the DW-MRI and ADC appearances of post-treatment fibrosis has yet to be fully characterized.

By contrast, when a lesion returns low signal intensity on the DW-MR image and appears bright on the ADC map, this usually signifies cystic or necrotic tissues (Fig. 3.9). This combination of appearances is encountered in benign cysts and cystic tumours, and further characterization may be aided by assessment of conventional morphologic imaging for internal lesion characteristics.

When a lesion appears to show high signal intensity restricted diffusion on the high *b*-value image, but is also bright on the ADC map, then T2 shine-through is the explanation. T2 shine-through occurs not infrequently in clinical practice, and may be observed in both benign and malignant conditions. Certain conditions demonstrate this phenomenon at imaging, including benign cysts and epidermoid tumours in the brain (CHEN et al. 2001).

When a lesion appears low signal intensity on the high *b*-value image, and appears dark on the ADC map, a few causes could be considered. Firstly, macroscopic fatty tissue can show such imaging characteristics, particularly when fat-suppressed single-shot echo-planar imaging DW-MRI technique is used for image acquisition (Fig. 3.10). Secondly, such an appearance can result from susceptibility artefacts from a variety of causes (e.g. iron deposition and haemorrhage). One good example is when there is haemochromatosis or haemosiderosis of the liver or spleen. The susceptibility effects induced by iron in tissues can result in errors in the DW-MRI measurements and ADC calculations in these organs. For these reasons, DW-MRI should be interpreted with care when macroscopic fat or haemorrhage is present within a lesion to avoid misinterpretation.

One important point to highlight when using DW-MR images and ADC maps for clinical or research applications is that, these images should not be read in isolation. It would be ideal to combine, where possible, the information from conventional morphologic imaging, DW-MRI *b*-value images, as well as the ADC maps to allow the best image interpretation to be made. The advantage of such an approach to image interpretation is illustrated in Fig. 3.4.

Visual appraisal of the DW-MR images and ADC map can also be helpful to gauge the response of tumours to treatment. With effective treatment, which results in a decrease in tumour cellularity, a responding tumour would typically show lower signal intensity on the DW-MR images (BYUN et al. 2002) and appear brighter on the ADC maps after treatment compared with the pretreatment imaging.

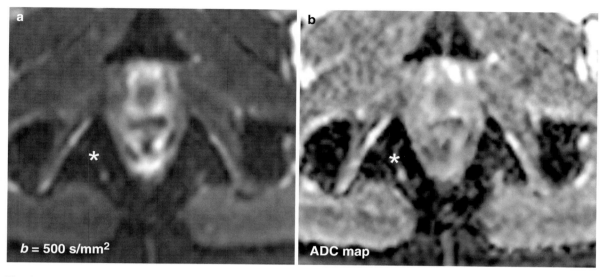

Fig. 3.10. Macroscopic fatty tissue returns low signal intensity on the higher *b*-value image and low ADC values. In this example, fat within the right ischiorectal fossa (*asterisk*) demonstrates this phenomenon

3.3

Quantitative ADC Evaluation

One of the unique advantages of DW-MRI is that the technique enables the quantitative ADC measurements of tissues to be recorded. The majority of radiological tools for disease assessment are qualitative, relying on the visual interpretation of imaging features. However, it is likely that quantitative imaging techniques will become increasingly important. Emerging quantitative imaging techniques in the body include dynamic contrast-enhanced MR imaging (DCE-MRI), positron emission tomography (PET) and DW-MRI. In oncology, each of these techniques can provide quantitative information that reflects a unique aspect of tumour biology, such as tumour vascularity, tumour metabolism and tumour cellularity; and are currently being investigated as potential imaging biomarkers for treatment response and prognosis.

3.3.1
Quantitative ADC Evaluation
by Regions of Interests

3.3.1.1
Summary Statistics

The simplest and most widely used method to quantify the ADC of tissues is by using summary statistics. The mean or median ADC value of a region of interest

(ROI) can be recorded and used to aid disease characterization and/or response assessment. As the lesion contour can be more difficult to define on the ADC map, it is customary to draw the ROI on the *b*-value image, and then copy this onto the ADC map to record their values. For this purpose, the higher *b*-value images are usually used as there is often better suppression of the background signal on these images. However, it may be possible to define the ROI on the morphological T1- or T2-weighted MR image, but this usually requires the matrix size and field-of-view to be equivalent across the DW-MR and morphological imaging.

In statistical terms, whether the mean or median ADC value of the ROI is recorded depends on the distribution of the voxel values within the ROI. If the ADC values are distributed normally within the ROI, then the mean value will reflect the central value. However, in the majority of tumours which are heterogeneous, the distribution of voxel values with the ROI is asymmetrical or even bimodal. In these instances, the median ADC value would be more reflective of the central tendency and is therefore usually recorded (Fig. 3.11).

3.3.1.2
Voxelwise Analysis

In the research or investigative setting, more sophisticated methods can be applied to evaluate the ADC. The ADC values can also be analysed on a voxel-by-voxel basis. Using such an approach, individual voxel ADC values within an ROI or the entire

Fig. 3.11. Quantitative ADC evaluation. The ADC of a tissue can be quantified by drawing a region of interest (ROI) around the target tissue. This is often done by drawing the outline on the *b*-value DW-MR image, which provides better delineation of the tissue outline, and then copy and paste this onto the ADC map. The summary ADC values recorded should ideally reflect the distribution of values within the ROI. In this example of peritoneal disease from ovarian cancer, the median value (*grey arrow*) is more indicative of the central value compared with the mean (*dark red arrow*) because of the asymmetric distribution of ADC values ($\times 10^{-3}$ mm^2/s) within the ROI as shown on this pixel histogram

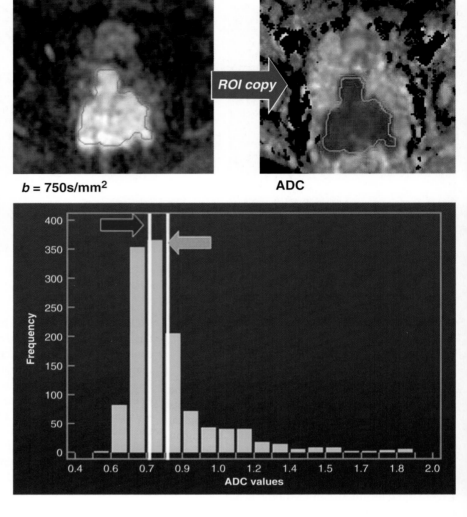

target volume is recorded. The distribution of the ADC values could be displayed using frequency or cumulative histograms. Changes in the distribution of the ADC values could be appreciated by comparing the histograms (Fig. 3.12) or by displaying the difference or cumulative histograms. More sophisticated methods of data analysis are currently being developed to track ADC changes of tumours in response to treatment, such as by the use of the so-called functional diffusion maps or threshold diffusion maps. Further details of these will be described in Chap. 10.

3.3.2
Software for ADC Calculation

The ADC is usually calculated on the vendor MR system, but it is perhaps worth remembering that the implementation of this calculation can vary to some

extent depending on the MR system or platform. It is customary for the ADC to be calculated using all the available *b*-values by default on most MR imaging systems. However, it may be possible to specify which *b*-values one would choose to include or exclude from the ADC calculations (e.g. the omission of the $b = 0$ s/ mm^2 image). In this way, it would be possible to fractionate the calculation of the ADC into a perfusion sensitive ADC and a perfusion insensitive ADC as previously described.

3.3.3
Applying Quantitative ADC
Values for Disease Characterization

The mean or median ADC values derived from ROIs drawn over target regions have been used to aid disease characterization. In oncology, it has been found

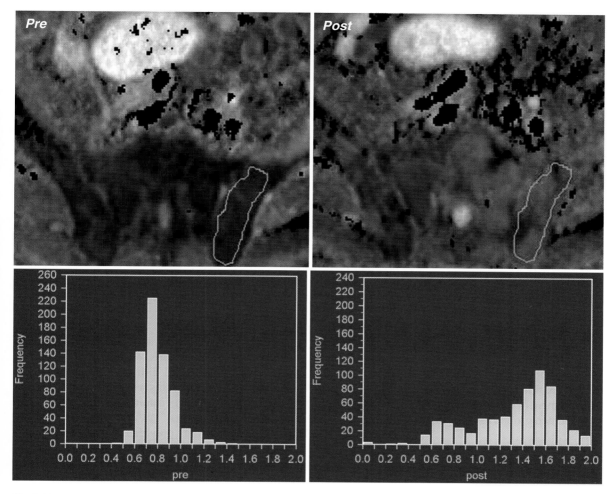

Fig. 3.12. Quantitative ADC assessment of treatment response. A 65-year-old man with metastatic bone disease from prostate cancer. ADC maps of the pelvis before and at 1 month after treatment using a novel targeted treatment. A region of interest (ROI) has been drawn around site of the disease in the left ilium (*green outline*). Visual assessment shows increase in ADC ($\times 10^{-3}$ mm^2/s) within disease area after treatment. Frequency histogram of the ADC voxel values within the ROI confirms an increase in the median value after treatment, with a shift of the histogram towards the right

that the ADCs of malignant lesions tend to be significantly lower compared with benign lesions. However, a few words of caution should be borne in mind.

Firstly, there is frequently substantial overlap in the ADCs between malignant and benign lesions. Hence, although ADC differences may be observed between cohorts of different types of lesions, it can be difficult to characterize individual lesions based on ADC values alone. Secondly, the mean or median ADC value does vary to some extent depending on the choice of *b*-values used for image acquisition and for ADC calculations (Koh et al. 2007). ADCs calculated using low *b*-values (e.g. <100 s/mm^2) are sensitive to micro-capillary perfusion effects, whereas ADCs calculated from using larger *b*-values are approaching pure diffusion.

Not surprisingly, reported ADC values of diseases derived from using only lower *b*-values are usually higher compared with those that are calculated using larger *b*-values or over a wide range of *b*-values. Hence, it is important to apply appropriate thresholds derived from similar MR systems and techniques (including *b*-values) when ADC is employed to aid disease evaluation. Thirdly, DW-MRI discriminates on the basis of tissue cellularity and not malignancy. Hence, a tumour and an abscess may both show low ADC values, and cannot be easily distinguished in this context. For this reasoning, it is important to emphasize the need to combine DW-MRI with other imaging techniques and clinical information to allow the best diagnosis to be made.

3.3.4
Measurement Reproducibility

There is now emerging evidence to suggest that ADC measurement obtained using a free-breathing DW-MRI technique is reproducible (KWEE et al. 2008). One study has demonstrated in normal volunteers that the ADC reproducibility is better using the free-breathing technique, compared with either breath-hold or respiratory-triggered techniques (KWEE et al. 2008). At 3T, the coefficient of variance for ADC measurement in the abdomen was found to be 14% (BRAITHWAITE et al. 2009). It has been shown that the ADC measurement variability across vendors and institutions when imaging the brain was in the region of about 6–10% (SASAKI et al. 2008). A recent two-centre clinical trial study has also shown that good measurement reproducibility could be achieved in this setting (KOH et al. 2009), with good reproducibility of the ADC and ADC high values (reproducibility coefficient of 14%). The readers are encouraged to explore the use of Bland–Altman statistics for the comparison of test–retest ADC results. An understanding of measurement reproducibility is important because it provides the level of confidence needed for changes in ADC following treatment or differences in the ADC measurements between two groups to be regarded as significant.

3.4
Image Display

A comprehensive imaging review of the DW-MR images should include evaluation of the b-value images, ADC maps and morphological images. Optimal display will help to facilitate image review.

3.4.1
Display of the b-Value DW-MR Images

Where possible, it is best to view the b-value images side-by-side, together with the ADC maps. A 2 × 2 layout allows the b-value images, ADC map and morphological series (e.g. T1- or T2-weighted image) to be simultaneously displayed for image assessment (Fig. 3.13).

In terms of image display, the b-value images are usually viewed as acquired, with areas of restricted diffusion appearing higher in signal intensity, compared with the background which appears black. However, it is sometimes advantageous to display the b-value images using an inverted grey scale. This results in areas of restricted diffusion appearing dark compared to the background that now appears white. Using the inverted grey scale for display, these images can superficially resemble PET or radionuclide imaging studies.

The ADC map is usually displayed in shades of grey, but on some MR systems a colour scale may be employed. A word of caution needs to be made when a colour scale is used to display ADC values. The eye perceives grey scale as a continuous range, but the perception of colours, depending on the colour scale employed, may render certain colours to be more striking to the eye than others, leading to false impression of the distribution of ADC values on these maps.

3.4.2
Image Fusion

On a high b-value DW-MR image, the background may be significantly suppressed, making it difficult to assess areas of restricted diffusion in relation to the anatomical features. For this reason, it can be advantageous to perform image fusion to combine the unique functional information of DW-MRI or ADC map with the anatomical details provided by the morphologic T1- or T2-weighted sequences. To do so, it is customary to ascribe a colour scale to the DW-MRI grey-scale display or ADC data, and then use this to fuse with the morphological image. The relative ease or difficulty in performing such image fusion is dependent to a large extent upon the vendor MR system and workstation available. Should this prove difficult on existing platforms, it should be relatively easy to transfer the data offline to an external computer, and use a third party imaging software (e.g. OSIRIX) to complete this task. Fusion of the DW-MR image or ADC map with the morphological image also allows areas of restricted diffusion to be directly compared with morphological changes on conventional imaging and can draw attention to subtle changes which may be unappreciated on the morphological images (Fig. 3.14). However, it is important to consider that when performing fusion imaging, the same colour scale should be used each time if possible. In addition, the window/width level and the degree/percentage of image fusion should be consistent where possible. This is because using a different colour scale, window display and percentage fusion each time can result in false perception and erroneous interpretation. The use of fusion imaging

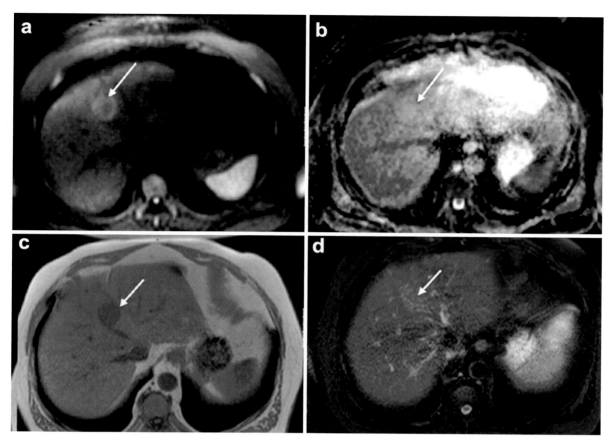

Fig. 3.13. Image Display. Optimal image display can aid disease assessment. In this example of a patient with a liver metastasis in the right lobe of the liver (*arrows*), the (**a**) $b = 750\,\text{s/mm}^2$ image and (**b**) ADC map are displayed, alongside the (**c**) morphological T1-weighted and (**d**) fat-suppressed T2-weighted image. Simultaneous display of DW-MR image, ADC map and morphologic images are advantageous for image viewing and assessment

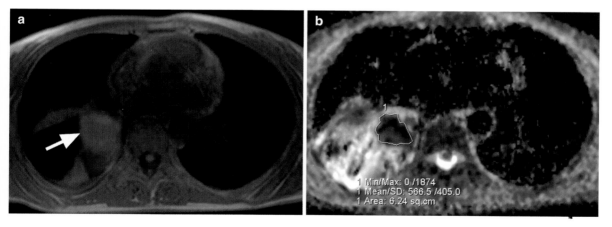

Fig. 3.14. (**a**) Fusion of the $b = 900\,\text{s/mm}^2$ image with the T1-weighted image in a patient with lung cancer enables the tumour which shows greater impeded diffusion (*arrow*) to be better discriminated from the collapsed lung. (**b**) Once the tumour is clearly identified, a region of interest was drawn and copied onto the ADC map to record its quantitative value ($0.57 \times 10^{-3}\,\text{mm}^2/\text{s}$)

has already been shown to be useful for the evaluation of bladder and uterine cancers (LIN et al. 2009; TAKEUCHI et al. 2009).

3.4.3
Diffusion-weighted Whole-body Imaging with Background Body Signal Suppression (DWIBS)

DWIBS is a whole-body diffusion-weighted imaging technique acquired as multiple axial image blocks, usually from the skull-base down to the level of the mid-thigh, using a high b-value (typically 900–1,000 s/ mm^2) to maximize background suppression. The images are stacked together and processed using radial maximum intensity projections in the coronal plane. These are then composed together for whole-body display using an inverted grey scale. DWIBS images resemble PET imaging, and for that reason the technique has also been known (albeit perhaps misleading) as MR PETography. For whole-body imaging, it is customary to assess the DWIBS images with morphological T1-weighted images, with or without short-tau inversion recovery (STIR) imaging. The technique is currently being widely evaluated for the detection of malignant or metastatic disease in a variety of tumours, both at 1.5 and 3 T.

3.5
Conclusions

DW-MRI b-value images and ADC maps may be visually assessed qualitatively, but the ADC maps can also be quantitatively evaluated, which is a major strength of the DW-MRI technique. The ADC value reflects tissue cellularity, and aids tissue characterization and response assessment. The DW-MR images, ADC maps and morphological images should be interpreted concurrently, to allow optimum assessment to be made. Attention to image display, including the use of fusion imaging, can aid image interpretation and disease assessment.

References

Bammer R, Auer M, Keeling SL et al (2002) Diffusion tensor imaging using single-shot SENSE-EPI. Magn Reson Med 48: 128–136

Braithwaite AC, Dale BM, Boll DT et al (2009) Short- and mid-term reproducibility of apparent diffusion coefficient measurements at 3.0-T diffusion-weighted imaging of the abdomen. Radiology 250: 459–465

Byun WM, Shin SO, Chang Y et al (2002) Diffusion-weighted MR imaging of metastatic disease of the spine: assessment of response to therapy. AJNR Am J Neuroradiol 23: 906–912

Chen S, Ikawa F, Kurisu K et al (2001) Quantitative MR evaluation of intracranial epidermoid tumors by fast fluid-attenuated inversion recovery imaging and echo-planar diffusion-weighted imaging. AJNR Am J Neuroradiol 22: 1089–1096

Fukuda Y, Ohashi I, Hanafusa K et al (2000) Anisotropic diffusion in kidney: apparent diffusion coefficient measurements for clinical use. J Magn Reson Imaging 11: 156–160

Gurses B, Kabakci N, Kovanlikaya A et al (2008) Diffusion tensor imaging of the normal prostate at 3 Tesla. Eur Radiol 18: 716–721

Koh DM, Collins DJ (2007) Diffusion-weighted MRI in the body: applications and challenges in oncology. AJR Am J Roentgenol 188: 1622–1635

Koh DM, Blackledge M, Collins DJ et al (2009) Reproducibility and ADC changes in response to CA4P and bevacizumab treatment in a two-centre phase I clinical trial. Eur Radiol

Koh DM, Takahara T, Imai Y et al (2008) Practical aspects of assessing tumors using clinical diffusion-weighted imaging in the body. Magn Reson Med Sci 6: 211–224

Kwee TC, Takahara T, Koh DM et al (2008) Comparison and reproducibility of ADC measurements in breathhold, respiratory triggered, and free-breathing diffusion-weighted MR imaging of the liver. J Magn Reson Imaging 28: 1141–1148

Le Bihan D, Breton E, Lallemand D et al (1988) Separation of diffusion and perfusion in intravoxel incoherent motion MR imaging. Radiology 168: 497–505

Lin G, Ng KK, Chang CJ et al (2009) Myometrial invasion in endometrial cancer: diagnostic accuracy of diffusion-weighted 3.0-T MR imaging–initial experience. Radiology 250: 784–792

Manenti G, Carlani M, Mancino S et al (2007) Diffusion tensor magnetic resonance imaging of prostate cancer. Invest Radiol 42: 412–419

Patterson DM, Padhani AR, Collins DJ (2008) Technology insight: water diffusion MRI–a potential new biomarker of response to cancer therapy. Nat Clin Pract Oncol 5: 220–233

Provenzale JM, Engelter ST, Petrella JR et al (1999) Use of MR exponential diffusion-weighted images to eradicate T2 "shine-through" effect. AJR Am J Roentgenol 172: 537–539

Ries M, Jones RA, Basseau F et al (2001) Diffusion tensor MRI of the human kidney. J Magn Reson Imaging 14: 42–49

Sasaki M, Yamada K, Watanabe Y et al (2008) Variability in absolute apparent diffusion coefficient values across different platforms may be substantial: a multivendor, multi-institutional comparison study. Radiology 249: 624–630

Sinha S, Sinha U (2004) In vivo diffusion tensor imaging of the human prostate. Magn Reson Med 52: 530–537

Takahara T, Imai Y, Yamashita T et al (2004) Diffusion weighted whole body imaging with background body signal suppression (DWIBS): technical improvement using free breathing, STIR and high resolution 3D display. Radiat Med 22: 275–282

Takeuchi M, Sasaki S, Ito M et al (2009) Urinary bladder cancer: diffusion-weighted MR imaging–accuracy for diagnosing T stage and estimating histologic grade. Radiology 251: 112–121

Thoeny HC, De Keyzer F (2007) Extracranial applications of diffusion-weighted magnetic resonance imaging. Eur Radiol 17: 1385–1393

Thoeny HC, De Keyzer F, Oyen RH et al (2005a) Diffusion-weighted MR imaging of kidneys in healthy volunteers and patients with parenchymal diseases: initial experience. Radiology 235: 911–917

Thoeny HC, De Keyzer F, Vandecaveye V et al (2005b) Effect of vascular targeting agent in rat tumor model: dynamic contrast-enhanced versus diffusion-weighted MR imaging. Radiology 237: 492–499

Xu J, Humphrey PA, Kibel AS et al (2009) Magnetic resonance diffusion characteristics of histologically defined prostate cancer in humans. Magn Reson Med 61: 842–850

Non-Oncological Applications in the Body

MR Neurography: Imaging
of the Peripheral Nerves

Taro Takahara and Thomas C. Kwee

CONTENTS

SUMMARY

Diffusion-weighted magnetic resonance neurography (DW-MR neurography) is a recently developed technique based on DW-MRI, and represents a ground-breaking step forward towards the selective imaging of peripheral nerves. DW-MR neurography uses conventional diffusion gradient encoding rather than diffusion-tensor imaging because the former results in superior visualization of the peripheral nervous system compared to the latter when the same image acquisition time is applied. DW-MR neurography allows for three-dimensional rendering of the peripheral nerves, hence has the potential to improve the diagnosis of peripheral nerve disorders, optimize lesion localization, and may also enable a faster and more straightforward evaluation of the extent of neural dysfunction compared with electrophysiological studies or conventional MR imaging sequences.

Taro Takahara, MD, PhD
Thomas C. Kwee, MD
Department of Radiology, University Medical Center Utrecht, Heidelberglaan 100, 3584 CX, Utrecht, The Netherlands

4.1

Introduction

Clinical history, neurological examination and electrophysiological studies are the mainstays for the evaluation of patients with peripheral neuropathy or plexopathy. However, in order to improve diagnostic accuracy, lesion localization and treatment planning of conditions that affect the peripheral nervous system, there is a need to develop non-invasive techniques that are able to visualize the peripheral nerves. As MR imaging produces images with excellent soft tissue contrast, it can be considered a primary candidate for the imaging of peripheral nerves.

Visualization of the peripheral nerves by MR imaging is termed MR neurography. MR neurography can be further categorized according to the type of MR technique used to acquire the images: conventional MR neurography and DW-MR neurography. Conventional MR neurography utilizes a variety of morphological imaging sequences, including short-tau inversion recovery (STIR), fat-suppressed T2-weighted imaging and T1-weighted imaging, performed in different anatomical planes (e.g. coronal, axial and oblique sagittal) to reveal normal peripheral nerves as linear or near-linear structures of intermediate-to-high (T2-weighted/ STIR) or intermediate-to-low (T1-weighted) signal intensities. By comparison, DW-MR neurography employs a thin-section DW-MR technique to interrogate an entire imaging volume, from which the high b-value dataset can be post-processed for three-dimensional neural visualization.

Both conventional and DW-MR neurography can be used to demonstrate the anatomical location of a neurogenic tumour, the relationship between a tumour and its nerve of origin, abnormal nerve thickening due to inflammatory processes and neural discontinuity resulting from traumatic injuries. Compared with DW-MR neurography, conventional MR neurography has lower nerve-to-background contrast, making peripheral nerves more difficult to identify from normal adjacent structures. As a result, image interpretation of conventional MR neurography can be time-consuming and precise lesion localization difficult. DW-MR neurography overcomes some of the intrinsic limitations of conventional MR neurography, in that it is able to more selectively demonstrate peripheral nerves over long trajectories.

In this chapter, we describe and illustrate the background, rationale and practical implementations of DW-MR neurography for the evaluation of the peripheral nervous system. We will discuss the normal anatomy of the main neural plexi revealed by DW-MR neurography and highlight the current and evolving clinical applications of the technique.

4.2
Concepts of MR Neurography

4.2.1
Conventional MR Neurography

The word "MR neurography" dates back to a 1993 Lancet article (FILLER et al. 1993). In that article, peripheral nerves were visualized using fat-suppressed T2-weighted images as high signal intensity structures. In radiological terms, an imaging technique post-fix by "graphy" usually implies that the imaging test is able to selectively highlight a particular anatomical structure or area of interest almost entirely and exclusively, including its three-dimensional orientation, with little or no superimposition of surrounding structures. For example, angiography allows for the selective three-dimensional visualization of vascular structures. However, the first MR neurography images could not fulfil this definition as the imaging technique applied could not specifically segmentate out the neural elements, but were in fact a series of anatomically orientated morphological images on which the peripheral nerves could be identified.

In most radiological departments, fat-suppressed T2-weighted (or STIR) images and (three-dimensional or thin-section two-dimensional) T1-weighted images are used for the evaluation of peripheral nerves. The combined uses of these MR imaging sequences constitute conventional MR neurography. Typically, fat-suppressed T2-weighted (or STIR) images are applied for the detection and delineation of disease, while T1-weighted images are used to aid diagnosis and anatomical description (MARAVILLA and BOWEN 1998, MOORE et al. 2001). Figure 4.1 shows a typical example of conventional MR neurography performed using STIR, T2-weighted and T1-weighted imaging. Three-dimensional gradient echo T1-weighted sequence has recently been shown to be able to provide clear visualization of the peripheral nerves of the brachial plexus because of the high spatial resolution thin-section partitions that can be achieved using this technique (ZHANG et al. 2008).

In patients with tumours of neurogenic and other origin, conventional MR neurography is being used to localize lesions in relation to specific nerve roots (MARAVILLA and BOWEN 1998, MOORE et al. 2001, DAILEY et al. 1997, HAYES et al. 1997). In patients with traumatic plexopathy, MR neurography can also help to define the level of injury to the peripheral nerves, to determine whether damage occurs at the level of the nerve roots or more distally (MARAVILLA and BOWEN 1998, MOORE et al. 2001, DAILEY et al. 1997, HAYES et al. 1997). In addition, in patients with peripheral neuritis, thickening of the brachial plexus can be seen when it is affected (MARAVILLA and BOWEN 1998, MOORE et al. 2001, DAILEY et al. 1997, HAYES et al. 1997). Thus, conventional MR neurography has enabled the visualization and anatomical localization of peripheral nerve pathologies, thereby improving diagnostic accuracy and treatment planning.

Fig. 4.1. Conventional MR neurography of the brachial plexus in a healthy subject using (**a**) coronal STIR, (**b**) T2-weighted imaging and (**c**) T1-weighted imaging. These images were obtained using a 16-channel head and neck receiver coil. All images show the brachial plexus (*arrows*) with high signal-to-noise ratio. Images with an even higher resolution can be obtained when using a microscopy coil or by applying a smaller field of view. However, it is difficult to depict the three-dimensional trajectory of these nerves, as the surrounding structures, such as cerebrospinal fluid, veins and fat tissue exhibit similar signal characteristics to the nerves on these images

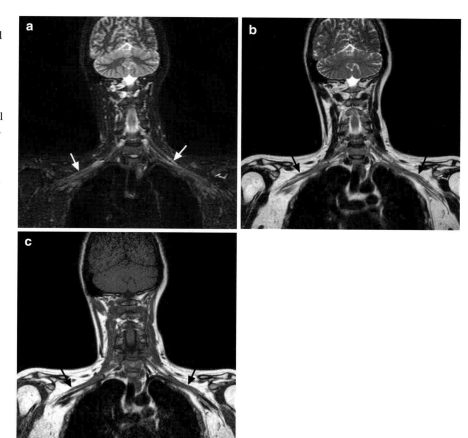

A major disadvantage of conventional MR neurography, however, is its inability to render three-dimensional or projectional images, such as by maximum intensity projection (MIP), to depict the path of peripheral nerves along the lengths of nerve sheaths, due to overlapping of structures from adjacent tissues. Furthermore, vascular structures, such as veins which frequently accompany peripheral nerves, can be difficult to distinguish from the neural elements (e.g. at the level of the brachial plexus) due to their similar signal characteristics on both T2- and T1-weighted imaging (Freund et al. 2007). For these reasons, image interpretation of conventional MR neurography images can be time consuming and precise lesion localization may be difficult. Figures 4.1 and 4.2 illustrate some of the drawbacks of conventional MR neurography.

4.2.2
Visualization of Nerves Using DW-MRI

DW-MRI appears to be a very effective method to visualize nerves of the peripheral nervous system. As is well known, the application of motion-probing gradients (MPGs) using DW-MRI results in signal suppression from structures with relatively unimpeded diffusion, such as blood vessels and cerebrospinal fluid. In structures with relatively impeded diffusion, the MR signal will be little suppressed by the MPGs and will appear relatively bright as the diffusion-sensitizing gradient increases.

Peripheral nerves consist of numerous neuronal fibres, across which diffusion is relatively impeded orthogonal to the long axis of the nerve fibres. Consequently, peripheral nerves exhibit high signal intensity at DW-MRI (Hajnal et al. 1991). The difference in water diffusivity being higher along the long axis of nerves compared to the orthogonal short axes is known as anisotropy. The degree of unequal water diffusion in relation to the axes of peripheral nerves can be quantified by calculating the fractional anisotropy (FA), and this value ranges from 0 to 1; where 0 represents fully isotropic water diffusion (i.e. no difference in water diffusion along any of the neural axes) and 1 represents fully anisotropic water diffusion. The FA of peripheral nerves has been reported to range between 0.599 and 0.80 (Kabakci et al. 2007, Khalil et al. 2008), suggesting that there is significantly less

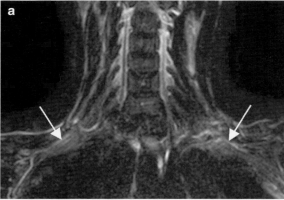

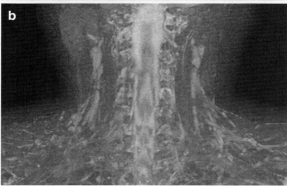

Fig. 4.2. Conventional MR neurography of the brachial plexus in a healthy subject performed using coronal (**a**) STIR imaging with the corresponding (**b**) maximum intensity projection (MIP) image. The STIR image reveals the nerves of the brachial plexus as moderately high signal intensity linear structures (*arrows*). However, note that when MIP was performed on the image set, other high signal intensity structures, such as cerebrospinal fluid and veins, are highlighted on the MIP image which obscures neural visualization

impeded water diffusion along the long axis of the nerves due to the orientation of the neuronal fibres. A variation of DW-MRI technique called diffusion tensor imaging (DTI) is required to measure FA, and DTI can also be used to track and map along the course of peripheral nerves (KABAKCI et al. 2007, KHALIL et al. 2008, TSUCHIYA et al. 2007). However, DTI is usually performed in the central nervous system and rarely used to image the peripheral nerves.

4.2.3
Difference Between Diffusion-Weighted MR Neurography and Diffusion Tensor Imaging/Tractography

The application of diffusion-sensitizing gradients for DW-MR neurography as first described is unique

(TAKAHARA et al. 2008). Although DW-MR neurography superficially resembles a DTI study, the two approaches are based on different concepts.

First, in contrast to DTI, DW-MR neurography does not require the application of MPGs in multiple directions. Typically, MPGs applied in three directions are sufficient, and peripheral nerve visualization may be even better by applying the MPG in only one direction (this will be discussed in a later section). Second, DW-MR neurography uses diffuse weighting as a contrast mechanism to visualize neural structures and does not attempt to perform neural "tracking" or "tractography". In other words, DW-MR neurography is simpler to perform and analyse than DTI, and does not attempt to study the directionality of water diffusion, but only aims to obtain a high-quality neurographic dataset for three-dimensional evaluation and image display.

As mentioned previously, DW-MRI highlights peripheral nerves as high signal intensity structures. However, DW-MR imaging sequences that were used for body imaging in the past could not be applied for three-dimensional image displays of peripheral nerves due to suboptimal image quality. In 2004, a new technique to acquire DW-MRI of the whole body, called DWIBS (diffusion-weighted whole-body imaging with background body signal suppression) (TAKAHARA et al. 2004a) was first described. The concept of DWIBS will be discussed in the next section. Applying the principles of DWIBS to DW-MRI neurography allows us to acquire thin-section datasets, which make it possible to produce three-dimensional images of peripheral nerves in virtually any part of the body.

4.2.4
DWIBS for Diffusion-Weighted MR Neurography

The imaging sequence for DW-MR neurography is identical to the one used for DWIBS (TAKAHARA et al. 2004a). Using this method, DW-MR images are obtained and handled like a three-dimensional dataset by acquiring multiple thin image sections (4–5 mm) rather than a series of two-dimensional thick image sections (8–10 mm). Thin image partitions are possible using this technique because of the long and efficient scan time afforded by performing the scan in free breathing. Although breath-hold or respiratory triggering were previously thought to be necessary for performing DW-MRI studies in the body, the application of MPGs results in significant signal attenuation only where there is significant water diffusion within the image voxel (i.e. intravoxel incoherent motion). By contrast, little signal attenuation is induced by respiratory motion because the phasic motion of breathing can be considered as a type of "coherent motion" during the short diffusion-encoding time of around 100 ms during which the MPGs are applied (Muro et al. 2005, Koh et al. 2008). For this reason, it is feasible to acquire thin image sections with excellent signal-to-noise during free breathing, which is one of the key features of DWIBS.

In addition, DWIBS as originally described, uses a STIR pre-pulse for fat suppression, in contrast to most prior DW-MRI studies in the body which used frequency selective (e.g. chemical shift selective, CHESS) fat-suppression techniques. It is well known that a STIR pre-pulse has the advantage of robust fat suppression over a larger field of view (FOV), even in areas of the body that may experience substantial magnetic field inhomogeneity. It has also been shown that the STIR pre-pulse is also effective when used with DW-MRI (Takahara et al. 2004a) to produce images with excellent background suppression. In this way, the images can be post-processed using MIPs with minimal image degradation from overlying imaging artefacts.

Hence, applying the concept of DWIBS enables DW-MRI to be effectively performed in the body, including regions such as the neck and shoulder, where both large magnetic field inhomogeneities and respiratory motion can substantially degrade image quality. Although the concept of DWIBS was primarily intended for cancer screening, the principles of image acquisition can be translated to improve peripheral nerve visualization (Takahara et al. 2004b, 2008). The key advantage of applying DWIBS for DW-MR neurography is that thin image sections with multiple signal averages can be obtained, thus providing a high-quality dataset for three-dimensional display of nerve trajectories. A further discussion about the theory and concepts of DWIBS can be found in Chap. 14. The readers may also want to refer to other review articles related to the subject (Koh et al. 2007, Kwee et al. 2008).

Table 4.1. Typical scan parameters for performing DW-MR neurography on a 1.5 T MR system

Sequence	SE-EPI
Acquisition plane	Axial
Field of view (mm)	350
Rectangular FOV percentage	80%
TR/TE (ms)	5,786/68
EPI factor (ETL)	47
SENSE factor	2
Acquisition matrix	160×256
Phase encode reduction	80%
Half Fourier scan factor	0.6
Slice thickness/gap (mm)	4/−1 (overlap)
Number of slices	60
Number of excitations	6
Type of fat suppression	STIR (or CHESS)

4.3

Technical Aspects

4.3.1
Basic Parameter Settings

Typical parameters for DW-MR neurography are shown in Table 4.1. The key points for the parameter settings are: (1) images should be acquired axially (with the phase-encoding in the anterior–posterior direction) rather than coronally, to minimize the FOV and reduce image distortion, (2) parallel imaging (e.g. SENSivitiy Encoding, GRAPPA) should be employed to reduce the number of echoes (i.e. the echo-planar imaging [EPI] factor or echo train length [ETL]), (3) STIR pre-pulse technique should be applied for robust fat suppression, which is especially important for imaging of the brachial plexus, and (4) to use thin (2–4 mm) but numerous image sections (60–80) across the imaging volume to enable three-dimensional visualization of the dataset. Generally, imaging using a 1.5 T-system is still preferred to a 3.0 T-system, because the latter still suffers from considerable image distortion and poor fat suppression. However, in the near future, 3.0 T may offer superior image quality when combined with improved fat-suppression schemes and further enhancements to the shimming technology.

4.3.2
Fat Suppression

When performing fat-suppressed studies in the body, a chemical shift selective technique (e.g. CHESS pre-pulse) is most often employed when performing DW-MRI in combination with a spin-echo (SE) EPI sequence. This technique works well in most standard two-dimensional axial image acquisitions. However, more robust fat suppression is often required in the neck and chest, especially when multiple image sections need to be acquired over a large FOV which would allow for three-dimensional image display. This is because unsuppressed fat signal in the peripheral regions over the large FOV (e.g. from the surface of the body) can obscure critical signal emanating from diseases in the central areas of the body. A STIR pre-pulse (a hyperbolic secant adiabatic inversion pulse) results in superior fat suppression compared with CHESS pre-pulse for fat suppression over an extended FOV (Figs. 4.3 and 4.4). Thus, a STIR-EPI DW-MRI sequence is generally recommended when performing DW-MR neurography, especially for visualization of the brachial plexus.

4.3.3
Post-Processing by Maximum Intensity Projection

Once the DW-MR neurography images are attained, they can be post-processed using slab (volume) MIP to visualize the anatomy and trajectory of the nerves roots and trunks. On certain vendor MR platforms, it is possible to make use of more sophisticated software to enhance the rendering and visualization of the neural elements. Using one particular MR system (Philips' Medical System, Best, The Netherlands), it is possible to employ a dedicated post-processing software, the so-called soap-bubble projection (Soap-Bubble, release 5.0; Philips Healthcare, Best) to improve the quality of the projection image. This software tool is implemented using Interactive Data Language release 5.2 (IDL, Research Systems, Boulder, CO), on a PC platform running Windows XP (Microsoft Corporation, Redmond, WA).

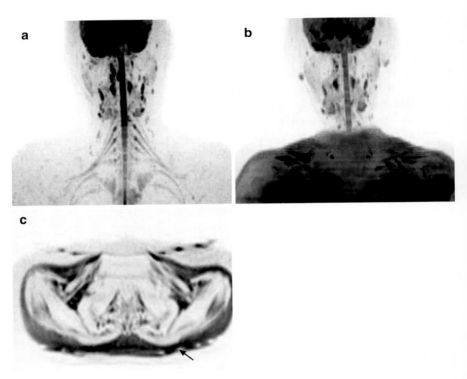

Fig. 4.3. Comparison of inverted grey-scale DW-MR neurographic images of the brachial plexus acquired using STIR fat suppression and CHESS fat suppression. Entire image volume maximum intensity projection (MIP) of the DW-MR neurographic images obtained using (**a**) STIR pre-pulse and (**b**) CHESS pre-pulse are shown. Note that using CHESS fat-suppression technique resulted in poor fat suppression in the subcutaneous areas, leading to the obscuration of the neural elements on the MIP image. If CHESS fat suppression is employed, post-processing would be necessary to remove the signal emanating from the body surface due to suboptimal fat suppression. The relatively poor fat suppression can be seen on the (**c**) high b-value axial inverted grey-scale DW-MRI source image (*arrow*)

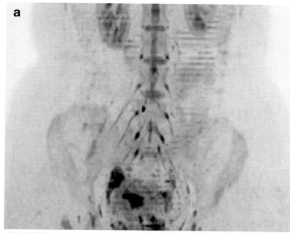

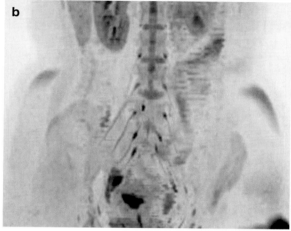

Fig. 4.4. Comparison of DW-MR neurographic images of the lumbosacral plexus acquired using STIR fat suppression and CHESS fat suppression. Entire image volume maximum intensity projections of DW-MR neurographic images obtained using (**a**) STIR pre-pulse and (**b**) CHESS pre-pulse. The magnetic field in the abdominal/pelvic region is more homogeneous compared to the neck/shoulder region. Therefore, in this case, there is less difference in the quality of the images obtained using either the STIR or CHESS fat-suppression technique

The soap-bubble software tool was originally developed for the visualization and quantitative analysis of three-dimensional coronary MR angiograms (WRAZIDLO et al. 1991, ETIENNE et al. 2002). Because of the complicated anatomical orientation, it is usually not possible to visualize all the coronary arteries in one plane, even by the use of curve or slab multi-planar reformats (MPRs). The soap-bubble software was designed to solve this problem. The name soap bubble originates from the idea that a volume to be rendered by MIP can be considered as an ellipsoid

or "soap bubble". By flattening the surface of this soap bubble, all the structures of interest within the image volume (e.g. the coronary arteries) can be projected down onto one plane. Since the anatomical orientation of nerves does not normally allow visualization of their course within a single plane using slab or curved MPRs, the soap-bubble procedure is thus also a post-processing procedure that can help neurological visualization and assessment.

From a practical point of view, the soap-bubble procedure is performed as follows: on the coronally reformatted DW-MR neurographic images, points are initially seeded on all visible nerve roots of the nerve plexus of interest. Sequential points along each nerve root are then automatically "seeded" by applying vessel-tracking function, in order to accelerate the rather time-consuming process of manual seed definition (Fig. 4.5). Unsatisfactory points of image seeding can be deleted and new ones manually inserted as necessary. Subsequently, a deformed plane containing all the defined seed points is created. This post-processing procedure typically takes up to about 10 min per nerve plexus, depending on the number of visualized nerve roots. Since the soap-bubble MIP can help to eliminate any surrounding or superimposing structures which also have a high signal at DW-MRI (such as lymph nodes and bone marrow), the utilization of the soap-bubble MIP function can thus enable better visualization and display of an entire nervous plexus compared with conventional slab or curved MIP (Fig. 4.6).

4.3.4
Unidirectionally Encoded Diffusion-Weighted MR Neurography

Although DW-MR neurography is used to visualize the peripheral nervous system, it was uncertain as to the number of MPGs or their directions of application that would be optimal for neural demonstration. DW-MR neurography using three orthogonal MPGs vs. MPGs applied in six directions was compared by TSUCHIYA et al. (2007) for the visualization of peripheral nerves originating from the cervical cord and thoracolumbar spinal cord in volunteers. They found that in a fair comparison (i.e. using similar image acquisition time and same effective number of excitations) between DW-MR neurography performed using three directions vs. six directions of MPGs, the former resulted in significantly better visualization

Fig. 4.5. Soap-Bubble MIP procedure. The *top left* window shows the seeding points being created along the nerves of the right brachial plexus. The *bottom window* shows the Soap-Bubble MIP image based on the seed points selected. The user can apply the neural tracking function with a free choice for the distance of tracking. This is usually set at about 20–30 pixels to achieve a balance between processing time and the accuracy of tracking

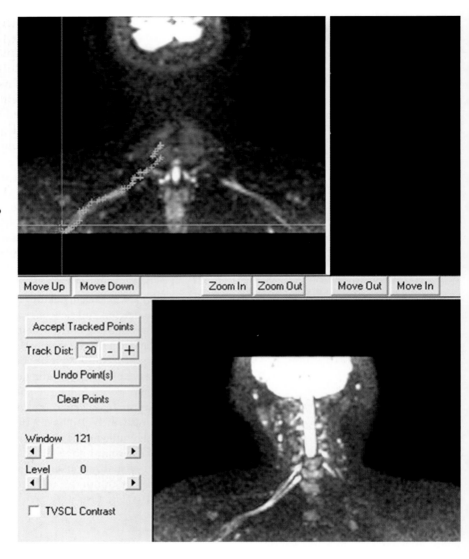

of the sacral plexus [personal communications]. In addition, and more importantly, DW-MR neurography with a MPG applied in just one direction proved to be even more superior to both DW-MR neurography using three or six motion probing directions when the same image acquisition time was used [personal communications]. This technique using just one MPG applied orthogonal to the long axis of the nerve was thus named unidirectionally encoded DW-MR neurography (or simply unidirectional imaging (UDI)) and this is the technique that we would currently recommend for the visualization of nerve roots and peripheral nerves (TAKAHARA et al. 2009a, b). Figure 4.7 demonstrate the effectiveness of the UDI techniques.

4.4
Normal Anatomy

4.4.1
General Image-Based Peripheral Nerve Anatomy

The peripheral nervous system resembles the vascular system in that it consists of tubular structures that branch peripherally. However, radiologists may not be well acquainted with the anatomy of the peripheral nervous system, especially those of the important neural plexi. Anatomy of the brachial and lumbosacral plexus is generally not described in

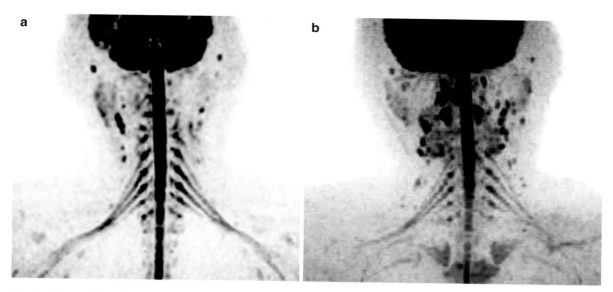

Fig. 4.6. Comparison of DW-MR neurographic images obtained using Soap-Bubble MIP and conventional slab MIP. (a) DW-MR neurographic image post-processed using Soap-Bubble MIP better depicts the entire nerve sheath of the brachial plexus compared with (b) conventional slab MIP post-processing procedure, which is degraded by superimposing objects such as bony structures and lymph nodes

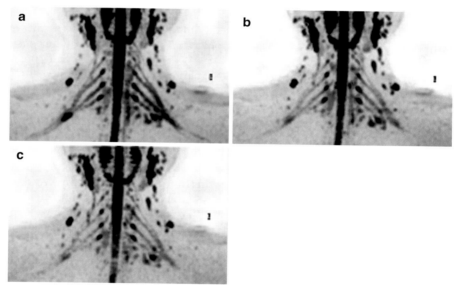

Fig. 4.7. Comparison of DW-MRI MIP neurographic images with (a) MPGs applied in one direction (i.e. unidirectionally encoded diffusion-weighted MR neurography or unidirectional imaging [UDI]), (b) three directions of MPGs and (c) six directions of MPGs (similar to DTI) at 1.5 T, using the same image acquisition time of 4 min and 3 s for each sequence. Note that the use of UDI results in the best visualization of the brachial plexus

standard radiological textbooks discussing image-based radiological anatomy. This is perhaps because until recently, these structures are not well demonstrated by conventional MR imaging. We would like to briefly review the anatomy of the two important neural plexi that can be now visualized using DW-MR neurography: the brachial plexus and the lumbosacral plexus.

4.4.2
Brachial Plexus

A DW-MR neurographic image and a schematic drawing of the brachial plexus are shown in Fig. 4.8 The brachial plexus is a somatic nerve plexus formed by intercommunications between the ventral rami of the lower four cervical nerves (C5–C8) and the first

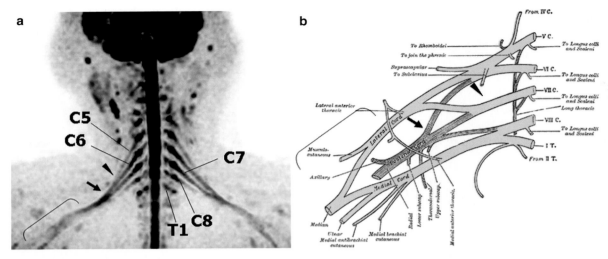

Fig. 4.8. Normal brachial plexus at (**a**) DW-MR neurography and (**b**) schematic drawing of the brachial plexus (Reprinted with permission from GRAY and LEWIS (1918)) The Brachial plexus consists of anterior rami of C5 to T1. C5 and C6 conjoint first (*arrowhead*), followed by a part of C7 (*arrow*), which forms the lateral trunk. However, at present, differentiation of lateral/medial/posterior trunks and their further courses (*bracket*) is not possible or unclear, because of limited spatial resolution. Also, fine nerve branches are not visible. The ganglia are well visualized from C3 to T1 in this image, which may aid in localizing the level of a neurogenic lesion. Note that the first large nerve that is well visualized is C5

thoracic nerve (T1). The plexus gives rise to the motor innervation of all the muscles in the upper limb except the trapezius and levator scapula muscles (MARAVILLA et al. 1998).

At DW-MR neurography, the pre-ganglionic part of the nerve roots is usually not visualized because of its small size and the variable cerebrospinal fluid flow which induces signal loss. The postganglionic portions of the C5 through C7 nerve roots are usually very well visualized, although visualization of the C8 and T1 nerves can be variable because of their small sizes (TAKAHARA et al. 2008). The nerve trunks resulting from the combination of nerve roots are usually well seen, but discrimination of the nerve divisions may be difficult. The DW-MR neurographic image in Fig. 4.8 was acquired using a cardiac coil with five receiver coil elements at 1.5 T, although a dedicated neurovascular receiver coil may allow even better image quality to be achieved.

4.4.3
Lumbosacral Plexus

The lumbar plexus is formed by the anterior divisions of the first to fourth lumbar (L1–L4) nerve roots, while the sacral plexus is formed by the lumbosacral trunk (LST, which comprises the anterior divisions of the fifth lumbar nerve root L5, with contribution from L4), the anterior division of the first sacral nerve root

(S1), and portions of the anterior divisions of the second to fourth sacral nerve roots (S2, S3 and S4).

The LST can be consistently found medial to the psoas muscle and enters the pelvis just anterior to the sacral ala, medial to the sacroiliac joint. As the LST enters the pelvis, it unites with the anterior division of S1 and portions of the anterior divisions of S2 and S3 to form a flattened band. Some parts of S2 to S4 join to form a small inferior band, but this is not visualized at DW-MR neurography because of its small size. The nerves of the sacral plexus continue as the sciatic nerve, which divides at the back of the lower thigh into the tibial and common peroneal nerves (MARAVILLA et al. 1998). The DW-MR neurographic image in Fig. 4.9 was obtained using a cardiac coil with five receiver coil elements at 1.5 T. Note the details of the lumbosacral plexus as described.

4.5
Clinical Applications of Diffusion-Weighted MR Neurography

4.5.1
Neurogenic Tumours

Tumours arising from peripheral nerves include benign and malignant peripheral nerve sheath tumours

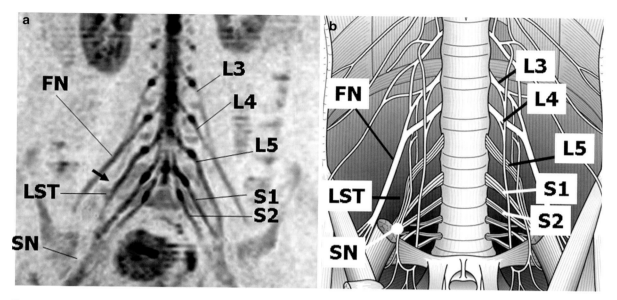

Fig. 4.9. Normal lumbosacral plexus at (**a**) DW-MR neurography and (**b**) schematic drawing of the lumbosacral plexus. The nerves of L4 and L5 join together to form the femoral nerve (FN). An inferior branch of L4 and L5 makes up the lumbosacral trunk (LST), which enters the pelvis, and joins the anterior divisions of S1 and S2, and S3 (not visualized on this image), extending to the sciatic nerve (SN). Note that the direction of travel of the L5 nerve shows a concavity/convexity that is different from that of S1 and S2

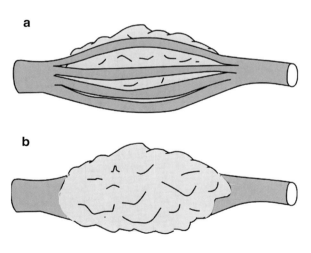

Fig. 4.10. Schematic drawings of the typical appearance of (**a**) schwannoma and (**b**) neurofibroma in long axis. (**a**) Schwannomas arise from the lining of the nerve, and nerve strands can be seen around the tumour. (**b**) Neurofibromas arise from the axons, resulting in a different appearance of the tumour. It is important to differentiate schwannoma from neurofibroma because the latter has a small risk of becoming malignant

(MPNSTs). Benign nerve sheath tumours are subdivided into two groups depending on the morphological and pathological characteristics: schwannoma (also known as neurilemoma or neurinoma) and neurofibroma. Malignant nerve sheath tumours include malignant schwannoma, nerve sheath fibrosarcoma and neurinosarcoma (WEBER et al. 2000).

Histologically, peripheral nerves are made up of two distinct components: the Schwann cells and the axons. Schwann cells are found in the innermost region of the nerve sheath, and these grow to wrap around neuronal axons, creating multiple bundles of nerve fibres or fascicles (WEBER et al. 2000).

Figure 4.10 shows the typical appearance of a schwannoma and a neurofibroma. Schwannomas tend to be located eccentrically to the axon, while neurofibromas tend to infiltrate the nerve and splay apart the individual nerve fibers. Schwannomas grow eccentrically displacing nerve fibres, whereas neurofibromas tend to infiltrate the nerve. The former may be surgically enucleated, while the latter often requires complete surgical resection of the involved nerve for complete removal (BALL and BIGGS 2007). MPNST can appear as an aggressive infiltrative tumour, and can show variable degrees of heterogeneity, enhancement and necrosis on conventional imaging.

DW-MR neurography can be helpful in demonstrating the relationship between the neurogenic tumour and the involved nerve (Fig. 4.11). By using a microscopy MR coil to perform small FOV imaging, the inner structures of a neurogenic tumour may be visualized, which can aid differentiation between a schwannoma and a neurofibroma (Fig. 4.12). Furthermore, DW-MR neurography is also very useful in showing the relationship between the tumour and surrounding structures on the composite maximum projection image "at a glance" (Fig. 4.13).

4.5.2
Trauma

Nerve injuries can occur due to severe trauma which leads to nerve avulsions or axonal damage. The most severe injury is the one of spinal cord, which can result in substantial motor paralysis in the body. Brachial plexus injury is one of the most common injuries of the peripheral nervous system, which can also result in considerable functional impairment of the affected upper limb. Imaging studies play an essential role in the differentiation between preganglionic and postganglionic injuries, a distinction that is critical for optimal treatment planning.

Conventional and CT myelography, as well as thin-section MR imaging using gradient echo sequences are useful for the diagnosis of preganglionic injuries (YOSHIKAWA et al. 2006). DW-MR neurographic images are not helpful for diagnosing preganglionic injuries, because the intradural region is difficult to visualize due to its small size at DW-MRI and also because of the flow of the cerebrospinal fluid. However, DW-MR neurography appears to be a useful technique to determine the location and extent of the injury outside the extradural space or outside the spine. These MR findings could be corroborated with the relevant electroneurography findings (Figs. 4.14 and 4.15). Nevertheless, a major drawback of this technique is that it is impossible to evaluate nerve injuries where there is a concomitant large haematoma (Fig. 4.16).

4.5.3
Mechanical Nerve Compression

The diagnosis of mechanical nerve compression is still a problem in diagnostic imaging, because the radiological diagnosis of "compression" does not always relate to the severity (e.g. the clinical symptoms) of presumed compression. DW-MR neurography is an imaging technique which also suffers from this uncer-

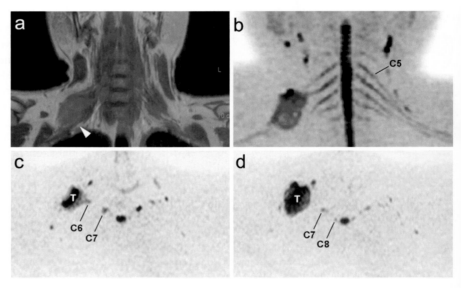

Fig. 4.11. Depiction of the relationship between tumour and the involved nerve (Reprinted, with permission, from TAKAHARA et al. 2008). A 32-year-old man with a pathologically proven schwannoma in the brachial plexus imaged at 1.5 T. (**a**) Coronal T1-weighted image shows a fusiform-shaped mass in the right supraclavicular region. (**b**) Inverted grey-scale diffusion-weighted MR neurographic image derived from using a Soap-Bubble MIP shows that the tumour originates from the C6 nerve root on the right. (**c**, **d**) Axial source images show multiple peripheral nerve roots and the connection between the tumour (T) and the right-sided C6 nerve. The C7 and C8 nerves are also visible

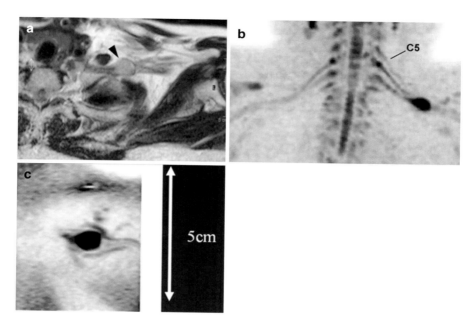

Fig. 4.12. Depiction of the inner structure of the tumour with use of a microscopy coil (Reprinted, with permission, from TAKAHARA et al. 2008). A 67-year-old woman with pathologically proven schwannoma in the brachial plexus imaged at 1.5 T. (**a**) Axial T2-weighted image shows a fusiform-shaped mass in the left supraclavicular region (*arrowhead*). (**b**) Inverted grey-scale diffusion-weighted MR neurographic image post- processed using Soap-Bubble MIP shows that the tumour arises from the left C7 nerve. (**c**) Close-up inverted grey-scale DW-MR image using the microscopy coil and post-processed using slab MIP clearly shows that the tumour does not infiltrate adjacent nerve fascicles, which aids in the discrimination of schwannoma from neurofibroma

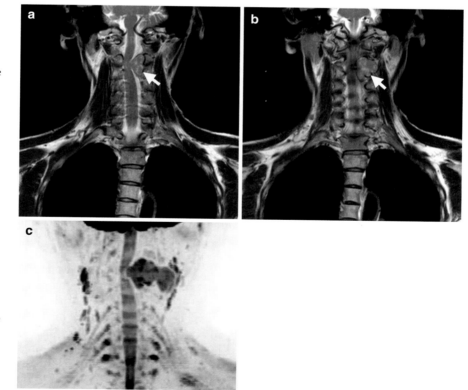

Fig. 4.13. Depiction of the relationship between the tumour and surrounding structures "at a glance". A 50-year-old woman with schwannoma in the brachial plexus imaged at 3.0 T. (**a**, **b**) Consecutive coronal T2-weighted images show a 48 mm intradural mass compressing the spinal cord, and extending to the left side of the neck through a left neural foramina (*arrows*). (**c**) DW-MR neurographic MIP image selectively demonstrates the neural elements and demonstrate the typical dumbbell shape of this neurogenic tumour and compression on the adjacent spinal cord on this single image ("at a glance")

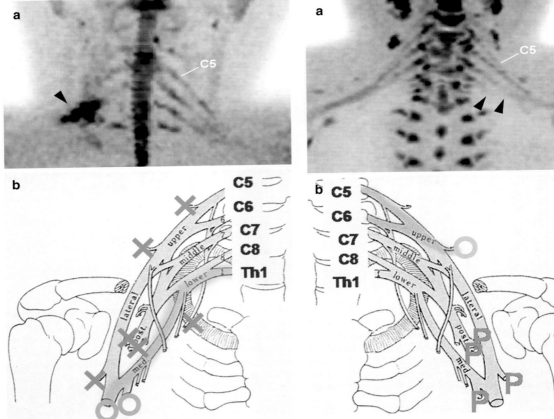

Fig. 4.14. Depiction of injury to the right brachial plexus (Reprinted, with permission, from Takahara et al. 2008). A 35-year-old man with right-sided brachial plexus injury, imaged at 1.5 T. Diffusion-weighted MR neurographic image (a) shows a haematoma (*arrowhead*) on the right side of the neck. Nerve roots of the C5 through C8 nerves are not clearly visible. Complete nerve injury was confirmed in the corresponding area by using electroneurography with electrical silence observed across the (X) involved nerve roots as shown in (b) the schematic diagram of the right brachial plexus (*O* normal; *X* no response)

Fig. 4.15. Distribution of nerve impairment following neural injury. A 26-year-old woman with left-sided brachial plexus injury imaged at 1.5 T. (a) DW-MR neurographic image shows asymmetric visualization of cervical nerves, with low signal intensity of the left-sided brachial plexus at the level of the left C7 and C8 nerves (*arrowheads*) compared with the contralateral side. (b) Partial nerve injury of this area was confirmed by electroneurography with findings of a polyphasic pattern on nerve stimulation study in regions shown on this schematic drawing (*O* normal response; *P* partial response)

tainty. However, in some cases, loss of the signal intensity or distortion of the nerve can be seen on the three-dimensionally rendered DW-MR neurographic images in case of suspected neural compression (Figs. 4.17 and 4.18). Nevertheless, the clinical significance of these imaging findings is still unknown.

4.5.4
Inflammatory Processes

Neuritis refers to an inflammation of the nerves, involving a single nerve or several nerves. The most frequent causes of neuritis are chronic acidosis, injury, certain infections such as tuberculosis or diphtheria, diabetes mellitus, poisoning and alcohol. MR imaging can show the areas of inflammation with regional/diffuse thickening and high signal intensity on the (fat-suppressed) T2-weighted images. The role of DW-MR neurography in this context is still unclear, but several cases with neuritis have exhibited increased signal intensity on the high *b*-value images using this technique (Fig. 4.19). Since DW-MRI is basically derived from a T2-weighted imaging sequence, where MPGs are applied to suppress structures with high diffusivity, it is plausible to hypothesize that MR neurography

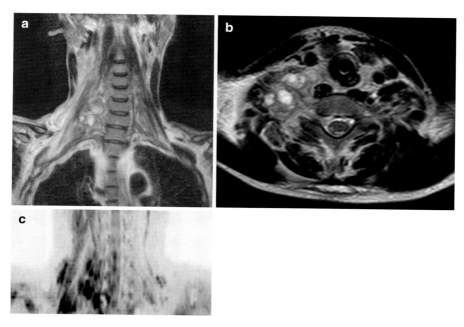

Fig. 4.16. Imaging of neural injury in the presence of a hematoma; a potential limitation of DW-MR neurography. A 30-year-old woman with brachial plexus injury and massive haematoma due to accompanying vertebral artery injury imaged at 1.5 T. (**a**) Coronal and (**b**) axial T2-weighted images show a multi-loculated inhomogeneous lesion at the root of the right neck consistent with haematoma. The right brachial plexus appears to be severely damaged. However, the haematoma returns high signal intensity even on the (**c**) DW-MR neurographic image leading to poor visualization of nerve injury. Hence, assessment of peripheral nerve can be difficult in the presence of a haematoma, which is a limitation of the technique

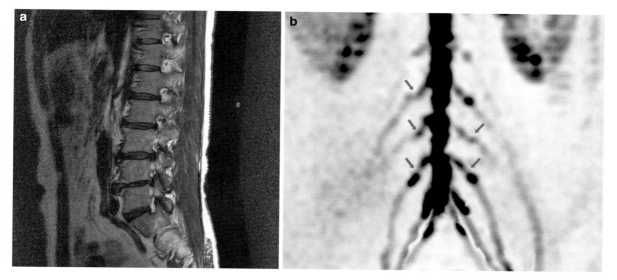

Fig. 4.17. Depiction of neural compression with signal loss on DW-MR neurography. A 72-year-old man with spondylosis deformans and disc herniations at the lumbar levels of L3/4 and L4/5 imaged at 3.0 T. (**a**) Parasagittal T2-weighted image shows relative neuroforaminal stenoses at the levels of L3/4 and L4/5 on the left. (**b**) DW-MR neurographic image post-processed with Soap-Bubble MIP visualizes areas of neural compression as regions of decreased signal intensity along the nerves (*arrows*) on the inverted grey-scale MIP image

Fig. 4.18. Depiction of nerve compression on maximum intensity projection (MIP) imaging. A 64-year-old man with left peroneal nerve paralysis due to severe scoliosis and neuroforaminal stenoses imaged at 1.5 T. (**a**) Conventional radiography shows prominent scoliosis with spondylosis deformans. (**b**) Sagittal T2-weighted image shows marked narrowing of the lumbar neuroforamina. However, it is difficult to appreciate the degree of neural compression in the presence of scoliosis. (**c**) Inverted grey-scale DW-MR neurographic MIP image shows the three-dimensional trajectory of the sacral plexus. Distortion of the L3, L4 and L5 roots could be observed (*arrows*), the changes on the left correspond to the clinical symptoms

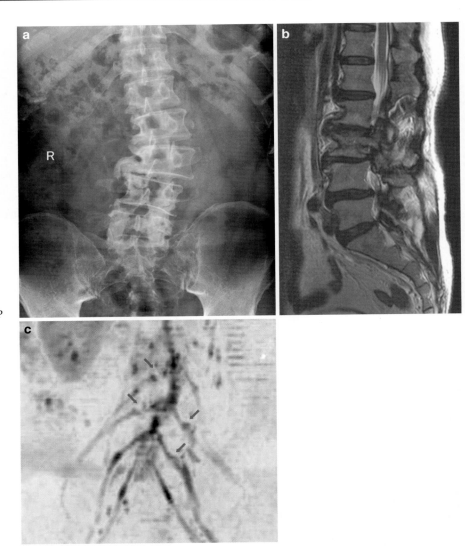

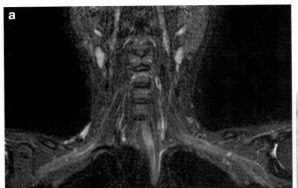

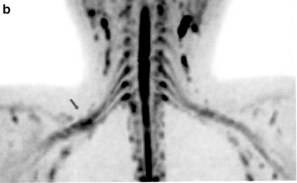

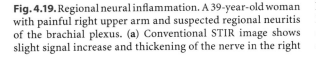

Fig. 4.19. Regional neural inflammation. A 39-year-old woman with painful right upper arm and suspected regional neuritis of the brachial plexus. (**a**) Conventional STIR image shows slight signal increase and thickening of the nerve in the right lateral segment of the brachial plexus. (**b**) Inverted grey-scale DW-MR neurographic maximum intensity projection image shows more striking increase in signal intensity in the corresponding area (*arrow*)

would be at least comparable to T2-weighted imaging for visualizing neuritis, and possibly superior because of the suppression of unwanted signals from surrounding structures. However, the role of DW-MR neurography for the patient with neuritis is currently still not established.

References

Ball JR, Biggs MT (2007) Operative steps in management of benign nerve sheath tumours. Neurosurg Focus 22:E7

Dailey AT, Tsuruda JS, Filler AG, Maravilla KR, Goodkin R, Kliot M. (1997) Magnetic resonance neurography of peripheral nerve degeneration and regeneration. Lancet 350: 1221–1222

Freund W, Brinkmann A, Wagner F, et al (2007) MR neurography with multiplanar reconstruction of 3D MRI datasets: an anatomical study and clinical applications. Neuroradiology 49:335–341

Etienne A, Botnar RM, Van Muiswinkel AM, Boesiger P, Manning WJ, Stuber M. (2002) "Soap-Bubble" visualization and quantitative analysis of 3D coronary magnetic resonance angiograms. Magn Reson Med 48:658–666

Filler AG, Howe FA, Hayes CE, et al (1993) Magnetic resonance neurography. Lancet 341:659–661

Gray H, Lewis WH (eds) (1918) Gray's anatomy, 20th edn. Lea & Febiger, Philadelphia, PA

Hajnal JV, Doran M, Hall AS, et al (1991) MR imaging of anisotropically restricted diffusion of water in the nervous system: technical, anatomic, and pathologic considerations. J Comput Assist Tomogr 15:1–18

Hayes CE, Tsuruda JS, Mathis CM, Maravilla KR, Kliot M, Filler AG (1997) Brachial plexus: MR imaging with a dedicated phased array of surface coils. Radiology 203:286–289

Kabakci N, Gürses B, Firat Z (2007) Diffusion tensor imaging and tractography of median nerve: normative diffusion values. AJR Am J Roentgenol 189:923–927

Khalil C, Hancart C, Le Thuc V, Chantelot C, Chechin D, Cotten A (2008) Diffusion tensor imaging and tractography of the median nerve in carpal tunnel syndrome: preliminary results. Eur Radiol 18:2283–2291

Koh DM, Takahara T, Imai Y, Collins D (2008) Practical aspects of clinical diffusion-weighted imaging in the body for tumour assessment. Magn Reson Med Sci 211–224

Kwee TC, Takahara T, Ochiai R, Nievelstein RA, Luijten PR (2008) Diffusion-weighted whole-body imaging with background body signal suppressions (DWIBS): features and potential applications in oncology. Eur Radiol 18: 1937–1952

Maravilla KR, Bowen BC (1998) Imaging of the peripheral nervous system: evaluation of peripheral neuropathy and plexopathy. AJNR Am J Neuroradiol 19:1011–1023

Moore KR, Tsuruda JS, Dailey AT (2001) The value of MR neurography for evaluating extraspinal neuropathic leg pain: a pictorial essay. AJNR Am J Neuroradiol 22:786–794

Muro I, Takahara T, Horie T, et al (2005) Influence of respiratory motion in body diffusion weighted imaging under free breathing (examination of a moving phantom). Nippon Hoshasen Gijutsu Gakkai Zasshi 61:1551–1558

Takahara T, Imai Y, Yamashita T, Yasuda S, Nasu S, Van Cauteren M (2004a) Diffusion weighted whole body imaging with background body signal suppression (DWIBS): technical improvement using free breathing, STIR, and high resolution 3D display. Radiat Med 22:275–282

Takahara T, Yamashita T, Yanagimachi N, Iino M, Koizumi J, Imai Y (2004b) Imaging of peripheral nerve disease using diffusion-weighted neurography (DWN) [abstract]. In: Radiological Society of North America scientific assembly and annual meeting program. Radiological Society of North America, Oak Brook, IL, 394p

Takahara T, Hendrikse J, Yamashita T, et al (2008) Diffusion-weighted MR neurography of the brachial plexus: feasibility study. Radiology 249:653–660

Takahara T, Kwee TC, Hendrikse J, et al (2009a) Selective visualization of peripheral nerves using diffusion-weighted MR neurography with unidirectional motion probing gradients. In: European Congress of Radiology. European Society of Radiology, Vienna, Austria, p C-730

Takahara T, Hendrikse J, Kwee TC, et al (2009b) Diffusion-weighted MR neurography of the sacral plexus with unidirectional motion probing gradients

Tsuchiya K, Imai M, Tateishi H, Nitatori T, Fujikawa A, Takemoto S (2007) Neurography of the spinal nerve roots by diffusion tensor scanning applying motion-probing gradients in six directions. Magn Reson Med Sci 6:1–5

Weber AL, Montandon C, Robson CD (2000) Neurogenic tumours of the neck. Radiol Clin North Am 38:1077–1090

Wrazidlo W, Brambs HJ, Lederer W, et al (1991) An alternative method of three-dimensional reconstruction from two-dimensional CT and MR data sets. Eur J Radiol 12:11–16

Zhang ZW, Song LJ, Meng QF, et al (2008) High-resolution diffusion-weighted MR imaging of the human lumbosacral plexus and its branches based on a steady-state free precession imaging technique at 3T. AJNR Am J Neuroradiol 29:1092–1094

Yoshikawa T, Hayashi N, Yamamoto S, et al (2006) Brachial plexus injury: clinical manifestations, conventional imaging findings, and the latest imaging techniques. Radiographics 26(Suppl 1):S133–143

Evaluation of Organ Function

5

Frederik de Keyzer and Harriet C. Thoeny

CONTENTS

Frederik de Keyzer, MSc
Department of Radiology, University Hospitals Leuven, Herestraat 49, 3000 Leuven, Belgium
Harriet C. Thoeny, MD
Institute of Diagnostic, Interventional and Pediatric Radiology, University and Inselspital, Freiburgstrasse 10, 3010 Bern, Switzerland

SUMMARY

As DW-MRI is mostly known for its ability to detect microstructural alterations in tissues, the current applications of this challenging technique are mostly located in the field of oncology, for tumour detection and monitoring of treatment response. However, the contrast generated in DW-MRI can also be used to provide information on the function of those organs that are related to production, displacement or excretion of fluid. Ideal targets for this kind of evaluation are the kidneys and the salivary glands. In the kidneys, the water mobility is generated through the filtration and diffusion of fluids, while gustatory stimulation can induce a large production and excretion of saliva in the salivary glands. With technical innovations allowing fast imaging with high signal-to-noise ratios, DW-MRI for the evaluation of liver and pancreas function, has also become feasible.

5.1

Introduction

Diffusion-weighted magnetic resonance imaging (DW-MRI) is a relatively novel technique, generating contrast based on differences in mobility of the water protons, with major contributing effects of cell density, extracellular extravascular space and tubular structures. Therefore, an interesting application of DW-MRI is to examine the function of those organs that exhibit production, displacement or excretion of fluid (Thoeny and De keyzer 2007). To date the organs whose function has been extensively investigated are the kidneys and the salivary glands. While fluid filtration and diffusion occur in the kidneys, the salivary glands can be stimulated to produce and excrete large amounts of saliva. With the technical innovations allowing fast imaging with high signal-to-noise ratios in recent years, the interest of the research community has expanded to include the liver and pancreas in the upper abdomen. In this chapter, we first discuss why comparisons of apparent diffusion coefficient (ADC) values between centres are difficult and depend strongly on the used b-values, exemplified by the parotid glands (THOENY et al. 2004). Thereafter, the different organs mentioned above are discussed in turn with an overview of the current status, guidelines and possible clinical applications.

5.2

Effect of *b*-Values

Comparison between ADC values of different studies and different centres is often complex due to varying sequence optimizations, study set-ups and image interpretation. However, one of the main causes of this problem is the use of different b-values between centres. This effect of the choice of b-values on the calculated ADC values has been demonstrated in the parotid glands (THOENY et al. 2004).

The differences in ADC values derived using different sets of b-value are due to the way ADC values are calculated. The measured signal intensities are fitted by a mono-exponential curve as follows:

$$S_i = S_0 * \exp(-b_i * \mathrm{ADC}) + n_i \,,$$

where S_i is the signal intensity measured on the native diffusion-weighted image acquired using b-value b_i. S_0 is a variable indicating the exact signal intensity for $b = 0\,\mathrm{s/mm^2}$, with the noise n_i adding to the signal.

Figure 5.1 demonstrates an example of a signal decay curve with increasing b-values. The dotted line is the best mono-exponential fit of the given dataset, using the native diffusion-weighted images acquired with b-values of 500, 750 and 1,000 s/mm². This mono-exponential curve fits the data at $b = 500$, 750 and 1,000 s/mm² reasonably well, but there is a strong deviation from this curve in the lower b-value ranges. This is due to the fact that in most normal tissues, the signal decay with increasing b-values is influenced not only by diffusion, but also by perfusion in microvessels (LE BIHAN et al. 1988) and compartmental subdivisions with different length scales of free diffusion

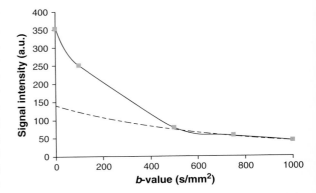

Fig. 5.1. Signal intensity decay curve with increasing b-values from a DW-MR acquisition (*solid line*). Least squares approximation of the three final data points for $b = 500$, $b = 750$, and $b = 1,000\,\mathrm{s/mm^2}$ (*dashed line*). The *dashed line* is extrapolated to illustrate the deviation from the fitted curve in the lower b-value range

(YABLONSKIY et al. 2003). These influences result in the bi-exponential pattern of signal attenuation, giving rise to the adoption of more advanced, bi-exponential fitting models, which aim to separate the fast- and slow-moving diffusion "pools". However, optimum bi-exponential data fitting requires the acquisition of many b-value images, which requires longer acquisition time, not to mention more time-consuming data post-processing. For these reasons, the mono-exponential model is still the most widely used. It can be easily seen that if a different b-value subset, such as $b = 0$, 50 and 100 s/mm² is used to calculate the ADC, the resulting value will be significantly different from the one calculated using b-values such as $b = 500$, 750 and 1,000 s/mm².

An example from the study by THOENY et al. (2004) illustrates the ADC values measured in the parotid glands in a group of eight healthy volunteers (Fig. 5.2). This clearly shows that ADC calculation derived from only higher ($>500\,\mathrm{s/mm^2}$) b-values leads to the lowest ADC values, while b-value sets containing only low b-values lead to the highest ADC values. ADC calculated using a b-value range that contains both low and high b-values will have an intermediate ADC value. Additionally, if more than two b-value images are used for the calculation of an ADC value, using the mono-exponential fitting method, the formula is usually rewritten to:

$$\ln(S_i) = -b_i * \mathrm{ADC} + \ln(S_0).$$

Using this formula, the more complex solution has been reduced to a linear regression. The difference

Fig. 5.2. Bar charts of signal intensity vs. different sets of *b*-values for exponential and logarithmic fits. These findings show that the higher the *b*-values the lower the ADC, and the lower the *b*-values the higher the ADC. It also shows the independence of the fit procedure ($p = 0.542$) (source: THOENY et al. 2004)

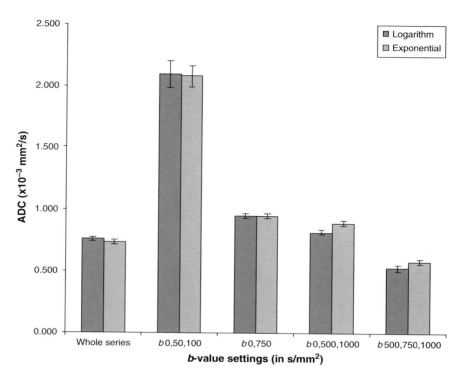

between the two fitting methods on the ADC values was never found to be significant in the dataset, meaning both methods can be used, depending on the available software and expertise on-site.

5.3

Salivary Glands

5.3.1
Introduction

The salivary glands are exocrine glands secreting saliva. The glandular acinar cells secrete fluid through transmembraneous transport from the intracellular space to the striated ducts, which ultimately drain into the mouth. Whereas the parotid glands are purely serous, the submandibular glands comprise both serous and mucinous acinar cells. As the salivary gland functionality is based on fluid production and transport, it is an ideal target for imaging by diffusion-weighted sequences. Using this technique, an estimation of the secretion of the salivary gland can be made, and can be used to assess altered saliva production in patients, e.g. after radiotherapy of the head and neck region.

5.3.2
Imaging at Rest

Several research groups have reported the ADC values derived from diffusion-weighted imaging in the salivary glands at rest (Table 5.1).

As can be seen, the ADC values of both the parotid and the submandibular glands differ substantially between centres. This can, in most cases, be attributed to the use of different range of *b*-values, scanner hardware and sequence parameters.

However, one consistent observation is that the ADC values of the submandibular glands are always higher than the parotid glands. In the unstimulated state, about two-thirds of the total saliva is produced by the submandibular glands, which could be a possible reason for the higher ADC. Also, the different histologic composition of the submandibular glands, with both serous and mucinous tissue, and the lower amount of adipose tissue that restricts diffusion, may account for the ADC difference.

5.3.3
Imaging During and After Stimulation

The ADC values at rest can give an indication of the functionality of the salivary glands. However, even in

Table 5.1. Overview of ADC values of the parotid and submandibular glands in literature

Group	Year	Population	No. included	b-Values (s/mm²)	ADC (×10⁻³ mm²/s) Parotid gland	Submandibular gland
Patel et al.	2004	Healthy patients	90	0 and 1,000	0.50 ± 0.28	–
Habermann et al.	2007	Healthy volunteers	27	0, 500, and 1,000	1.12 ± 0.08 (1.5 T)	–
Sumi et al.	2002	Healthy volunteers	36	500 and 1,000	0.28 ± 0.01	0.37 ± 0.01
Yoshino et al.	2001	Patients without salivary disease	18	0 and 771	0.62 ± 0.15	0.98 ± 0.26
Zhang et al.	2001	Patients before RT	21	10, 50, 100, and 150	2.42 ± 0.56	2.54 ± 0.64
Thoeny et al.	2005	Healthy volunteers	12	400, 600, 800, and 1,000	0.88 ± 0.09	1.30 ± 0.11

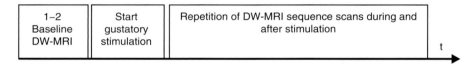

Fig. 5.3. Example time course of a typical diffusion-weighted examination of salivary gland function. One or two baseline scans have to be performed to acquire a good baseline measurement; thereafter, stimulation is started and identical scans as the baseline scan(s) are repeated as fast as possible. The exact timing depends strongly on the type of stimulation and on the scan sequence used

cases of xerostomia, where there is impairment of saliva production, the saliva production at rest is usually sufficient to keep the mouth hydrated. However, saliva production is impaired when the glands are stimulated during speech, swallowing or eating. The salivary glands cannot produce enough saliva for these functions which can lead to nutritional deficiencies and decreased quality of life. Xerostomia is also prone to infections in the oral cavity and increases dental caries. The condition can result from autoimmune disorders, such as Sjögren's disease, following radiotherapy for head and neck cancers or may be drug induced.

To optimally assess glandular function, it will be beneficial to estimate the amount of saliva produced during stimulation, which poses additional imaging challenges compared with DW-MRI at rest. For imaging of the salivary glands during stimulation, a faster sequence is needed, with high enough quality that can be repeated during the entire stimulation period.

The time course of a diffusion-weighted examination of salivary gland function is shown in Fig. 5.3. The acquisition time for each diffusion-weighted sequence is typically between 1.5 and 3 min, with a total follow-up time of 15–25 min after the start of stimulation. This time frame allows examination of the early stimulation-induced effects, but also of the later effects, such as a normalization of the saliva production, or possibly a return to baseline values. Each diffusion-weighted sequence should cover the entire parotid glands, and if possible include the submandibular glands, with good resolution and enough slices through the glands to exclude partial volume effects. The patient should be fixed in the coil by light strapping to avoid any movement over the entire examination period.

Using such a set-up, it has been shown that the ADC values of salivary glands change over the time course of gustatory stimulation (Thoeny et al. 2005a; Habermann et al. 2007; Dirix et al. 2008). Thoeny et al. (2005a) and Dirix et al. (2008) described a biphasic response to salivary stimulation in volunteers, both in the parotid glands and the submandibular glands (Figs. 5.4 and 5.5). In the parotid gland, although the inter-patient variability of baseline ADC

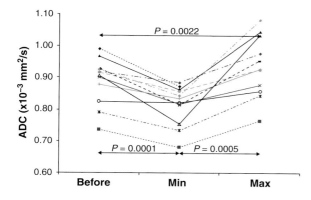

Fig. 5.4. ADC of the parotid glands in 12 volunteers before and during gustatory stimulation. A significant decrease in ADC during the first 5–7 min of salivary stimulation (between *before* and *min*) ($p = 0.0001$) is demonstrated and a significant increase during the following 15–20 min when compared with the previous dip (between *min* and *max*) ($p = 0.0005$) and baseline (between *before* and *max*) ($p = 0.0022$) values (source: THOENY et al. 2005)

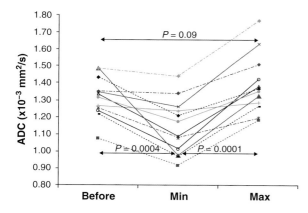

Fig. 5.5. ADC of the submandibular glands in 12 volunteers before and during gustatory stimulation. During the first 5–7 min of salivary stimulation, a significant decrease (between *before* and *min*) ($p = 0.0004$) in ADC could be observed; however, the increase during the following 20 min was only significant when compared with the lowest ADC value (between *min* and *max*) ($p = 0.0001$), but not compared with the baseline value (between *before* and *max*) ($p = 0.09$) (source: THOENY et al. 2005)

values was quite large, there was still an observable significant decrease to a minimal ADC value in almost all volunteers within the first 5 min after the start of stimulation. Thereafter, in the following 15 min, a steady increase to a maximal ADC value was seen, and this maximal value was significantly higher than both the minimal value and the baseline value (Fig. 5.4). According to clinical studies, these findings might be attributed to emptying of stored

saliva during the early phase of stimulation, reflected by decreased ADC; followed by an increase in ADC corresponding to active saliva production.

A similar change was observed in the submandibular glands, with a biphasic response to initially a minimum ADC value, and a subsequent increase to a maximum ADC value, in the same time frame as the parotid glands (Fig. 5.5). The minimum value was also significantly lower than the baseline value, and the maximal value was significantly higher than the minimal value. However, the maximum value was not significantly higher than the baseline value.

By contrast, the research of HABERMANN et al. (2007) did not show a decrease of ADC in the first minutes after the start of stimulation, but only a small but significant ADC increase in the first 2 min after the stimulation. The difference with the study by THOENY et al. could be due to the different type of salivary stimulation used or to the different *b*-value sets, highlighting a different effect of the gustatory stimulation.

5.3.4
Comparison with Salivary Gland Scintigraphy

Functional evaluation of the salivary glands by DW-MRI has been compared to scintigraphy in several studies (DIRIX et al. 2008; ZHANG et al. 2001). In a group of patients treated with radiotherapy for head and neck cancer, ZHANG et al. (2001) examined salivary gland function using a scintigraphy scan after injection of 370 MBq of ^{99m}Tc sodium pertechnetate tracer and saliva production was stimulated using lemon juice. They also performed a routine MR examination with an added DW-MRI sequence without gustatory stimulation. The parameters evaluated at salivary gland scintigraphy were the uptake ratio (UR) and maximum accumulation (MA), which were compared to the signal intensity ratios (SIR) on T1- and T2-weighted images and to the ADC values from the DW-MRI. In that study (ZHANG et al. 2001), they could not find a correlation between any of the SGS parameters and the SIR on T1- or T2-weighted MR images. However, the ADC values show a strong significant positive correlation with the UR and the MA values. Moreover, when subdividing the glands into a dysfunctional and a functional group, the functional glands had a significantly higher ADC than the dysfunctional glands (2.44×10^{-3} and 1.91×10^{-3} mm^2/s, respectively), whereas none of the SIR values showed a difference. Therefore, a single DW-MRI examination, even without gustatory stimulation, appeared to inform on the functionality of the salivary glands.

In another study, DIRIX et al. (2008) applied DW-MRI combined with gustatory stimulation in patients undergoing radiotherapy of the head and neck, again confirming the value of ADC in assessing salivary gland function under pathological conditions. In that study, a parotid-sparing radiotherapy scheme was applied, resulting in a lower dose irradiation on the contralateral parotid gland with the aim of preserving parotid gland function. After radiotherapy, a higher ADC value before stimulation was found for the parotid gland which received the highest dose irradiation, while in the contralateral gland, the baseline ADC value was preserved. This difference could be due to radiotherapeutically induced inflammation or even to necrosis formation in the irradiated gland. Before radiotherapy, a biphasic ADC response with an initial decrease and a subsequent increase was seen in both parotid glands, when the patient received gustatory stimulation with a tablet of ascorbic acid (THOENY et al. 2005a). After radiotherapy, this biphasic response was still present in the spared parotid gland, but was absent in the parotid gland included in the high-dose radiation field.

5.3.5
Practical Issues

Due to the high inter-patient variability, a number of practical concerns should be addressed prior to imaging. Attention to these will allow better comparison between studies and in the interpretation of the results.

5.3.5.1
Patient Inclusion/Preparation

Many factors influence the amount of saliva that is produced by gustatory stimulation. These include the sex of the patient as well as smoking or medication (BERK et al. 2005). In addition, the time of the day and the season have an effect on saliva production. The influence from these factors cannot be excluded from any examination, and as such should be described or systemized as far as possible. It is, for instance, optimal for any comparative study to use control groups that are age- and sex-matched, and also matched for the number of smokers and drug-users. These studies should also preferably be performed at the same time of day. Hence, any saliva stimulation study should take into account the possible effects of various patient factors in order to draw the appropriate conclusions.

One important factor that can alter saliva production is the hydration state of the patient. While severely dehydrated patients are incapable of producing any saliva, slightly dehydrated patients will display a lower saliva production than those who are normally hydrated (BERK et al. 2005). In most recent publications, the effect of hydration state is minimized by enforcing an eating/drinking scheme in the hour(s) preceding the examination. In the studies by THOENY et al. and DIRIX et al., the investigators asked the patients or volunteers not to drink or eat for at least 1 h prior to the examination, thereby minimizing the effects of mastication and hydration state (THOENY et al. 2005a; DIRIX et al. 2008). An alternative approach is the one adopted by HABERMANN et al. (2007) which placed the patients on a strict hydration diet in order to minimize the hydration-induced variability. In their recently published study, they allowed all volunteers to drink 1.5 L of water in the 4 h preceding the examination.

5.3.5.2
Magnetic Resonance Scans

Most studies estimating saliva production have been performed on 1.5 T MR systems. However, investigations at higher field strengths are also feasible. HABERMANN et al. (2007) have made a comparative study at 1.5 and 3 T. The mean gland ADC values (±standard deviation, $^*10^{-3}$ mm^2/s) before stimulation on 1.5 T was 1.12 ± 0.08, which was comparable to the value at 3 T (1.14 ± 0.04). Also, the gustatory stimulation caused an increase in ADC at both field strengths up to 1.18 ± 0.09 and 1.17 ± 0.05, respectively. Imaging at 3 T seemed to display slightly smaller ADC effect after stimulation, but showed lower variability. Currently, the choice of 1.5 or 3 T does not seem important as the results are very similar. Further studies might show the advantages of imaging at either field strength, and will help to determine the optimal setup for the gustatory stimulation studies.

An appropriate coil selection is necessary for optimal acquisition of DW-MR images. If only a single parotid gland is examined, a surface carotid coil would be best in view of the very high signal-to-noise ratio that can be achieved. However, when both parotid glands and/or both submandibular glands, and theoretically the sublingual glands, need to be imaged, a head coil, either circularly polarized or phased-array, would be ideal. The phased-array head coils have the added benefit of allowing parallel acquisition techniques which permit faster imaging during stimulation studies. Unfortunately, the phased-array head coils from most providers are made for brain examination, and do not provide enough coverage to obtain high signal images from the submandibular glands. The newer neurovascular coils, which have been available more recently, do provide the needed coverage. A viable alternative is to use a combination of the posterior part of the head coil, with a flexible neck coil (Yoshino et al. 2001; Habermann et al. 2007).

Most studies to date use summary statistics of the mean or median ADC value in region of interest (ROI)-based analysis of the images, and therefore do not require perfect immobilization of the patient during the entire examination. However, future studies should aim at assessing the heterogeneity of saliva production in the different areas of the salivary glands, especially in the light of intensity-modulated radiotherapy. A voxel-per-voxel analysis of the gustatory stimulation-induced changes is then required and minimizing motion, such as by solid fixation, becomes important. For all salivary stimulation examinations, head support cushions should be used to immobilize the head as much as possible, while providing maximum comfort to the patient. If available, a bite bar attached to the head coil could provide extra fixation, minimize motion and therefore allow voxel-by-voxel analysis without separate coregistration software.

The DW-MRI sequence parameters may differ from centre to centre. These sequences can be subdivided into two groups. Firstly, there is a DW-MRI scan with good anatomical information which can be also used for oncological applications (see Chap. 7). This is also the most convenient scan to co-register with a T1- or T2-weighted acquisition, or even with a CT scan. In the framework of organ function evaluation this type of sequence is often used for imaging at rest, when not providing the patients with gustatory stimulation. As time limitations are not so stringent in these applications, the DW-MR images are usually acquired using a lower bandwidth, more slices, more averages and so on. This yields attractive images with very high signal-to-noise ratios. Often, it is also preferable to acquire more b-values in this acquisition in order to better calculate the ADC maps. Secondly, there are the faster single-shot DW-MRI sequences which are used for gustatory stimulation studies. Using these faster sequences prevents image degradation that may result

Table 5.2. Frequently used DW-MRI sequence parameters for salivary gland examinations at 1.5 T

Sequence parameter	Imaging at rest	Imaging during stimulation
Field of view (mm)	180–240	180–240
Matrix	$(96-128) \times (128-160)$	$(60-96) \times 128$
Slice thickness (mm)	3–5	4–5
Number of slices	10–40	6–20
TR/TE (ms)	$\infty/70-90$	$\infty/70-90$
Maximal b-value (s/mm²)	500–1,000	500–1,000
Number of b-values	2–10	2–4
Number of excitations	4–8	3–5
Bandwidth (Hz/Px)	1,502	1,502
Orientation	Axial	Axial
Total scan time (min)	3–6	1–3

from motion during the longer stimulation study. Examples of DW-MRI parameters for both types of imaging approaches are shown in Table 5.2.

5.3.5.3
Types of Saliva Stimulation

The most common means of saliva stimulation used in these studies are either a continuous drip of lemon juice or a tablet of ascorbic acid (vitamin C tablet). As these have a completely different physical state when administered (fluid vs. dry tablet), one might speculate that the stimulation effect will also be different. This might indeed explain the different stimulation effects found in the studies by Habermann et al. (2007) and Thoeny et al. (2005a). In the study by Habermann et al. (2007), an immediate ADC increase was evidenced after administering 5 mL of lemon juice. By comparison, Thoeny et al. used a tablet of ascorbic acid for gustatory stimulation, and they found a significant early decrease of ADC, followed by an increase. The reason for the difference could be because the tablet induced drainage of the remaining saliva into the mouth for digestion of the tablet, even before new saliva was produced, while this did not happen with the lemon juice.

Although the set-up for lemon juice administration is a bit more complex than giving a vitamin C tablet to the patient during scanning, it has a few potential benefits. Firstly, it will allow more precise control on how much stimulation is given to the patient. A vitamin C tablet dissolves in the mouth at different rates in different people, while the lemon juice can be administered at exact doses, and for an exact duration. Secondly, the lemon juice drip can be put in place during the initial patient positioning and does not require further movement to put the tablet into the mouth at the correct time. This allows for a faster continuation of the scan, and more importantly, movement of the patient at the start of the stimulation is minimized.

Some salivary gland scintigraphy studies use carbachol injection to induce saliva production. This is a cholinergic agonist which results in glandular stimulation. If used in MR imaging studies, it would facilitate comparison with scintigraphy results and, as this substance is injected, would make dosing easier. This theoretical advantage may help in the standardization of MR examination for the evaluation of salivary gland function, but to date no literature can be found describing the use of carbachol in this setting.

5.4
Kidneys

5.4.1
Introduction

As the main kidney functions are related to water transport, such as glomerular filtration, active and passive tubular reabsorption or secretion, diffusion characteristics may provide useful insight into functional and structural consequences of various renal diseases, including renal parenchymal disease, acute and chronic renal failure, inflammatory diseases and obstructive uropathy.

Since the first published reports on DW-MRI of the human kidneys in the early 1990s (MÜLLER et al. 1994b), most of the subsequent articles were focused on *animal studies* or were performed in *healthy volunteers* investigating the feasibility of DW-MRI and addressing technical issues. It is only recently that a few studies have been performed in patients to show the potential correlation of DW-MRI parameters with renal function and to apply this new technique to evaluate diffuse renal pathologies as a result of structural and functional changes.

5.4.2
Technical Considerations

When performing DW-MRI of the kidneys several technical considerations have to be taken into account.

In contrast to DW-MRI of the brain where motion is usually restricted to single-pixel or even sub-pixel movements, imaging in the upper abdominal region is challenging because of massive respiratory motion, arterial pulsations and intestinal peristalsis. Minimization of the movement effects is mandatory, and can be achieved by using free-breathing or breath-hold sequences.

When using free-breathing sequences, respiratory triggering and cardiac gating should be applied whenever possible. There are several advantages over breath-hold sequences: free breathing allows for acquisition of multiple averages with consequent high signal-to-noise ratio, and at the same time multiple b-values can be applied with coverage of the entire kidneys. The drawback of using free-breathing sequences, with triggering and entire kidney coverage, is that the measurement time is quite long (>5 min).

On the other hand, breath-hold sequences have the advantage of being much faster (<25 s); however, fewer b-values and fewer averages can be applied in this limited time with consequent lower signal-to-noise ratio. In severely ill patients and children, breath-hold might be difficult or even impossible, and in such cases respiratory triggering with free breathing is recommended.

A further reduction in motion and especially in susceptibility artefacts can also be obtained using parallel imaging techniques and the shortest possible echo times (TE). Parallel imaging techniques allow reduction in the echo-train length in the DW-MRI readout, yielding a reduction in scan time and a subsequent lower movement effect. This echo-train length reduction minimizes the sampling on the free induction decay curve, and subsequently lowers the sensitivity to susceptibility influences.

In some cases it may be useful to administer antiperistaltic drugs to reduce bowel motion artefacts to minimize susceptibility artefacts due to air in the bowels.

Breath-hold sequences usually do not allow enough time to apply the diffusion-sensitizing gradients in three orthogonal directions, and the most representative direction needs to be taken. This should be decided before the scan and should be kept constant between scans, in order to minimize the inter-scan variability. In sequences with free breathing, application of the diffusion-sensitizing gradients in three orthogonal directions, and subsequent calculation of the trace image is feasible and even strongly recommended to minimize the effect of diffusion anisotropy. In some applications, however, diffusion anisotropy is a useful parameter to examine kidney structure and function. This can be assessed using diffusion-tensor imaging (DTI). Hereby, the diffusion-sensitizing gradients are applied in 6–12 directions, taking into account that the structure of the medulla of the human kidney has a tendency towards a radial orientation (RIES et al. 2001). However, this radial symmetry shows large inter-individual variations and is therefore difficult to exploit in clinical practice (RIES et al. 2001). Furthermore, the imaging analysis is more complicated and therefore this technique is currently more applicable for scientific research than routine clinical practice.

When imaging at higher field strengths (e.g. 3 T), it can be beneficial to use dielectric cushions to reduce the signal loss occurring due to wavelength effects (DIETRICH et al. 2008).

5.4.3
DW-MRI in Experimental Settings

In *experimental settings*, DW-MRI has been applied for the evaluation of renal artery stenosis (RAS) and ureteral obstruction in pigs (MÜLLER et al. 1994a) which showed a decrease of the ADC resulting from both pathologic conditions. In another study on pigs, DW-MRI was able to differentiate acute and chronic unilateral ureteral obstruction (PEDERSEN et al. 2003). In *acute* unilateral ureteral obstruction the ADC in the medulla was significantly *reduced* 24 h after ligation of the ureter, with similar findings in the cortex but to a lesser extent. In contrast to these observations, the renal ADC in pigs with partial *chronic* ureteral obstruction was *increased* in renal medulla and cortex. Diabetic rats with cellular oedema showed significantly lower ADC values in the kidneys than the control group; the results correlated with histopathological findings (RIES et al. 2003). A decrease in ADC in dog kidneys following ischaemia induced by renal artery ligation has been described (LIU and XIE 2003). These results of DW-MRI in kidneys observed in animal studies under different pathological conditions suggest promise in applying such measurements to humans.

5.4.4
DW-MRI in Healthy Native Kidneys

5.4.4.1
Kidneys of Foetuses and Children

DW-MRI might be a helpful tool in the non-invasive prenatal diagnosis of renal pathologies and in the detection of kidney diseases in children. In this setting, early detection of renal infection is very important to start the appropriate treatment. DW-MRI is an ideal method to provide information on structural alterations and has the advantages of neither ionizing radiation nor the administration of contrast media in comparison with conventional techniques such as contrast-enhanced CT or MR imaging. However, knowledge of the normal findings is a prerequisite for further application of this promising technique.

Foetal renal development was evaluated by DW-MRI in very few studies (CHAUMOITRE et al. 2007; WITZANI et al. 2006; SAVELLI et al. 2007). ADC values of the foetal kidneys were found to decrease between 17 and 28 weeks of gestation, while no significant change was observed between 28 and 36 weeks. However, there is large scattering of the ADC values for the respective gestational age and, therefore, the interpretation of pathological values has to be made with caution. These large variations in ADC values might also be attributed to motion artefacts, which are a major problem in foetal MR imaging.

During childhood, an age-related change in the renal ADC could be observed with increase in age due to physiological changes in the kidney, the greatest changes being seen in the first years of life (JONES and GRATTAN-SMITH 2003). These findings are explained by the fact that the glomerular filtration rate (GFR) in newborns is below adult levels and because of the high vascular resistance, the foetal kidneys receive less than 5% of the cardiac output compared to 20% in adults. With the development of the glomerular basement membrane in parallel with an increase in renal blood flow, there is a 20-fold increase in GFR reflected by an increasing ADC over time.

Hence, the knowledge of normal ADC values is important for the detection and interpretation of bilateral diffuse renal pathologies. However, visual analysis of the ADC map or the high b-value image can already be helpful to notice focal changes in the kidneys or unilateral signal changes, e.g. in patients with unilateral pyelonephritis (Fig. 5.6). The regions affected by pyelonephritis reveal higher signal intensity on the high b-value images whereas the corresponding ADC map shows areas of hypointensity.

5.4.4.2
Kidneys of Healthy Volunteers

The feasibility and reproducibility of DW-MRI of the kidneys in healthy volunteers have already been demonstrated in several studies (Table 5.3).

However, there is ongoing controversy as to whether the ADC values are higher in the renal cortex

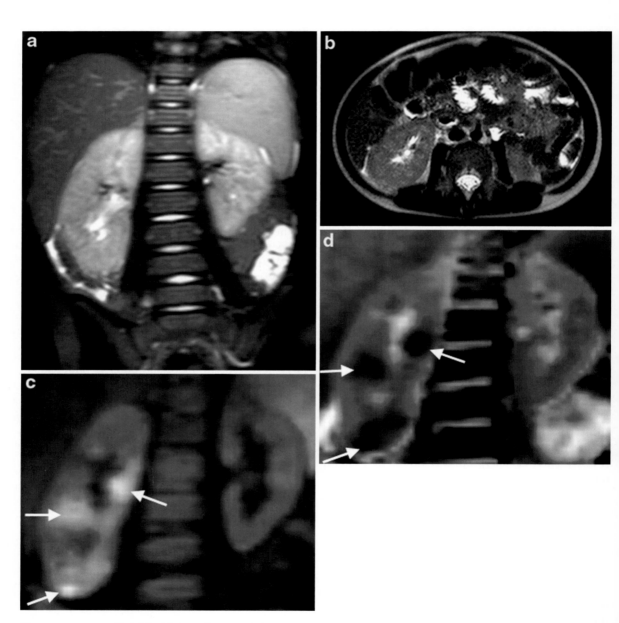

Fig. 5.6. A 4-year-old child with fever for several days. Conventional MR imaging in the coronal (**a**) and axial (**b**) plane reveals an enlarged right kidney without evidence of focal alterations. DW-MRI shows focal areas of hyperintensity (arrows) on the $b = 900\,s/mm^2$ image (**c**) and focal hypointense areas on the corresponding ADC map (**d**) suggestive of pyelonephritis

Table 5.3. Overview of literature ADC values of the cortex and medulla in native healthy kidneys

Group	Year	b-Values (s/mm²)	ADC ($\times 10^{-3}$ mm²/s)		
			Cortex	Medulla	Overall
MÜLLER et al.	1994	2, 8, 22, 32, 57, 89, 176, 395	–	–	3.54 ± 0.47
NAMIMOTO et al.	1999	20, 300	2.55	2.84	–
THOENY et al.	2005	0, 100, 150, 200, 250, 300, 500, 750, 1,000	2.03 ± 0.09	1.87 ± 0.08	–
COVA	2004	0, 500	–	–	1.72 ± 2.65
SIEGEL et al.	1995	73, 370	2.95 ± 0.58	2.43 ± 0.60	–
CHOW et al.	2001	10, 300	2.58 ± 0.53	2.09 ± 0.55	–
RIES et al.	2001	0, 195, 390	2.89 ± 0.28	2.18 ± 0.36	–
YAMADA et al.	1999	30, 300, 900, 1,100	–	–	1.55 ± 0.27
MÜRTZ et al.	2002	50, 300, 700, 1,000, 1,300	1.63 ± 1.40	–	–
ICHIKAWA et al.	1999	1.6, 16, 55	–	–	5.76 ± 1.36
XU et al.	2007	0, 500	–	–	2.87 ± 0.11

or the medulla. While several studies found higher ADC values in the medulla than in the cortex (MÜLLER et al. 1994a; PRASAD and PRIATNA 1999; NAMIMOTO et al. 1999), more recent studies including our own work found just the opposite (RIES et al. 2001; CHOW et al. 2003; YANG et al. 2004; THOENY et al. 2005b). Some researchers did not differentiate between cortex and medulla due to the lower spatial resolution of the DW-MRI studies and consequent difficulties in ROI placement. Very different ADC values have been reported for control (normal) kidneys ranging from 1.63×10^{-3} mm²/s (MÜRTZ et al. 2002) to 5.76×10^{-3} mm²/s (ICHIKAWA et al. 1999). These differences are primarily due to the selected b-value ranges and hamper easy comparisons between studies. Therefore, when performing DW-MRI for quantitative analysis of the ADC values, attention has to be paid to the underlying b-factors, as well as other technical considerations such as respiratory triggering, cardiac gating and breath-hold sequences, as these also have a bearing on the calculated ADC.

5.4.5
DW-MRI in Patients

In patients with acute and chronic renal failure, ADC values in the cortex and medulla were signifi-

cantly lower than those of the normal kidneys with ADC values being lowest for patients with chronic renal failure (NAMIMOTO et al. 1999; THOENY et al. 2005b). Similarly, in patients with RAS the ADC values in the cortex, but not in the medulla, were significantly lower than those of normal and contralateral kidneys. Furthermore, a linear correlation between renal ADC values and serum creatinine level has been observed. Other investigators have described similar findings (THOENY et al. 2005b; FUKUDA et al. 2000). A moderate correlation between renal ADC values and the split GFR obtained by renal scintigraphy showed significantly lower ADC values in impaired kidneys (XU et al. 2007). However, no significant difference in renal ADCs between moderate and severe impairment groups could be observed.

DW-MRI may be applied for the differentiation of pyonephrosis from hydronephrosis (CHAN et al. 2001) with ADC values of the renal pelvis in patients with pyonephrosis being significantly lower than those of patients with hydronephrosis. Another study (TOYOSHIMA et al. 2000) showed that ADC values of kidneys in hydronephrosis were reduced only if it was accompanied by renal dysfunction. In pregnant women and also in patients suffering from renal calculi, such information can be very helpful in deciding between treatment of immediate intervention or watchful waiting.

Fig. 5.7. ADC map of a normal transplanted kidney (**a**) with homogeneous signal intensity of the entire renal allograft. On the contrary, a diffuse hypointensity extends from the medulla into the cortex in the ADC map on the right (**b**), which corresponded to a severe case of pyelonephritis

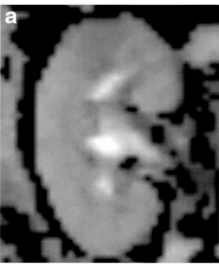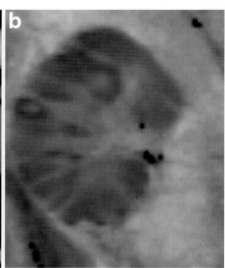

In patients with acute unilateral ureteral obstruction, a decrease in the perfusion fraction or ADC$_{low}$ dependent on the degree and duration of obstruction can be observed (THOENY et al. 2005b). Mechanical obstruction to urinary outflow causes a rise in luminal pressure and dilatation of the collecting system, with consequent increase in the interstitial pressure in the cortex and medulla, as well as a decrease in renal blood flow, which is reflected in decreased perfusion fraction. However, the influence of medication has to be taken into account when analysing the DW-MRI results of patients with acute obstruction.

In patients with acute pyelonephritis, visual analysis of the ADC map or a high b-value image can help to confirm the suspected diagnosis by showing a hypointense kidney on one side or focal areas of hypointensity on the ADC map corresponding to hyperintensity on the high b-value image (Fig. 5.7). As pyelonephritis is often observed in young women or children, DW-MRI is potentially of greatest value in these patient subgroups as there is no need to expose patients to ionizing radiation or administration of contrast medium.

It has been assumed that the ADC values of the kidneys are influenced by the hydration state of the patient (MÜLLER et al. 1994a). A recent study, however, found that the ADC values are independent of the fluid intake (DAMASIO et al. 2008). This is an important practical issue for renal imaging since it is nearly impossible to control hydration state of the patient in daily clinical routine prior to imaging studies.

A summary of literature reports on ADC changes in pathological kidneys is given in Table 5.4.

5.4.6
DW-MRI in Transplanted Kidneys

Accurate, safe and early detection of allograft dysfunction after kidney transplantation remains a major challenge. For this purpose, functional MR imaging methods appear promising as non-invasive approaches to detect early functional impairment (KNESPLOVA and KRESTIN 1998; GRENIER et al. 2003; PRASAD and PRIATNA 1999, HUANG et al. 2003).

DW-MRI has been performed on transplanted kidneys in an animal study (YANG et al. 2004). In this experimental transplant rejection model, ADC values in the cortex and medulla decreased significantly, suggesting the potential of this method for monitoring early graft rejection. Furthermore, the feasibility and reproducibility of DW-MRI in normal renal allografts in humans has been demonstrated reporting similar ADC values in cortex and medulla in contrast to native kidneys (THOENY et al. 2006). These different ADC values in native and transplanted kidneys might be attributed to the fact that transplanted

Table 5.4. Summary of published articles on renal DW-MRI

Pathology	ADC changes		
	Cortex	Medulla	Overall
Chronic renal failure	↓↓[H]	↓↓[H]	–
Acute renal failure	↓[H]	↓[H]	–
Renal artery occlusion/acute ischemia	↓[D]	↓[D]	–
Renal artery stenosis	↓[H]	nc[H]	↓[P]
Chronic ureteric obstruction	↑[P] ↓[H]	↑[P] ↓[H]	–
Acute ureteric obstruction	↓[P] ↓[H]	↓↓[P] ↓[H]	↓[P]
Diabetes mellitus	↓[H]	↓[H]	↓[R]
	If creatinine is raised	If creatinine is raised	Only if oedema
Pyonephrosis	–	–	↓↓[H]
			In renal pelvis
Pyelonephritis	↓[H]	↓[H]	–
Diuretics (furosemide)	–	–	nc[R]
Hydration after dehydration	–	–	↑↑[H]
Acute tubular necrosis	B↓[R]	↓[R]	–
Drug toxicity	↓[R]	↓[R]	–

H humans; *D* dogs; *P* pigs; *R* rats; *nc* no change

kidneys are denervated, which leads to alterations in the renal haemodynamics. In addition, medication may also have an effect on the ADC values of renal transplant recipients. Examples of a healthy transplanted kidney and a severe case of pyelonephritis are given in Fig. 5.7.

In contrast to native kidneys, evaluation of transplanted kidneys is a major challenge because the contralateral native kidney cannot be used as control. Thus, knowledge of the baseline ADC values of the transplanted kidneys is therefore of utmost importance to detect eventual pathological changes and attention has to be paid to the *b*-values used in the initial and subsequent studies, so that meaningful comparison can be made. The fitting method is another important issue to address. When using biexponential fitting, information on the perfusion fraction and the diffusion coefficient can be calculated separately, providing additional information on the pathophysiological changes in the renal allografts. DW-MRI in transplanted human kidneys is a very sensitive method to detect early changes in patients with various underlying diseases; however, its specificity has to be defined in larger studies comparing the ADC values to changes on histopathological specimens.

5.5
Upper Abdominal Applications

5.5.1
Introduction

Upper abdominal applications of DW-MRI are strongly hampered by the large amount of air–tissue boundaries, due to the presence of air in the lungs and often in the stomach or bowels. Moreover, due to the close proximity of the heart and prevalence of large arteries, strong time-of-flight effects and vascular pulsatility can occur, leading to artefacts which degrade image quality. Most importantly, respiratory motion is very large, with through-plane motion of at least 5 cm during inspiration compared with expiration.

These drawbacks have limited the use of DW-MRI in the upper abdomen to evaluate organ function, although some potentially useful applications of DW-MRI have already been investigated in the last couple of years. In the following sections, we will give a short overview of the use of DW-MRI in the liver and the pancreas.

5.5.2
DW-MRI for Functional Evaluation of the Liver

Most complications from chronic liver disease result from progressive hepatic fibrosis. Detection of occult early and intermediate stages of liver fibrosis might help in the risk stratification of patients and might predict prognosis of the individual patient with chronic liver disease.

To date, liver biopsy is the gold standard for diagnosing and quantifying hepatic fibrosis, with classification into five stages: F0 (no fibrosis), F1 (portal fibrosis), F2 (periportal fibrosis), F3 (bridging fibrosis) and F4 (cirrhosis). However, liver biopsy is invasive with the inherent risk of procedure-related complications and is also prone to sampling errors (Di Sario et al. 2004; Bedossa et al. 2003).

As DW-MRI is able to assess restricted diffusion in the interstitial space due to fibrosis and also to evaluate decrease in hepatic perfusion as suspected in patients with increasing degree of fibrosis its application seems to be promising to non-invasively detect and quantify liver fibrosis. Depending on the choice of the underlying b-factors, the calculated ADC value provides different information on diffusion and perfusion which is of additional help in this specific setting.

The mean ADC in patients with cirrhosis has been reported to be lower compared to the ADC values in healthy volunteers (Boulanger et al. 2003; Girometti et al. 2007; Aubé et al. 2004). Recently, a correlation of DW-MRI parameters and the degree of fibrosis has been shown, observing a decrease in ADC with increasing degrees of liver fibrosis (Koinuma et al. 2005; Taouli et al. 2007; Taouli et al. 2008; Lewin et al. 2007). DW-MRI of the liver appears to non-invasively allow early detection of hepatic fibrosis and monitoring disease in this group of patients. Furthermore, focal liver lesions might be detected at the same time as patients with

liver cirrhosis are at risk of developing hepatocellular carcinoma.

A more detailed account of the current innovations, clinical implications and pitfalls of the quantification of liver fibrosis is provided in Chap. 6.

5.5.3
DW-MRI in the Pancreas

The pancreas contains both endocrine and exocrine tissue. The endocrine pancreas secretes insulin and other hormones. The exocrine pancreas contains pancreatic acini, producing pancreatic juices, which is secreted into the duodenum to aid digestion. In cases of chronic pancreatitis, the pancreatic structure and function is irreversibly damaged, resulting in lower secretion of enzymes, in turn leading to digestive dysfunction, abdominal pain and even diabetes. The most common cause of chronic pancreatitis is alcohol abuse.

Diagnosis of chronic pancreatitis is often delayed due to the low sensitivity and specificity of current imaging modalities, and the high incidence of complications associated with pancreatic biopsies (Mitchell et al. 2003). Due to the glandular nature and the abundant fluid secretion of the pancreas, DW-MRI could potentially detect glandular dysfunction. To date, however, only one interesting study on the use of DW-MRI for the evaluation of pancreatic function has been published (Erturk et al. 2006).

Erturk et al. (2006) used a single-shot spin-echo echo-planar imaging DW-MRI sequence which they repeated before and several times after an intravenous administration of secretin. Secretin is a hormone which acts on the pancreatic duct cells, causing the production and secretion of a large fluid volume, with a resulting expected increase in ADC due to the higher proton mobility of fluids. This study was performed on 38 patients without pancreatic disease, 16 patients without chronic pancreatitis but with a history of alcohol abuse (the at-risk group), and nine patients diagnosed with chronic pancreatitis. The patients without pancreatic disease, as expected, showed a median increase in ADC value of the pancreas of 75%, which occurred between 90 s and 4 min after the administration of secretin. A similar increase was found for the at-risk group, but the time when this occurred was significantly higher, ranging from 4 to 8 min after the administration. This was indicative of a functional pancreas, but already with a slightly impaired response to stimulation. The group of patients with a chronic pancreatitis, however, did not show any significant ADC increase in the entire follow-up period (8 min), which would indicate either non-responsive or at least strongly delayed pancreatic function. This interesting study highlights the possible use of DW-MRI for the non-invasive and accurate detection of early changes in chronic pancreatitis, and even for the identification of patients at highest risk of developing chronic pancreatitis (ERTURK et al. 2006).

Acknowledgement The authors would like to thank Peter Vermathen (PhD) for his valuable insight and contributions to this manuscript.

References

Aubé C, Racineux PX, Lebigot J et al (2004) Diagnosis and quantification of hepatic fibrosis with diffusion weighted MR imaging: preliminary results. J Radiol 85: 301–306

Bedossa P, Dargère D, Paradis V (2003) Sampling variability of liver fibrosis in chronic hepatitis C. Hepatology 38: 1449–1457

Berk LB, Shivnani AT, Small W Jr (2005) Pathophysiology and management of radiation-induced xerostomia. J Support Oncol 3: 191–200

Boulanger Y, Amara M, Lepanto L et al (2003) Diffusion-weighted MR imaging of the liver of hepatitis C patients. NMR Biomed 16: 132–136

Chan JH, Tsui EY, Luk SH et al (2001) MR diffusion-weighted imaging of kidney: differentiation between hydronephrosis and pyonephrosis. Clin Imaging 25: 110–113

Chaumoitre K, Colavolpe N, Shojai R et al (2007) Diffusion-weighted magnetic resonance imaging with apparent diffusion coefficient (ADC) determination in normal and pathological fetal kidneys. Ultrasound Obstet Gynecol 29: 22–31

Chow LC, Bammer R, Moseley ME et al (2003) Single breath-hold diffusion-weighted imaging of the abdomen. J Magn Reson Imaging 18: 377–382

Cova M, Squillaci E, Stacul F et al (2004) Diffusion-weighted MRI in the evaluation of renal lesions: preliminary results. Br J Radiol 77: 851–857

Damasio MB, Tagliafico A, Capaccio E et al (2008) Diffusion-weighted MRI sequences (DW-MRI) of the kidney: normal findings, influence of hydration state and repeatability of results. Radiol Med 113: 214–224

Dietrich O, Reiser MF, Schoenberg SO (2008) Artifacts in 3-T MRI: physical background and reduction strategies. Eur J Radiol 65: 29–35

Dirix P, De Keyzer F, Vandecaveye V et al (2008) Diffusion-weighted magnetic resonance imaging to evaluate major salivary gland function before and after radiotherapy. Int J Radiat Oncol Biol Phys 71: 1365–1371

Di Sario A, Feliciangeli G, Bendia E et al (2004) Diagnosis of liver fibrosis. Eur Rev Med Pharmacol Sci 8: 11–18

Erturk SM, Ichikawa T, Motosugi U et al (2006) Diffusion-weighted MR imaging in the evaluation of pancreatic exocrine function before and after secretin stimulation. Am J Gastroenterol 101: 133–136

Fukuda Y, Ohashi I, Hanafusa K et al (2000) Anisotropic diffusion in kidney: apparent diffusion coefficient measurements for clinical use. J Magn Reson Imaging 11: 156–160

Girometti R, Furlan A, Bazzocchi M et al (2007) Diffusion-weighted MRI in evaluating liver fibrosis: a feasibility study in cirrhotic patients. Radiol Med 112: 394–408

Grenier N, Basseau F, Ries M et al (2003) Functional MRI of the kidney. Abdom Imaging 28: 164–175

Habermann CR, Gossrau P, Kooijman H et al (2007) Monitoring of gustatory stimulation of salivary glands by diffusion-weighted MR imaging: comparison of 1.5T and 3T. AJNR Am J Neuroradiol 28: 1547–1551

Huang AJ, Lee VS, Rusinek H (2003) MR imaging of renal function. Radiol Clin North Am 41: 1001–1017

Ichikawa T, Haradome H, Hachiya J et al (1999) Diffusion-weighted MR imaging with single-shot echo-planar imaging in the upper abdomen: preliminary clinical experience in 61 patients. Abdom Imaging 24: 456–461

Jones RA, Grattan-Smith JD (2003) Age dependence of the renal apparent diffusion coefficient in children. Pediatr Radiol 33: 850–854

Knesplova L, Krestin GP (1998) Magnetic resonance in the assessment of renal function. Eur Radiol 8: 201–211

Koinuma M, Ohashi I, Hanafusa K et al (2005) Apparent diffusion coefficient measurements with diffusion-weighted magnetic resonance imaging for evaluation of hepatic fibrosis. J Magn Reson Imaging 22: 80–85

Le Bihan D, Breton E, Lallemand D et al (1988) Separation of diffusion and perfusion in intravoxel incoherent motion MR imaging. Radiology 168: 497–505

Lewin M, Poujol-Robert A, Boëlle PY et al (2007) Diffusion-weighted magnetic resonance imaging for the assessment of fibrosis in chronic hepatitis C. Hepatology 46: 658–665

Liu AS, Xie JX (2003) Functional evaluation of normothermic ischemia and reperfusion injury in dog kidney by combining MR diffusion-weighted imaging and Gd-DTPA enhanced first-pass perfusion. J Magn Reson Imaging 17: 683–693

Mitchell RM, Byrne MF, Baillie J (2003) Pancreatitis. Lancet 361: 1447–1455

Müller MF, Prasad PV, Bimmler D et al (1994a) Functional imaging of the kidney by means of measurement of the apparent diffusion coefficient. Radiology 193: 711–715

Müller MF, Prasad P, Siewert B et al (1994b) Abdominal diffusion mapping with use of a whole-body echo-planar system. Radiology 190: 475–478

Mürtz P, Flacke S, Träber F et al (2002) Abdomen: diffusion-weighted MR imaging with pulse-triggered single-shot sequences. Radiology 224: 258–264

Namimoto T, Yamashita Y, Mitsuzaki K et al (1999) Measurement of the apparent diffusion coefficient in diffuse renal disease by diffusion-weighted echo-planar MR imaging. J Magn Reson Imaging 9: 832–837

Patel RR, Carlos RC, Midia M et al (2004) Apparent diffusion coefficient mapping of the normal parotid gland and parotid involvement in patients with systemic connective tissue disorders. AJNR Am J Neuroradiol 25: 16–20

Pedersen M, Wen JG, Shi Y et al (2003) The effect of unilateral ureteral obstruction on renal function in pigs measured by diffusion-weighted MRI. APMIS Suppl 109: 29–34

Prasad PV, Priatna A (1999) Functional imaging of the kidneys with fast MRI techniques. Eur J Radiol 29: 133–148

Ries M, Jones RA, Basseau F et al (2001) Diffusion tensor MRI of the human kidney. J Magn Reson Imaging 14: 42–49

Ries M, Basseau F, Tyndal B et al (2003) Renal diffusion and BOLD MRI in experimental diabetic nephropathy. Blood oxygen level-dependent. J Magn Reson Imaging 17: 104–113

Savelli S, Di Maurizio M, Perrone A et al (2007) MRI with diffusion-weighted imaging (DWI) and apparent diffusion coefficient (ADC) assessment in the evaluation of normal and abnormal fetal kidneys: preliminary experience. Prenat Diagn 27: 1104–1111

Siegel CL, Aisen AM, Ellis JH et al (1995) Feasibility of MR diffusion studies in the kidney. J Magn Reson Imaging 5: 617–620

Sumi M, Takagi Y, Uetani M et al (2002) Diffusion-weighted echoplanar MR imaging of the salivary glands. AJR Am J Roentgenol 178: 959–965

Taouli B, Tolia AJ, Losada M et al (2007) Diffusion-weighted MRI for quantification of liver fibrosis: preliminary experience. AJR Am J Roentgenol 189: 799–806

Taouli B, Chouli M, Martin AJ et al (2008) Chronic hepatitis: role of diffusion-weighted imaging and diffusion tensor imaging for the diagnosis of liver fibrosis and inflammation. J Magn Reson Imaging 28: 89–95

Thoeny HC, De Keyzer F (2007) Extracranial applications of diffusion-weighted magnetic resonance imaging. Eur Radiol 17: 1385–1393

Thoeny HC, De Keyzer F, Boesch C et al (2004) Diffusion-weighted imaging of the parotid gland: influence of the choice of b-values on the apparent diffusion coefficient value. J Magn Reson Imaging 20: 786–790

Thoeny HC, De Keyzer F, Claus FG et al (2005a) Gustatory stimulation changes the apparent diffusion coefficient of salivary glands: initial experience. Radiology 235: 629–634

Thoeny HC, De Keyzer F, Oyen RH et al (2005b) Diffusion-weighted MR imaging of kidneys in healthy volunteers and patients with parenchymal diseases: initial experience. Radiology 235: 911–917

Thoeny HC, Zumstein D, Simon-Zoula S et al (2006) Functional evaluation of transplanted kidneys with diffusion-weighted and BOLD MR imaging: initial experience. Radiology 241: 812–821

Toyoshima S, Noguchi K, Seto H et al (2000) Functional evaluation of hydronephrosis by diffusion-weighted MR imaging. Relationship between apparent diffusion coefficient and split glomerular filtration rate. Acta Radiol 41:642–646

Witzani L, Brugger PC, Hörmann M et al (2006) Normal renal development investigated with fetal MRI. Eur J Radiol 57: 294–302

Xu Y, Wang X, Jiang X (2007) Relationship between the renal apparent diffusion coefficient and glomerular filtration rate: preliminary experience. J Magn Reson Imaging 26: 678–681

Yablonskiy DA, Bretthorst GL, Ackerman JJ (2003) Statistical model for diffusion attenuated MR signal. Magn Reson Med 50: 664–669

Yamada I, Aung W, Himeno Y et al (1999) Diffusion coefficients in abdominal organs and hepatic lesions: evaluation with intravoxel incoherent motion echo-planar MR imaging. Radiology 210: 617–623

Yang D, Ye Q, Williams DS et al (2004) Normal and transplanted rat kidneys: diffusion MR imaging at 7T. Radiology 231: 702–709

Yoshino N, Yamada I, Ohbayashi N et al (2001) Salivary glands and lesions: evaluation of apparent diffusion coefficients with split-echo diffusion-weighted MR imaging – initial results. Radiology 221: 837–842

Zhang L, Murata Y, Ishida R et al (2001) Functional evaluation with intravoxel incoherent motion echo-planar MRI in irradiated salivary glands: a correlative study with salivary gland scintigraphy. J Magn Reson Imaging 14:223–229

DW-MRI Assessment of Diffuse Liver Disease

6

Jignesh Patel and Bachir Taouli

CONTENTS

SUMMARY

MR imaging plays an increasingly important role in the evaluation of patients with chronic liver disease, due to its high contrast resolution, lack of ionizing radiation, and the possibility of performing functional imaging. With advances in MR imaging hardware and coil systems, DW-MRI can now be applied to liver imaging applications with good image quality. In this chapter, we will review available DW-MRI data for the diagnosis and quantification of liver fibrosis, and for the detection of hepatocellular carcinoma. We will also discuss limitations and future directions of DW-MRI for the assessment of patients with chronic liver disease.

6.1

Background

6.1.1
Epidemiology of Chronic Liver Disease

Fibrosis and cirrhosis are the end result of many chronic liver diseases including viral infections, alcohol abuse, non alcoholic steatohepatitis (NASH), primary sclerosing cholangitis, primary hemochromatosis, Wilson disease, and autoimmune disease. In the United States, chronic hepatitis C virus (HCV) infection accounts for approximately 40% of all chronic liver diseases, resulting in estimated 8,000–10,000 deaths annually, and is the most frequent indication for liver transplantation (ALTER et al. 1999; KIM et al. 2001; LAUER et al. 2001). Furthermore, patients with viral hepatitis have one of the highest risks for developing hepatic fibrosis and cirrhosis, which can lead to end-stage liver disease, portal hypertension, and hepatocellular carcinoma (HCC).

JIGNESH PATEL, MD
BACHIR TAOULI, MD
Department of Radiology, New York University Langone
Medical Centre, New York, NY 10016, USA

Simulations in the United States for 2010–2019 suggest that morbidity and mortality associated with HCV will increase dramatically, resulting in 165,900 deaths from chronic liver disease, 27,200 deaths from HCC and $10.7 billion in direct medical costs (WONG et al. 2000; DAVIS et al. 2003; DEUFFIC-BURBAN et al. 2007). Antiviral treatment of chronic hepatitis C can eradicate the infection, increase patient survival, and reduce the need for liver transplantation, making it a cost-effective strategy (BUTI et al. 2005). The current standard of care for chronic HCV is the combination of pegylated interferon α and ribavirin, with an overall sustained response between 54 and 63%, depending on the genotype (genotypes 2 and 3 are more likely to respond than genotype 1), viral load, and degree of fibrosis (patients with advanced fibrosis and cirrhosis have a low response to treatment) (MANNS et al. 2001; FRIED et al. 2002; HADZIYANNIS et al. 2004).

6.1.2
Histopathological Classification of Liver Fibrosis

Most classification systems recognize five stages of fibrosis, graded as F0 (no fibrosis), F1 (portal fibrosis), F2 (periportal fibrosis), F3 (bridging fibrosis), and F4 (cirrhosis). Clinically significant fibrosis is generally defined by F2 involvement or greater. Currently, evaluation of disease severity relies on histological findings obtained at liver biopsy performed to assess degree of fibrosis (stage) and necroinflammatory changes (grade) (METAVIR et al. 1994; BATTS et al. 1995). Although liver biopsy is a relatively safe procedure when performed by experienced clinicians, liver biopsy has poor patient-acceptance and is not risk-free. Previous studies have suggested a risk of hospitalization of 1–5%, a 0.57% risk of severe complications, and a mortality rate of 1:1,000–1:10,000 (FROEHLICH et al. 1993; JANES et al. 1993; CADRANEL et al. 2000). Liver biopsy is also prone to inter-observer variability and sampling error (MAHARAJ et al. 1986; REGEV et al. 2002; BEDOSSA et al. 2003). In addition, liver biopsy is not easily repeatable, and therefore not a suitable tool for drug trials assessing new antiviral and antifibrotic drugs.

6.1.3
Non-invasive Diagnosis of Liver Fibrosis and Cirrhosis

The development of non-invasive biomarkers of liver fibrosis would reduce biopsy-related risk/costs and facilitate earlier diagnosis, thus improving the monitoring of the progression of chronic viral hepatitis. A number of serological markers of liver fibrosis have been developed recently. These include simple tests such as serum transaminases AST/ALT ratio, platelet count, and the prothrombin index, or more complex tests such as the Fibrotest developed by Imbert-BISMUTH et al. (2001), which is based on a combination of basic serum markers. This test panel performed with 75% sensitivity and 85% specificity for the diagnosis of METAVIR fibrosis stage ≥F2 (BEDOSSA et al. 1996). In a subsequent publication, the same group reported a lower performance of the Fibrotest and Actitest (activity index, which incorporates ALT) in chronic HCV treated patients, with area under the curve (AUC) of 0.76 ± 0.03 (POYNARD et al. 2003).

Other recently developed methods such as sonographic transient elastography (FibroScan) (CASTERA et al. 2005; ZIOL et al. 2005; ROUVIERE et al. 2006), MR perfusion-weighted imaging (ANNET et al. 2003; HAGIWARA et al. 2008), and MR elastography (HUWART et al. 2006; ROUVIERE et al. 2006; HUWART et al. 2007; YIN et al. 2007a, b) have also shown promise for prediction of advanced liver fibrosis and cirrhosis.

6.2
Role of Conventional MR Imaging for the Diagnosis of Liver Fibrosis and Cirrhosis

MR imaging has become an increasingly important imaging modality for the investigation of patients with chronic liver disease. However, it has a limited role in the evaluation of disease activity in chronic hepatitis. SEMELKA et al. (2001) have described two parenchymal enhancement patterns in chronic hepatitis using gadolinium-enhanced MR imaging, an early patchy enhancement correlating with liver inflammatory changes, and a late linear enhancement correlating with the presence of fibrosis. In addition, several morphologic criteria have been described (ITO et al. 2000, 2003; AWAYA et al. 2002). However, these findings are limited in sensitivity and specificity, and subject to inter-observer variability.

6.3
Diffusion-Weighted Imaging for the Diagnosis and Quantification of Liver Fibrosis

DW-MRI is based on intravoxel incoherent motion (IVIM), and provides non-invasive quantification of water diffusion and capillary/blood perfusion

(LE BIHAN 1990). DW-MRI is a non-contrast-enhanced imaging sequence, which is attractive in patients with renal dysfunction at risk for nephrogenic systemic fibrosis (THOMSEN et al. 2008).

6.3.1
DW-MRI Acquisition/Processing/Quantification for Liver Disease

6.3.1.1
DW-MRI Acquisition

DW-MRI is performed optimally on 1.5 or 3 T MR systems with high performance gradients, most frequently using a single-shot echoplanar imaging (SS EPI) sequence with diffusion gradients applied in three orthogonal directions [frequency-encoding (x), phase-encoding (y), section-select directions (z)]. EPI provides ultrafast imaging times minimizing the effect of gross physiological motion from respiration and cardiac motion. Suggested acquisition parameters are listed in Table 6.1. The finger pulse trigger acquisition suggested in earlier studies to decrease motion artefacts from cardiac pulsation (MURTZ et al. 2002) is not routinely used in our practice. Frequency selective fat saturation is used to reduce chemical shift artefacts. Imaging is preferably obtained before contrast medium injection to avoid the potential

T1-shortening effects of contrast enhancement on the apparent diffusion coefficient (ADC) values. Breath-hold, free-breathing, or respiratory-triggered EPI sequences can be performed in conjunction with parallel imaging to improve image quality (TAOULI et al. 2004). A free-breathing or respiratory-triggered acquisition allows the use of multiple b-values in a single acquisition, which improves image quality compared to breath-hold acquisition, however at the expense of longer acquisition time (KWEE et al. 2008). The selection of b-values should be based on a compromise between image quality and adequate diffusion-weighted contrast (TAOULI et al. 2003). The choice of higher or lower b-values affects SNR and image quality. Higher b-values require longer TEs with subsequent lower SNR and more EPI related distortion. Conversely, lower b-values have less diffusion weighting and more perfusion contamination with higher SNR. In addition, at least three b-values should be used to obtain a good fit for ADC calculation. A recent study (GIROMETTI et al. 2007) suggested that a more accurate assessment of liver fibrosis is obtained when using intermediate b values (400 s/mm^2) rather than higher values. The use of higher b-values (>400 s/mm^2) to make the ADCs approach the true diffusion coefficient and minimize perfusion contribution and T2 shine-through effect is recommended (BURDETTE et al. 1999).

Table 6.1. Proposed parameters for routine liver fat-suppressed SS EPI diffusion acquisition (using a multichannel 1.5 T system)

Parameter	Values
Acquisition plane	Axial
TR (ms)	1,800–2,500
TE (ms)	Minimum
FOV (cm)	36–40
b-Values (s/mm^2)	0-50--500 or 1,000
Matrix	192 × 192
Slice thickness/gap (mm)	7–8/0.8
Number of averages	2 (BH)-4 (RT)
Parallel imaging acceleration factor	2
EPI factor	192
Acquisition time (s)	<25 (BH)[a]-at least 120 (RT)

[a]Two packages are usually necessary to cover the whole liver

6.3.1.2
DW-MRI Processing

The diffusion data can be evaluated on voxel-based ADC maps which may be obtained on any commercial workstation. Liver ADC values should be calculated in multiple locations within the liver (excluding the lateral left lobe which could be affected by cardiac-related artefacts) by placing regions of interest (ROI) to measure mean and SD of ADC values.

6.3.2
Results in Liver Fibrosis and Cirrhosis

The diagnosis of fibrosis/inflammation is difficult using only conventional imaging sequences. Both processes can have normal appearance on conventional imaging. Several studies have demonstrated that the ADC of cirrhotic liver is lower than that of normal liver (NAMIMOTO et al. 1997; AMANO et al. 1998; ICHIKAWA et al. 1998; KIM et al. 1999; TAOULI et al. 2003; AUBE et al. 2004) (Fig. 6.1).

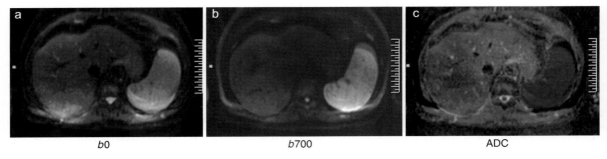

a	b	c
$b0$	$b700$	ADC

Fig. 6.1. Patient with chronic HCV infection without liver fibrosis on biopsy. Diffusion-weighted images at (**a**) $b = 0\,s/mm^2$ (*b0*) and (**b**) $b = 700\,s/mm^2$ (*b700*) with (**c**) corresponding ADC map. The calculated ADC was high $1.6 \times 10^{-3}\,mm^2/s$ (according to the ADC values described by Taouli et al. 2007)

Table 6.2. Summary of recent studies utilizing DW-MRI for the analysis of chronic liver disease

Study	*b*-Values	*N*	ADC[a] results
Girometti et al. (2007)	0, 150, 250, 400, 600, 800	57 (28 cirrhotic, 29 normal)	1.14 cirrhosis, 1.54 normal
Aube et al. (2004)	200, 400, 600, 800	27 (13 cirrhotic, 14 normal)	2.05 cirrhosis, 2.9 normal
Koinuma et al. (2005)	0, 128	163 (34 normal)	Decreasing ADC with increasing fibrosis
Lewin et al. (2007)	0, 200, 400, 800	74 (54 with fibrosis, 20 normal)	Decreasing ADC with increasing fibrosis
Boulanger et al. (2003)	50, 100, 150, 200, 250	28 (18 fibrosis, 10 normal)	2.3 hepatitis C, 1.79 normal
Taouli et al. (2008)	0, 500	44 (31 with fibrosis, 13 normal)	Decreasing ADC with increasing fibrosis
Taouli et al. (2007)	50, 300, 500, 700, 1,000	30 (23 chronic, 7 normal)	Decreasing ADC with increasing fibrosis

[a]ADC ($\times 10^{-3}\,mm^2/s$)

Koinuma et al. (2005) evaluated a large population of patients ($N = 163$) with DW-MRI using a low *b*-value ($128\,s/mm^2$). Thirty-one of these patients underwent liver biopsy. The results demonstrated a significant negative correlation between hepatic ADC and fibrosis score. There was, however, no correlation between ADC and the grades of liver inflammation. Lewin et al. (2007) investigated the role of DW-MRI (using *b*-values of 0, 200, 400, 800 s/mm²) compared to FibroScan and serum markers (APRI: aspartate aminotransferase to platelet ratio index, FibroTest, and Forns index) in a large series of HCV patients ($n = 54 + 20$ healthy volunteers), and demonstrated an excellent performance of DW-MRI for prediction of moderate and severe fibrosis (Table 6.2). Patients with moderate-to-severe fibrosis (F2–F4) had hepatic ADC values lower than those without or with mild fibrosis (F0–F1) and healthy volunteers: the mean ADC values being 1.10 ± 0.11, 1.30 ± 0.12 and $1.44 \pm 0.02 \times 10^{-3}\,mm^2/s$ respectively. In

addition, they found a significant relationship between ADC and the inflammation scores, and suspected a possible influence of steatosis on reducing the ADC values.

Girometti et al. (2007) reported lower ADC values in cirrhotic livers compared to healthy controls (1.11 ± 0.16 vs. $1.54 \pm 0.12 \times 10^{-3}\,mm^2/s$), and showed an AUC of 0.96, with a sensitivity of 92.9%, specificity of 100%, positive predictive value of 100%, negative predictive value of 99.9% and accuracy of 96.4%, for diagnosing cirrhosis, using an ADC cutoff value of $1.31 \times 10^{-3}\,mm^2/s$ (using $b = 0, 150, 250$ and $400\,s/mm^2$).

However, in addition there have been reports showing little value of DW-MRI for the diagnosis of liver fibrosis and cirrhosis. For example, Boulanger et al. (2003) explored 18 HCV patients and 10 control subjects with DW-MRI, using *b*-values of $50–250\,s/mm^2$, and observed no significant difference between HCV patients and the control subjects (mean ADC values of

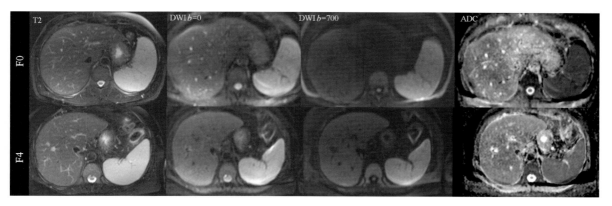

Fig. 6.2. Patient with chronic hepatitis C without evidence of fibrosis at liver biopsy (F0-*top row*), and patient with cirrhosis secondary to chronic hepatitis C (F4-*bottom row*). Breath-hold fat-suppressed TSE T2-weighted image (T2) and breath-hold fat-suppressed single-shot echoplanar diffusion-weighted images for $b = 0\,mm^2/s$ (DWI $b = 0$) and $b = 700\,mm^2/s$ (DWI $b = 700$) and ADC map (using $b = 0$ and 700 mm²/s) are shown. In the

patient without fibrosis, hepatic ADC was within normal range, measuring $1.6 \times 10^{-3}\,s/mm^2$, the liver appearing brighter than the spleen (which is known to have low ADC). In the cirrhotic patient, T2-weighted image shows minimal morphologic changes in relation with cirrhosis. However, hepatic ADC was decreased (reaching the spleen ADC), measuring $1.0 \times 10^{-3}\,s/mm^2$ (according to the ADC values described by TAOULI et al. 2007)

2.30 ± 1.28 and 1.79 ± 0.25 × $10^{-3}\,mm^2/s$ respectively). The ADC values of patients with hepatitis were even higher than those from the control subjects. A potential explanation for these findings is that the differences between fibrotic and non-fibrotic liver cannot be demonstrated using small b-values (<300 s/mm²) because of a significant amount of perfusion contamination in the ADC measurements (YAMADA et al. 1999) (Fig. 6.2).

In our experience, in an earlier study, we also observed a decrease in the mean liver ADC value in cirrhosis compared with the normal liver (TAOULI et al. 2003) in 23 patients (including 9 cirrhotic patients) using DW-MRI at 1.5 T (with two imaging sequences and b-values of 0, 500 and 0, 134, 267, 400 s/ mm²). More recently, we have found ADC to be a significant predictor of fibrosis stage ≥1 (sensitivity 88.5% and specificity 73.3%) and inflammation grade ≥1 (sensitivity 75% and specificity 78.6%) (TAOULI et al. 2008). In another study, we observed a decrease in liver ADC in significant and severe fibrosis using b-values ≥500 s/mm² (TAOULI et al. 2007) at DW-MRI, with the best correlation between ADC value and liver fibrosis demonstrated using $b = 700$ s/mm². The ADC value was a found to be a predictor of moderate-to-severe fibrosis (stage ≥2), which is clinically essential, since only patients with fibrosis stage ≥2 should receive antiviral treatment (KIM et al. 2005; YEE et al. 2006), because of the potential toxicity, cost, and limited efficacy of the treatment.

The mechanism of impeded water diffusion appears to be multifactorial in patients with liver fibrosis and

cirrhosis. It is possibly related to the presence of increased connective tissue in the liver (which is proton-poor) and to decreased blood flow. A recent animal study (ANNET et al. 2007) showed that rats with hepatic fibrosis demonstrate reduced ADC values in vivo, but not when DW-MRI was performed ex vivo, thus favoring a significant perfusion effect on the ADC measurement. Recent work by LUCIANI et al. (2008), based on IVIM MR (LE BIHAN 1988; LE BIHAN et al. 1988, 1989, 1991; TURNER et al. 1990), has also suggested that impeded diffusion observed in patients with cirrhosis reflects diminished capillary perfusion, and to a much lesser extent, on pure molecular diffusion. Their analysis of 37 patients demonstrated globally lower ADC values between cirrhotics and normal cases (ADC = 1.23 ± 0.4 vs. 1.39 ± 0.2 × $10^{-3}\,mm^2/s$) which they have attributed primarily to a reduction in perfusion in cirrhotic livers.

6.4

Diffusion-Weighted Imaging for the Diagnosis of Hepatocellular Carcinoma

We have shown that HCC detection is improved with DW-MRI compared to fat-suppressed breath-hold T2-weighted imaging in 24 cirrhotic patients (80.5 vs. 53.9%) (Fig. 6.3) (PARIKH et al. 2008). Typical cases of HCC demonstrate reduced tissue diffusivity (increased signal at higher b-values, and decreased

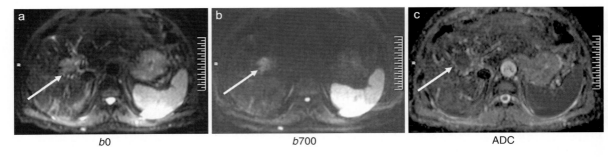

$b0$ $b700$ ADC

Fig. 6.3. Patient with chronic HCV infection and cirrhosis. Diffusion-weighted images obtained at (**a**) $b = 0 \, s/mm^2$ ($b0$) and (**b**) $b = 700 \, s/mm^2$ ($b700$) with (**c**) corresponding ADC map. The calculated liver ADC was $1.1 \times 10^{-3} \, mm^2/s$ (according to the ADC values described by Taouli et al. 2007). The patient was found to have an incidental HCC (*arrow*) in the right lobe which demonstrates high signal intensity on the $b = 700 \, s/mm^2$ image, with corresponding low ADC, compatible with restricted diffusion

ADC values) unless they are well differentiated or treated by chemoembolization, in which case they can fail to show bright diffusion signal. There is no published data comparing the detection rates of HCC using DW-MRI compared to Gadolinium-enhanced sequences.

Bruegel et al. (2008) have recently applied respiratory-triggered DW-MRI (using b-values of 50, 300 and 600 s/mm²) to discriminate benign from malignant lesions, and more specifically HCC, with a reported sensitivity of 90%, specificity of 86%, and accuracy of 88%. They found a significantly lower ADC value in HCC ($1.05 \pm 0.09 \times 10^{-3} \, mm^2/s$) compared with benign lesions (focal nodular hyperplasia, haemangiomas and cysts). Our experience was similar by comparison. Using a breath-hold DW-MRI acquisition technique (with b-values 0–500 s/mm²), we found that HCC had returned a low mean ADC value ($1.33 \pm 0.13 \times 10^{-3} \, mm^2/s$), which was significantly lower than that of benign lesions, but not significantly different from those measured in liver metastases ($0.94 \pm 0.60 \times 10^{-3} \, mm^2/s$) (Taouli et al. 2003). The ADC values of HCCs reported in the literature range between 0.99 and $3.84 \times 10^{-3} \, mm^2/s$, depending on the b-value and the sequence parameters employed (Muller et al. 1994; Namimoto et al. 1997; Ichikawa et al. 1998; Kim et al. 1999; Taouli et al. 2003; Bruegel et al. 2008).

6.5

Limitations of DW-MRI

Multiple aspects of DW-MRI need to be addressed for the evaluation of chronic liver disease before it can be utilized in clinical practice. Studies with a larger number of patients are needed to improve the statistical power of the current observation, since only studies in relatively small number of patients have been performed in selected populations. The use of different imaging sequence parameters and hardware has made it difficult to compare between studies and DW-MRI requires further standardization so that clinicians can understand the results of the study. For example, factors such as fatty infiltration and iron deposition may alter the measurement of tissue diffusivity, making ADC values difficult to interpret. Other technical factors such as cardiac motion can limit the evaluation of the left hepatic lobe and respiratory motion affecting ADC values in the right lobe may need to be addressed with respiratory-gated techniques.

6.6

Future Directions

In the future, the use of 3 T imaging can provide higher SNR in a single breath-hold allowing for improved image quality. However, at higher fields, there is an increased susceptibility to local field inhomogeneity using EPI technique, which may limit the use of higher b-values (Fig. 6.4). The utilization of other DW-MRI sequences such as multishot EPI or non-EPI sequences with higher spatial resolution could be explored as a potential solution to such obstacles.

A multiparametric MR imaging approach to functional liver imaging may provide the most robust information on the presence of liver fibrosis and inflammation. Incorporating conventional MR imaging, perfusion-weighted MR imaging, MR spectroscopy, and MR elastography (Huwart et al. 2006, 2007;

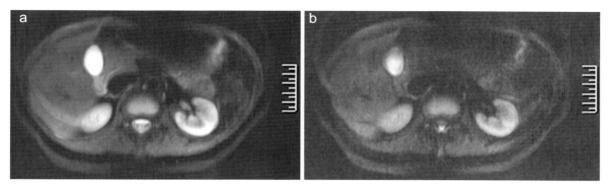

Fig. 6.4. 3T SS EPI DW-MR images in a normal volunteer obtained using b-values of (**a**) $b = 0\,s/mm^2$ and (**b**) $b = 200\,s/mm^2$. The images show good signal-to-noise ratio, however increased ghosting artefact has degraded image quality

Rouviere et al. 2006; Yin et al. 2007a, b) may eventually provide a comprehensive approach to chronic liver imaging.

More work is also needed to evaluate the reproducibility of DW-MRI measurements, which needs to be rigorously assessed before validating ADC as a potential biomarker of liver fibrosis or cirrhosis.

References

Alter MJ, Kruszon-Moran D, Nainan OV et al (1999) The prevalence of hepatitis C virus infection in the United States, 1988 through 1994. N Engl J Med 341: 556–562

Amano Y, Kumazaki T, Ishihara M (1998) Single-shot diffusion-weighted echo-planar imaging of normal and cirrhotic livers using a phased-array multicoil. Acta Radiol 39: 440–442

Annet L, Materne R, Danse E et al (2003) Hepatic flow parameters measured with MR imaging and Doppler US: correlations with degree of cirrhosis and portal hypertension. Radiology 229: 409–414

Annet L, Peeters F, Abarca-Quinones J et al (2007) Assessment of diffusion-weighted MR imaging in liver fibrosis. J Magn Reson Imaging 25: 122–128

Aube C, Racineux PX, Lebigot J et al (2004) [Diagnosis and quantification of hepatic fibrosis with diffusion weighted MR imaging: preliminary results]. J Radiol 85: 301–306

Awaya H, Mitchell DG, Kamishima T et al (2002) Cirrhosis: modified caudate-right lobe ratio. Radiology 224: 769–774

Batts KP, Ludwig J (1995) Chronic hepatitis. An update on terminology and reporting. Am J Surg Pathol 19: 1409–1417

Bedossa P, Dargere D, Paradis V (2003) Sampling variability of liver fibrosis in chronic hepatitis C. Hepatology 38: 1449–1457

Bedossa P, Poynard T (1996) An algorithm for the grading of activity in chronic hepatitis C. The METAVIR Cooperative Study Group. Hepatology 24: 289–293

Boulanger Y, Amara M, Lepanto L et al (2003) Diffusion-weighted MR imaging of the liver of hepatitis C patients. NMR Biomed 16: 132–136

Bruegel M, Holzapfel K, Gaa J et al (2008) Characterization of focal liver lesions by ADC measurements using a respiratory triggered diffusion-weighted single-shot echo-planar MR imaging technique. Eur Radiol 18: 477–485

Burdette JH, Elster AD, Ricci PE (1999) Acute cerebral infarction: quantification of spin-density and T2 shine-through phenomena on diffusion-weighted MR images. Radiology 212: 333–339

Buti M, San Miguel R, Brosa M et al (2005) Estimating the impact of hepatitis C virus therapy on future liver-related morbidity, mortality and costs related to chronic hepatitis C. J Hepatol 42: 639–645

Cadranel JF, Rufat P, Degos F (2000) Practices of liver biopsy in France: results of a prospective nationwide survey. For the Group of Epidemiology of the French Association for the Study of the Liver (AFEF). Hepatology 32: 477–481

Castera L, Vergniol J, Foucher J et al (2005) Prospective comparison of transient elastography, Fibrotest, APRI, and liver biopsy for the assessment of fibrosis in chronic hepatitis C. Gastroenterology 128: 343–350

Davis GL, Albright JE, Cook SF et al (2003) Projecting future complications of chronic hepatitis C in the United States. Liver Transpl 9: 331–338

Deuffic-Burban S, Poynard T, Sulkowski MS et al (2007) Estimating the future health burden of chronic hepatitis C and human immunodeficiency virus infections in the United States. J Viral Hepat 14: 107–115

Fried MW, Shiffman ML, Reddy KR et al (2002) Peginterferon alfa-2a plus ribavirin for chronic hepatitis C virus infection. N Engl J Med 347: 975–982

Froehlich F, Lamy O, Fried M et al (1993) Practice and complications of liver biopsy. Results of a nationwide survey in Switzerland. Dig Dis Sci 38: 1480–1484

Girometti R, Furlan A, Bazzocchi M et al (2007) Diffusion-weighted MRI in evaluating liver fibrosis: a feasibility study in cirrhotic patients. Radiol Med (Torino) 112: 394–408

Hadziyannis SJ, Sette H Jr, Morgan TR et al (2004) Peginterferon-alpha2a and ribavirin combination therapy in chronic hepatitis C: a randomized study of treatment duration and ribavirin dose. Ann Intern Med 140: 346–355

Hagiwara M, Rusinek H, Lee VS et al (2008) Advanced liver fibrosis: diagnosis with 3D whole-liver perfusion MR imaging–initial experience. Radiology 246: 926–934

Huwart L, Peeters F, Sinkus R et al (2006) Liver fibrosis: non-invasive assessment with MR elastography. NMR Biomed 19: 173–179

Huwart L, Sempoux C, Salameh N et al (2007) Liver fibrosis: noninvasive assessment with MR elastography versus aspartate aminotransferase to-platelet ratio index. Radiology 245: 458–466

Ichikawa T, Haradome H, Hachiya J et al (1998) Diffusion-weighted MR imaging with a single-shot echoplanar sequence: detection and characterization of focal hepatic lesions. AJR Am J Roentgenol 170: 397–402

Imbert-Bismut F, Ratziu V, Pieroni L et al (2001) Biochemical markers of liver fibrosis in patients with hepatitis C virus infection: a prospective study. Lancet 357: 1069–1075

Ito K, Mitchell DG, Gabata T (2000) Enlargement of hilar periportal space: a sign of early cirrhosis at MR imaging. J Magn Reson Imaging 11: 136–140

Ito K, Mitchell DG, Kim MJ et al (2003) Right posterior hepatic notch sign: a simple diagnostic MR finding of cirrhosis. J Magn Reson Imaging 18: 561–566

Janes CH, Lindor KD (1993) Outcome of patients hospitalized for complications after outpatient liver biopsy. Ann Intern Med 118: 96–98

Kim AI, Saab S (2005) Treatment of hepatitis C. Am J Med 118: 808–815

Kim T, Murakami T, Takahashi S et al (1999) Diffusion-weighted single shot echoplanar MR imaging for liver disease. AJR Am J Roentgenol 173: 393–398

Kim WR, Gross JB Jr, Poterucha JJ et al (2001) Outcome of hospital care of liver disease associated with hepatitis C in the United States. Hepatology 33: 201–206

Koinuma M, Ohashi I, Hanafusa K et al (2005) Apparent diffusion coefficient measurements with diffusion-weighted magnetic resonance imaging for evaluation of hepatic fibrosis. J Magn Reson Imaging 22: 80–85

Kwee TC, Takahara T, Koh DM et al (2008) Comparison and reproducibility of ADC measurements in breathhold, respiratory triggered, and free-breathing diffusion-weighted MR imaging of the liver. J Magn Reson Imaging 28: 1141–1148

Lauer GM, Walker BD (2001) Hepatitis C virus infection. N Engl J Med 345: 41–52

Le Bihan D (1988) Intravoxel incoherent motion imaging using steady-state free precession. Magn Reson Med 7: 346–351

Le Bihan D (1990) Diffusion/perfusion MR imaging of the brain: from structure to function. Radiology 177: 328–329

Le Bihan D, Breton E, Lallemand D et al (1988) Separation of diffusion and perfusion in intravoxel incoherent motion MR imaging. Radiology 168: 497–505

Le Bihan D, Turner R (1991) Intravoxel incoherent motion imaging using spin echoes. Magn Reson Med 19: 221–227

Le Bihan D, Turner R, MacFall JR (1989) Effects of intravoxel incoherent motions (IVIM) in steady-state free precession (SSFP) imaging: application to molecular diffusion imaging. Magn Reson Med 10: 324–337

Lewin M, Poujol-Robert A, Boelle PY et al (2007) Diffusion-weighted magnetic resonance imaging for the assessment of fibrosis in chronic hepatitis C. Hepatology 46: 658–665

Luciani A, Vignaud A, Cavet M et al (2008) Liver cirrhosis: intravoxel incoherent motion MR imaging–pilot study. Radiology 249: 891–899

Maharaj B, Maharaj RJ, Leary WP et al (1986) Sampling variability and its influence on the diagnostic yield of percutaneous needle biopsy of the liver. Lancet 1: 523–525

Manns MP, McHutchison JG, Gordon SC et al (2001) Peginterferon alfa-2b plus ribavirin compared with interferon alfa-2b plus ribavirin for initial treatment of chronic hepatitis C: a randomised trial. Lancet 358: 958–965

The French METAVIR Cooperative Study Group (1994) Intraobserver and interobserver variations in liver biopsy interpretation in patients with chronic hepatitis C. The French METAVIR Cooperative Study Group. Hepatology 20: 15–20

Muller MF, Prasad P, Siewert B et al (1994) Abdominal diffusion mapping with use of a whole-body echo-planar system. Radiology 190: 475–478

Murtz P, Flacke S, Traber F et al (2002) Abdomen: diffusion-weighted MR imaging with pulse-triggered single-shot sequences. Radiology 224: 258–264

Namimoto T, Yamashita Y, Sumi S et al (1997) Focal liver masses: characterization with diffusion-weighted echo-planar MR imaging. Radiology 204: 739–744

Parikh T, Drew SJ, Lee VS et al (2008) Focal liver lesion detection and characterization with diffusion-weighted MR imaging: comparison with standard breath-hold T2-weighted imaging. Radiology 246: 812–822

Poynard T, McHutchison J, Manns M et al (2003) Biochemical surrogate markers of liver fibrosis and activity in a randomized trial of peginterferon alfa-2b and ribavirin. Hepatology 38: 481–492

Regev A, Berho M, Jeffers LJ et al (2002) Sampling error and intraobserver variation in liver biopsy in patients with chronic HCV infection. Am J Gastroenterol 97: 2614–2618

Rouviere O, Yin M, Dresner MA et al (2006) MR elastography of the liver: preliminary results. Radiology 240: 440–448

Semelka RC, Chung JJ, Hussain SM et al (2001) Chronic hepatitis: correlation of early patchy and late linear enhancement patterns on gadolinium-enhanced MR images with histopathology initial experience. J Magn Reson Imaging 13: 385–391

Taouli B, Chouli M, Martin AJ et al (2008) Chronic hepatitis: Role of diffusion-weighted imaging and diffusion tensor imaging for the diagnosis of liver fibrosis and inflammation. J Magn Reson Imaging 28: 89–95

Taouli B, Martin AJ, Qayyum A et al (2004) Parallel imaging and diffusion tensor imaging for diffusion-weighted MRI of the liver: preliminary experience in healthy volunteers. AJR Am J Roentgenol 183: 677–680

Taouli B, Tolia AJ, Losada M et al (2007) Diffusion-weighted MRI for quantification of liver fibrosis: preliminary experience. AJR Am J Roentgenol 189: 799–806

Taouli B, Vilgrain V, Dumont E et al (2003) Evaluation of liver diffusion isotropy and characterization of focal hepatic lesions with two single-shot echo-planar MR imaging sequences: prospective study in 66 patients. Radiology 226: 71–78

Thomsen HS, Marckmann P, Logager VB (2008) Update on nephrogenic systemic fibrosis. Magn Reson Imaging Clin N Am 16: 551–560

Turner R, Le Bihan D, Maier J et al (1990) Echo-planar imaging of intravoxel incoherent motion. Radiology 177: 407–414

Wong JB, McQuillan GM, McHutchison JG et al (2000) Estimating future hepatitis C morbidity, mortality, and costs in the United States. Am J Public Health 90: 1562–1569

Yamada I, Aung W, Himeno Y et al (1999) Diffusion coefficients in abdominal organs and hepatic lesions: evaluation with intravoxel incoherent motion echo-planar MR imaging. Radiology 210: 617–623

Yee HS, Currie SL, Darling JM et al (2006) Management and treatment of hepatitis C viral infection: recommendations from the department of veterans affairs hepatitis C resource center program and the national hepatitis C program office. Am J Gastroenterol 101: 2360–2378

Yin M, Talwalkar JA, Glaser KJ et al (2007a) Assessment of hepatic fibrosis with magnetic resonance elastography. Clin Gastroenterol Hepatol 5: 1207–1213.e2

Yin M, Woollard J, Wang X et al (2007b) Quantitative assessment of hepatic fibrosis in an animal model with magnetic resonance elastography. Magn Reson Med 58: 346–353

Ziol M, Handra-Luca A, Kettaneh A et al (2005) Noninvasive assessment of liver fibrosis by measurement of stiffness in patients with chronic hepatitis C. Hepatology 41: 48–54

Oncological Applications in the Body

DW-MRI for Disease Detection

Dow-Mu Koh

SUMMARY

DW-MRI is increasingly recognized as an imaging technique which can increase the contrast between normal and tumour tissues, thus facilitating their detection. High b-value (e.g. $b = 750$–$1,000 \, s/mm^2$) DW-MRI increases signal suppression of normal and background tissue, allowing foci of cellular tumour tissues to be identified as areas of high signal intensity. However, the contrast between tumour and its surrounding tissue is influenced by the histology of the tumour, as well as the nature of the tissue in which the tumour resides. In some instances, ADC maps may prove more valuable for disease identification. DW-MRI has been applied for tumour detection in the neck, chest, abdomen and pelvis. The clinical utility of the imaging technique and potential pitfalls are discussed.

7.1

Introduction

The application of DW-MRI in oncology is growing due to recognition that this imaging technique provides unique insight into tissue cellularity, tissue organization, integrity of cells and membranes, as well as the tortuosity of the extracellular space, which can be helpful for detecting malignant diseases, and for distinguishing tumour tissues from non-tumour tissues (Koh et al. 2007; Thoeny et al. 2007).

Tumour tissues, because of their poorly regulated cell growth, are frequently more cellular compared with the native tissues they arise from, and thus demonstrate high signal intensity impeded diffusion on high b-value DW-MRI and return low apparent diffusion coefficients (ADCs). Thus, by applying DW-MRI,

Dow-Mu Koh, MD, MRCP, FRCR
Royal Marsden NHS Foundation trust, Department of Diagnostic Radiology, Downs Road, Sutton, Surrey SM2 5PT, UK

a unique contrast mechanism can be harnessed to detect cellular tumour tissues. However, because the imaging technique discriminates lesions on the basis of tissue diffusivity rather than malignancy, there are also potential pitfalls that can occur when applying DW-MRI for the detection of malignancies. This chapter discusses the principles of applying DW-MRI to aid tumour detection in the body, including the potential limitations and pitfalls. The current and emerging applications of DW-MRI for tumour detection in oncological practice are reviewed.

7.2
Principles of DW-MRI for Lesion Detection in Oncology

For disease to be visible on DW-MRI, there has to be a differential in the signal intensity of the disease vs. the background when imaging is performed at a selected b-value. Ideally, the signal from the background should be relatively suppressed compared with the signal returned from the tumour tissue, thus allowing the pathological process to be clearly distinguished. Since benign and normal tissues tend to show greater signal attenuation at high b-values (e.g. 750–1,000 s/mm^2) compared with cellular tumours, the use of high b-value DW-MRI has been recognized as a method to increase the radiological contrast between tumours and normal tissue. This method of disease assessment relies primarily on the visual assessment of the high b-value DW-MR images to identify potential pathological tissue as high signal intensity areas of impeded diffusion (Fig. 7.1) against the relatively darkened background. Whilst this approach seems to be effective for a large range of tumours located at different anatomical sites in the body, and is used as the basis for the whole-body diffusion-weighted MR imaging with background suppression (DWIBS) technique, potential false positives and false negatives can occur due to factors related to the underlying pathology and/or the anatomical background in which the disease resides. Hence, effective utilization of DW-MRI in the body for disease detection requires a clear understanding of the pathological process being investigated and the behaviour of normal tissue at the anatomical sites in which the disease is located. As such, the usefulness of high b-value DW-MR images is not invariable and the imaging approach should take these factors into consideration.

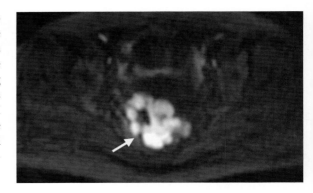

Fig. 7.1. High b-value ($b = 1,000$ s/mm^2) axial DW-MR image obtained through the pelvis showing a multi-lobulated mass (*arrow*) which was histologically confirmed to be an ovarian carcinoma. Note that the mass returns hyperintense signal, whereas the signal from the background is relatively suppressed with diminished anatomical detail

7.2.1
Influence of Pathology on Disease Detection

Tumours vary widely in their tissue composition and organization, which in turn can influence their appearances on DW-MRI. The relationship between tumour cellularity and their tissue diffusivity is not straightforward, although it has been shown that there is a correlation between tissue cellularity or the histological subtypes with the measured ADC in tumour such as gliomas (FILIPPI et al. 2001; GUO et al. 2002), soft tissue sarcomas (NAGATA et al. 2008), renal (MANENTI et al. 2008), prostate (TAMADA et al. 2008; ZELHOF et al. 2009) and breast carcinomas (YOSHIKAWA et al. 2008). These tumours show varying degrees of high signal intensity impeded diffusion on the high b-value DW-MR image. However, less cellular tumours (e.g. cystic, mucinous or necrotic tumours) can show significant signal attenuation with increasing b-value, making them difficult to detect against the background tissue on the high b-value DW-MR image. Thus, if only the high b-value DW-MR images are surveyed at evaluation, lesions such as these may be missed. Figure 7.2 illustrates a male patient with metastatic renal cell carcinoma to the spine. As a result of the underlying histology, the metastasis in the vertebral body shows significant signal attenuation on the $b = 800$ s/mm^2 image, such that it is no longer discernible. However, the metastasis can be clearly seen on the $b = 0$ s/mm^2 image and the ADC map.

The administration of treatment, such as chemotherapy, can also make tumours less visible on

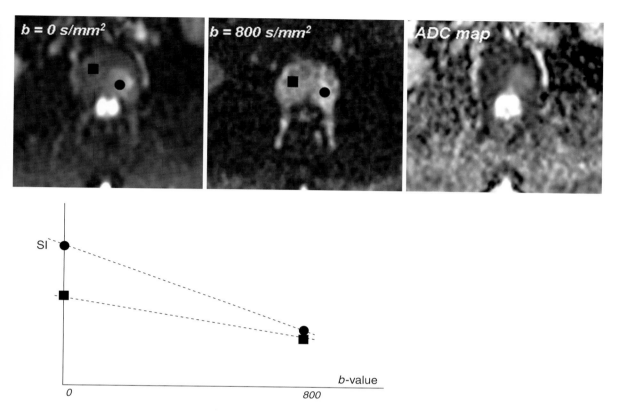

Fig. 7.2. A 48-year-old man with metastatic renal cell carcinoma to the spine. Axial DW-MR images obtained at $b = 0$ and $b = 800$ s/mm^2 show a metastasis (indicated by *black circle*) in the third lumbar vertebra. While the metastasis appears mildly hyperintense on the $b = 0$ s/mm^2 image, it is barely perceptible on the $b = 800$ s/mm^2 image, compared with surrounding bone (*black square*). Simplified schematic plots of the signal intensity vs. b-values show differential signal attenuation of the metastasis (*circle*) vs. the normal vertebral bone (*square*), illustrating the reason for the reduced contrast between lesion and background at higher b-value. The metastasis could easily have been overlooked if only the higher b-value image was used for disease evaluation. The ADC map showed increased water diffusivity in the metastasis

DW-MRI. Effective chemotherapy leads to tumour cell death and tissue necrosis, and consequently an increase in tumour ADC. As a result, a tumour can appear of lower signal intensity post-treatment on the high b-value DW-MR image compared with the pretreatment images. Consequently, small foci of disease (<1 cm) can be more difficult to identify after treatment on DW-MRI (Fig. 7.3).

It has to be remembered that the hyperintense signal returned on a high b-value DW-MR image is not pathognomonic of malignancy, as other cellular processes can result in a similar appearance. For example, cellular abscess collection can show hyperintense signal intensity on a high b-value image (YOSHIDA et al. 2008) and return low ADC values (Fig. 7.4), thus mimicking malignant disease. However, the clinical presentation of patients with sepsis is usually different from those with malignant disease. Hence, it is important to interpret DW-MR images with reference to the clinical context.

The presence of material within tissues that causes strong susceptibility effects on DW-MRI can also confound disease detection, especially when echo-planar imaging is used for DW-MRI measurements. Hence, pathological processes that contain blood degradation products and those resulting in significant iron deposition within tissues can cause significant susceptibility artefacts in the tissue of interest on DW-MRI, leading to reduced signal intensity observed on the high b-value images, which can impact upon disease detection.

7.2.2
Influence of Background Tissue on Disease Detection

The ability of DW-MRI to detect disease also depends on the nature of the background tissue in which the tumour resides. In the body, the normal spleen, lymph

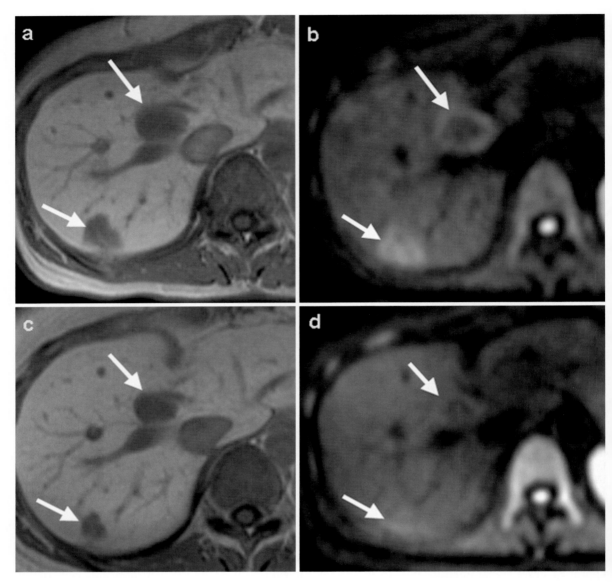

Fig. 7.3. Chemotherapy can reduce lesion conspicuity on DW-MRI. Pre-chemotherapy. (**a**) T1-weighted post-Gd-EOB-DTPA contrast and (**b**) DW-MR $b = 750\,s/mm^2$ images show two metastases in the liver (*arrows*). One metastasis shows near uniform hyperintensity and the other rim hy- perintensity on the DW-MR image. Following 12 weeks of chemotherapy, (**c**) T1-weighted post-Gd-EOB-DTPA contrast showed some reduction in size of the metastases. However, the metastases now appear much less conspicuous on the (**d**) $b = 750\,s/mm^2$ DW-MR image

nodes, testes, ovaries, kidneys, endometrium and spinal cord appear hyperintense on high b-value DW-MR images. The spleen, in particular, is a highly cellular organ which shows marked hyperintensity on high b-value DW-MRI. Hence, one of the potential pitfalls of DW-MRI is for the identification of disease adjacent to or within the spleen (Fig. 7.5). Using DW-MRI, lymph nodes whether malignant or benign, will show hyperintensity on high b-value DW-MRI. Thus,

detecting malignant disease within lymph nodes using DW-MRI is challenging and DW-MR imaging strategies are being investigated to improve nodal staging. This will be discussed in detail in Chap. 13.

There is now increasing interest in utilizing DW-MRI for the detection of bone metastases and malignant marrow infiltration. In the elderly, where the normal bone marrow is largely replaced by fat, any signal arising from the normal bone marrow will

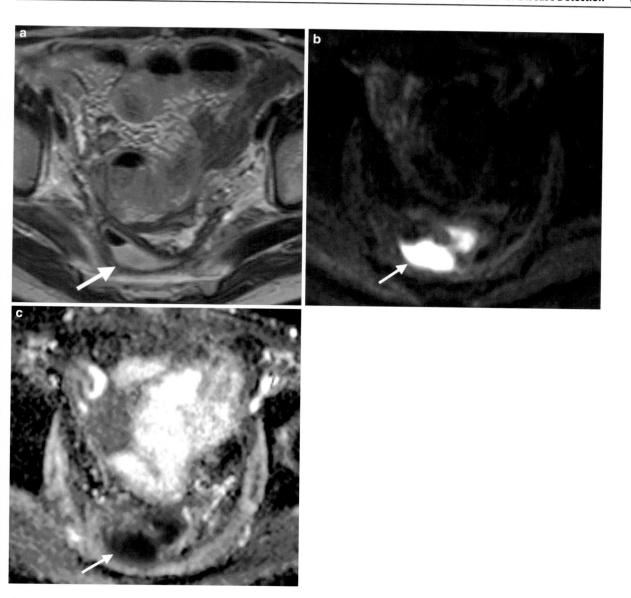

Fig. 7.4. Pelvic abscess in a 56-year-old woman with a history of abdomino-perineal resection for rectal cancer presented with pelvic pain. (**a**) T2-weighted axial image shows a high signal intensity abscess containing air-fluid level in the presacral space (*arrow*). (**b**) The abscess (*arrow*) demonstrates hyperintensity on the DW-MRI $b = 900\,\text{s/mm}^2$ image and return low ADC value on the ADC map (**c**)

be effectively suppressed using fat-suppressed echo-planar DW-MRI. Hence, studies conducted with older study populations have shown the diagnostic value of DW-MRI for the detection of skeletal metastases. However, DW-MRI may be less successful in detecting metastatic disease in patients of a younger age group since residual hypercellular red marrow will appear hyperintense on the high b-value DW-MR image, which may be indistinguishable from foci of disease.

When performing DW-MRI in the body, considerations for image quality and signal-to-noise restrict the use of very high b-values for imaging (e.g. $b = 2,000\,\text{s/mm}^2$) (Kitajima et al. 2008). Most DW-MRI examinations in the body utilize b-values between 0 and $1,000\,\text{s/mm}^2$. Within this range of b-values, the peripheral zone of the prostate gland frequently still appears hyperintense on the high b-value DW-MR image, which is due to the relatively long T2 relaxation time of the glandular tissue. This may be viewed upon

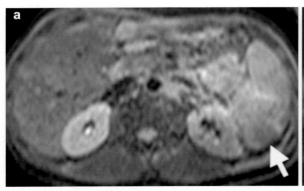
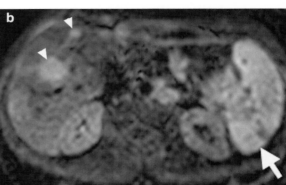

Fig. 7.5. A 38-year-old man with metastatic melanoma. (**a**) Fat-suppressed T2-weighted axial imaging shows a mildly hypointense lesion within the spleen (*arrow*). (**b**) The lesion is poorly visualized on the DW-MRI $b = 750\,\text{s/mm}^2$ image (*arrow*) as the normal splenic tissue is also hyperintense on the diffusion-weighted image. Note further metastases within the liver (*arrowheads*)

as a "T2 shine-through effect" (see also Chap. 3) which can confound disease detection. For this reason, it has been found that reviewing the ADC maps of the prostate is more useful for the detection of disease within the peripheral zone of the prostate gland.

From the above discussions, it is clear that successful application of DW-MRI for tumour detection in the body will require an understanding of the underlying pathology and the anatomical region to which the imaging is applied. It is also important to emphasize that good conventional morphological imaging should always be performed, to enable abnormalities detected on DW-MRI to be correlated with the morphological imaging, allowing the best image interpretation to be made.

7.3
Applications of DW-MRI for Tumour Detection in the Body

DW-MRI has been applied for tumour detection in the body for both clinical evaluation and research. DW-MRI has been employed at many sites in the abdomen and pelvis to detect tumours including the liver, prostate, uterine-cervix, peritoneum, pancreas, colon, kidneys and urinary bladder. Above the diaphragm, DW-MRI has also been utilized for tumour detection in the oesophagus, lung, breast and head and neck region. Of these, there is now significant evidence to recommend the clinical use of DW-MRI for lesion detection in the liver (Table 7.1) (Ichikawa et al. 1998; Naganawa et al. 2005; Nasu et al. 2006; Bruegel et al. 2008; Coenegrachts et al. 2008;

Goshima et al. 2008; Koh et al. 2008; Parikh et al. 2008; Zech et al. 2008). Although DW-MRI is also showing substantial promise for the detection and evaluation of bone pathologies, this will be discussed in a separate chapter.

7.3.1
Focal Liver Lesions

DW-MRI has proved valuable for the detection of focal liver lesions. Applying a small diffusion weighting (e.g. $50\text{–}100\,\text{s/mm}^2$) results in nulling of the high signal from intra-hepatic vasculature, enabling focal liver lesions to be visualized as hyperintense foci against the liver parenchyma (Fig. 7.6). As the application of diffusion-weighting suppresses signal from the intra-hepatic vasculature, DW-MRI in the liver has also been termed as a "black-blood" technique. The range of b-values employed for imaging the liver typically varies between 50 and $800\,\text{s/mm}^2$. Recent studies have shown that DW-MRI, whether performed in breath-hold, free-breathing or respiratory-triggering, were superior to conventional T2-weighted MR imaging sequences for the detection of focal hepatic lesions (Table 7.1).

In patients with colorectal liver metastases it was found that DW-MRI combined with conventional unenhanced T1- and T2-weighted imaging was superior to SPIO enhanced T2-weighted MR imaging for the detection of liver metastases (Nasu et al. 2006). In another study in patients with suspected colorectal liver metastases, the combination of DW-MRI with liver specific contrast MnDPDP-enhanced T1-weighted imaging of the liver, resulted in the highest diagnostic

Table 7.1. Published studies employing DW-MRI for the detection of focal liver lesions

Year	Authors	Journal	Number	Comparison	Findings
2008	COENEGRACHTS et al.	EJR	25	SPIO enhanced MRI and TSE T2-weighted MRI	Non-contrast single-shot EPI DE-MRI best for lesion detection
2008	PARIKH et al.	Radiology	53	Breath-hold T2-weighted MRI	DW-MRI better than T2-weighted MRI for lesion detection
2008	KOH et al.	Eur Radiol	33	T1-weighted MnDPDP-enhanced MRI	Adding DW-MRI to MnDPDP-enhanced T1-weighted MRI resulted in highest detection rate for colorectal liver metastases
2008	BRUEGEL et al.	AJR	52	T2-weighted imaging	Respiratory-triggered DW-MRI had the highest sensitivity for lesion detection
2008	ZECH et al.	Invest Rad	20	T2-weighted imaging	Higher rate of lesion detection using DW-MRI
2008	GOSHIMA et al.	JMRI	76	To investigate optimal b-value for lesion detection	$b = 100\,s/mm^2$ found to be optimal for lesion detection
2007	COENEGRACHTS et al.	BJR	24	TSE T2-weighted MRI	DW-MRI increased lesion conspicuity
2006	NASU et al.	Radiology	24	SPIO-enhanced T2-weighted MRI	DW-MRI together with unenhanced T1 and T2-weighted imaging resulted in highest detection rate compared with SPIO-enhanced imaging
2005	NAGANAWA et al.	JMRI	6	DW-MRI with SPIO enhancement	DW-MRI after SPIO administration increased the contrast-to-noise ratio of malignant lesions
1998	ICHIKAWA et al.	AJR	46		Using echo-planar DW-MRI increased detection of malignancy

accuracy (ROC area under the curve Az = 0.95) for the detection of liver metastases compared with either technique on its own (KOH et al. 2008). The improved diagnostic accuracy of combining DW-MRI with MnDPDP-enhanced imaging could be attributed to complementary detection and localization of disease within the liver. DW-MRI improved the detection of small metastases that mimicked intra-hepatic vasculature on contrast-enhanced imaging, while MnDPDP-enhanced MR imaging identified disease missed by DW-MRI in the periphery of the liver or in areas where there were imaging artefacts (Fig. 7.7).

In patients with chronic liver disease, it has also been reported that the addition of DW-MRI to conventional dynamic gadolinium contrast-enhanced MR imaging can improve the detection of hepatocellular carcinomas (XU et al. 2009). However, in the presence of liver cirrhosis, cirrhotic and regenerative nodules can exhibit a range of signal intensities on DW-MRI, making the detection of hepatocellular carcinoma using DW-MRI against these background liver changes more challenging. The role of DW-MRI for the detection of cholangiocarcinoma is also being evaluated.

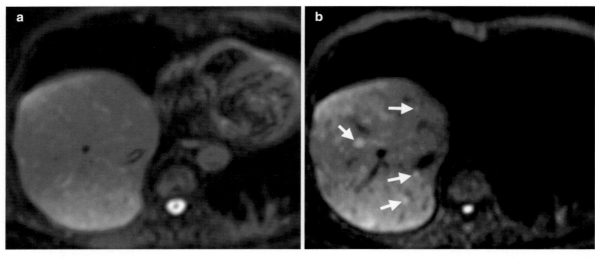

Fig. 7.6. A 52-year-old man with metastatic colorectal cancer. Axial DW-MR images acquired at *b*-values of (**a**) $b = 0\,s/mm^2$ and (**b**) $b = 100\,s/mm^2$. By applying a diffusion weighting, there is suppression of the signal within the intra-hepatic vasculature, allowing the small hyperintense liver metastases to be identified (*arrows*)

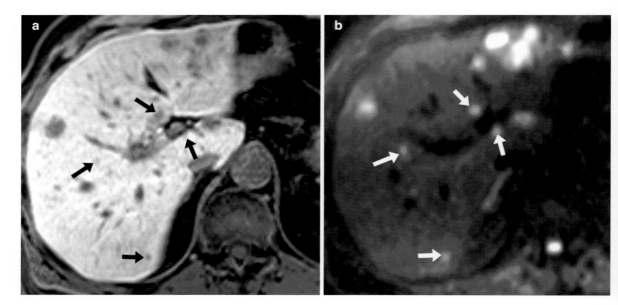

Fig. 7.7. Combining DW-MRI with hepatocyte-selective contrast-enhanced MR imaging can improve the detection of colorectal liver metastases. (**a**) Fat-suppressed T1-weighted imaging performed in the liver phase of contrast enhancement after Gd-EOB-DTPA administration. In this phase, both the intra-hepatic vasculature and liver metastases are hypointense to the avidly enhancing liver parenchyma. Small metastases may be easily overlooked (*arrows*). However, these are clearly demonstrated on the (**b**) DW-MRI $b = 750\,s/mm^2$ image. (Reproduced with permission from Cancer Imaging)

7.3.2
Prostate Cancer

In the male pelvis, parametric ADC maps of the prostate gland have been used to improve the detection of prostate cancer. In the prostate gland, the addition of DW-MRI to T2-weighted MR imaging has been shown to improve the detection of prostatic carcinoma in the peripheral zone of the prostate gland (Fig. 7.8) (HAIDER et al. 2007; MORGAN et al. 2007). The addition of DW-MRI to T2-weighted imaging was also found to be helpful for lesion localization in patients that had both

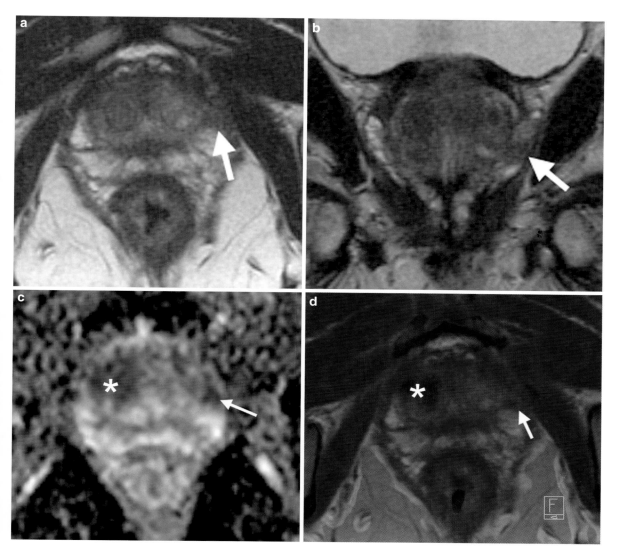

Fig. 7.8. A 69-year-old man with prostate cancer. T2-weighted (**a**) axial and (**b**) coronal images show low signal intensity focus in the periphery of the left prostate gland towards the glandular apex (arrows), which may be overlooked, particularly on axial imaging. (**c**) The focus returns low ADC value on the ADC map (arrow). The abnormality can be clearly detected on (**d**) created by the fusion of the ADC map with the morphological T2-weighted image (arrow). Sextent biopsy of the area confirmed carcinoma of the prostate. In the example, benign prostatic hypertrophy in the central gland (asterisk) also returned low ADC values

previous negative transrectal ultrasound-guided biopsy and persistently elevated serum prostate specific antigen levels before a repeated biopsy was undertaken (PARK et al. 2008).

Recently, it was shown that the combination of dynamic contrast-enhanced MR imaging with DW-MRI may also improve the detection of carcinoma arising from the transitional zone (YOSHIZAKO et al. 2008). Interestingly, the combination of DW-MRI with metabolic ratios derived from 3D proton spectroscopy was reported to improve the detection and char-

acterization of prostate cancer (MAZAHERI et al. 2008). However, the detection of prostate cancer in the transitional zone of the prostate gland remains challenging. The use of diffusion-tensor imaging, which allows for the evaluation of tissue anisotropy, is showing promise for the detection of cancer arising within the transitional zone or central gland of the prostate but requires further investigation (MANENTI et al. 2007; XU et al. 2009; ZELHOF et al. 2009). In patients who have received radiotherapy treatment, DW-MRI when added to T2-weighted imaging also improved the ability to discriminate between recurrent disease and post-therapy changes (KIM et al. 2009).

7.3.3
Uterine and Cervical Cancer

In the female pelvis, DW-MRI has been shown to be an accurate technique for the detection of uterine (TAMAI et al. 2007) and cervical malignancies (MCVEIGH et al. 2008). In the endometrium and cervix, as the ADC of the normal endometrium and cervix are significantly higher than that of malignant tissue, parametric ADC maps are useful for detecting the presence of cancers (MCVEIGH et al. 2008; INADA et al. 2009). When gadolinium contrast medium is not administered during the examination, DW-MRI has also been found to be a sensitive technique, when used in conjunction with T2-weighted imaging, for the detection of uterine malignancy (INADA et al. 2009). In particular, the use of fusion images combining high b-value DW-MR images with morphological T2-weighted images can aid the identification of uterine malignancies and determine the depth of myometrial invasion by uterine carcinomas (Fig. 7.9) (INADA et al. 2009; LIN et al. 2009). The use of fusion images (DW-MRI and T2-weighted) significantly improved the accuracy of assessing the depth of myometrial invasion by uterine cancers compared with T2-weighted and contrast-enhanced MR imaging (LIN et al. 2009).

DW-MRI appears to have a more limited role for the identification of ovarian malignancy since normal ovary appears hyperintense on high b-value DW-MR images (FUJII et al. 2008). However, there is interest in the application of the technique for the characterization of adnexal masses which are detected at imaging (THOMASSIN-NAGGARA et al. 2009).

7.3.4
Peritoneal Disease

One of the areas in the body where DW-MRI has shown substantial promise is in the detection of peritoneal disease (FUJII et al. 2008). Conventional imaging is reliant on delayed fat-suppressed contrast-enhanced T1-weighted imaging for the identification of peritoneal metastases (LOW et al. 1997; LOW 2007). Peritoneal disease appears as enhancing peritoneal thickening or nodules on delayed post-contrast T1-weighted MR imaging. However, DW-MRI is also a useful technique for the identification of small volume peritoneal disease (LOW et al. 2007). Peritoneal deposits typically appear as hyperintense foci against the signal-suppressed peritoneal fat on high b-value DW-MR images. In one study (FUJII et al. 2008) it was found that applying DW-MRI has 90% sensitivity and 96% specificity for the detection of peritoneal metastases in patients with gynaecological cancers (Fig. 7.10).

7.3.5
Pancreatic Tumours

High b-value ($b = 1,000\,\text{s/mm}^2$) DW-MR imaging can aid the detection of pancreatic tumours in patients (ICHIKAWA et al. 2007) (Fig. 7.11). DW-MRI may detect pancreatic cancers at an earlier stage of disease,

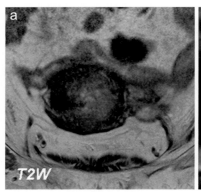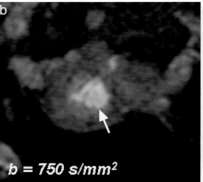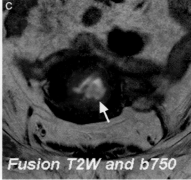

Fig. 7.9. A 63-year-old woman with endometrial cancer. (**a**) Para-axial T2-weighted image shows an intermediate signal intensity mass which appears to infiltrate into the outer half of the myometrium on the left. (**b**) DW-MRI at $b = 750\,\text{s/mm}^2$ depicts the mass arising from the endometrium as a high signal intensity lesion (arrow). (**c**) Fusion of the DW-MR image (coloured) with the T2-weighted image confirms that the depth of tumour invasion is limited to the inner myometrium (arrow). The disease extent was proven at histopathology

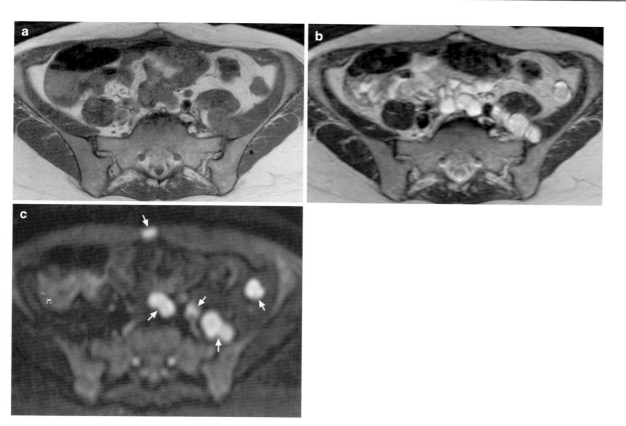

Fig. 7.10. A 55-year-old woman with peritoneal disease. The sites of disease are difficult to localize on the unenhanced (**a**) T1-weighted and (**b**) T2-weighted images. (**c**) High *b*-value (*b* = 900 s/mm²) DW-MRI clearly depicts sites of peritoneal, retroperitoneal and anterior abdominal wall disease as hyperintense foci against the signal-suppressed peritoneal fat (*arrows*)

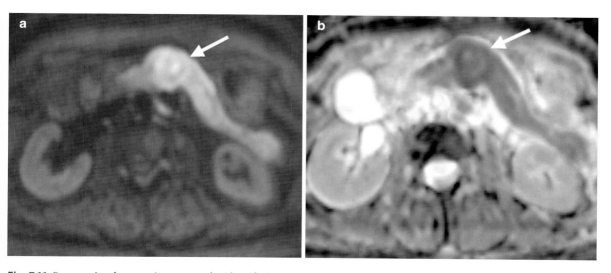

Fig. 7.11. Pancreatic adenocarcinoma may be identified as a focal mass lesion (arrows) of variable hyperintensity on (**a**) high *b*-value (*b* = 900 s/mm²), and return lower ADC value compared with the rest of the pancreas on the ADC map (**b**)

Fig. 7.12. Colorectal cancers demonstrate hyperintense signal on (**a**) high *b*-value ($b = 900\,s/mm^2$) DW-MR image, thus facilitating their detection (*arrow*). (**b**) The image generated by fusion of the DW-MR image (colour) and the T2-weighted image shows the posterior anatomical location of the tumour within the rectum (*shaded red and arrowed*). However, a villous adenoma may also demonstrate similar features

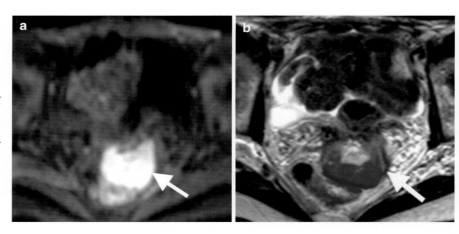

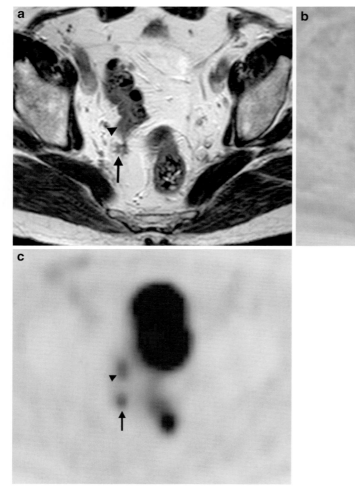

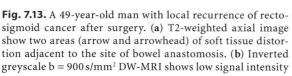

Fig. 7.13. A 49-year-old man with local recurrence of rectosigmoid cancer after surgery. (**a**) T2-weighted axial image show two areas (arrow and arrowhead) of soft tissue distortion adjacent to the site of bowel anastomosis. (**b**) Inverted greyscale $b = 900\,s/mm^2$ DW-MRI shows low signal intensity areas of reduced tissue diffusivity (*arrow and arrowhead*). The findings are corroborated with (**c**) 19FDG-PET imaging showing two hypermetabolic foci corresponding to the sites of the DW-MRI abnormalities (*arrow and arrowhead*), consistent with local disease recurrence

thus affording the patient the potential for surgical cure (SHINYA et al. 2008). DW-MRI has also been shown to be promising for distinguishing pancreatic carcinoma from mass-forming pancreatitis (TAKEUCHI et al. 2008). The application of DW-MRI for the characterization of pancreatic masses will be discussed in greater detail in Chap. 8.

7.3.6
Colorectal Cancers

High *b*-value DW-MRI has also been used to detect colorectal cancer. In clinical practice, CT colonography is used to detect colonic polyps and cancers. However, colorectal cancers and polyps also show hyperintense impeded water diffusion on the high *b*-value DW-MR images (ICHIKAWA et al. 2006) which has been used as the basis for tumour evaluation (Fig. 7.12). One study comparing DW-MRI with fluorodeoxyglucose positron emission tomography (FDG-PET) found DW-MRI to be inferior to FDG-PET for the detection of primary tumour, but superior to FDG-PET for the detection of nodal disease (ONO et al. 2009). In addition to the assessment of the primary tumour, there is also interest in applying the technique for the evaluation of disease recurrence after initial treatment (Fig. 7.13).

7.3.7
Renal Tumours

DW-MRI is currently being investigated as a technique for characterizing renal masses (ZHANG et al. 2008; KIM et al. 2009; TAOULI et al. 2009). In patients with congenital or acquired cystic disease of the kidneys, detection of renal cancers can be challenging. The potential value of high *b*-value DW-MRI in the context of detecting renal cancers in patients with cystic diseases of the kidneys has been shown (KITAZUME et al. 2009). DW-MRI may help to identify tumours in apparently cystic or poorly enhancing lesions of the kidneys; however, this requires further investigation (Fig. 7.14).

7.3.8
Bladder Tumours

Tumours arising from the urinary bladder are usually seen as hyperintense masses on high *b*-value DW-MR images (MATSUKI et al. 2007). In patients presenting with haematuria, DW-MRI has been shown to have a high sensitivity (98.1%), specificity (92.3%), positive predictive value (100%), negative predictive value (92.3%) and accuracy (97.0%) for identifying bladder tumours (ABOU-EL-GHAR et al. 2009). The correlation between DW-MRI and cystoscopic findings was found to be excellent (kappa = 0.94) (ABOU-EL-GHAR et al. 2009). In another study (EL-ASSMY et al. 2009), DW-MRI was found to have a higher staging accuracy for bladder cancers compared with T2-weighted imaging. The staging accuracy using DW-MRI and T2-weighted imaging was 63.6 vs. 6.1% in differentiating superficial from invasive tumours, and 69.6 vs. 15.1% for diagnosing organ-confined from non-organ-confined tumours. Another independent

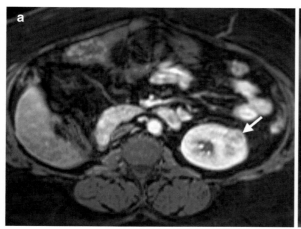
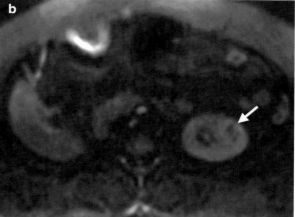
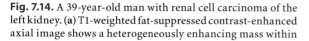

Fig. 7.14. A 39-year-old man with renal cell carcinoma of the left kidney. (**a**) T1-weighted fat-suppressed contrast-enhanced axial image shows a heterogeneously enhancing mass within the left kidney (arrow). (**b**) The mass demonstrates rim hyperintensity on the *b* = 900 s/mm² DW-MR image. Clear cell carcinoma of the kidney was confirmed after surgery

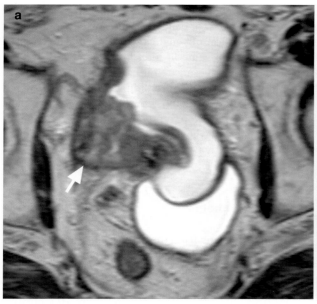 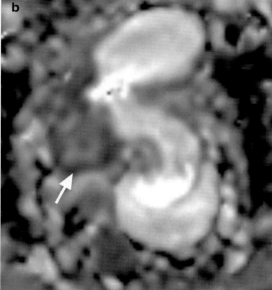

Fig. 7.15. A 57-year old man with bladder cancer (arrows). (a) T2-weighted MR image showing a large mass arising from the right bladder wall, resulting in significant distortion of the bladder contour. (b) ADC map of the pelvis shows reduced tissue diffusivity and low ADC values returned from the tumour

observation was that using high *b*-value DW-MRI with conventional T2-weighted MR imaging resulted in a higher diagnostic accuracy (88%) for the local T-staging of bladder cancers compared with T2-weighted imaging alone (67%) or T2-weighted imaging with dynamic contrast-enhanced imaging (79%) (Takeuchi et al. 2009). Combining T2-weighted imaging, DW-MRI and dynamic contrast-enhanced MR imaging resulted in the highest diagnostic accuracy of 92% (Takeuchi et al. 2009), demonstrating the incremental value of DW-MRI for tumour detection in clinical practice (Fig. 7.15).

7.3.9
Oesophageal and Gastric Cancers

When performing DW-MRI of the oesophagus and stomach, imaging of the gastro-oesophageal junction may pose technical issues because of respiratory, cardiac and peristaltic motion. Anti-peristaltic agent is typically administered prior to imaging. Initial experience using DW-MRI has shown limited sensitivity (40%) (Sakurada et al. 2009) in the detection of oesophageal cancers; although, the technique has been shown to be feasible for the evaluation of gastric tumours (Shinya et al. 2007).

Improvements in imaging technology, with the combined use of respiratory and cardiac triggering may in future improve the diagnostic accuracy of the technique for the detection of oesophageal cancers (Fig. 7.16).

7.3.10
Lung Cancers

DW-MRI in the chest can be technically challenging because of the need to overcome the effects of respiratory and cardiac motion. Nevertheless, DW-MRI of the chest is now feasible using breath-hold, free-breathing or respiratory-triggered imaging acquisitions. DW-MRI has now been applied for the detection (Qi et al. 2009) and characterization of focal pulmonary lesions (Matoba et al. 2007; Uto et al. 2009).

In patients presenting with lung collapse, DW-MRI has been shown to be helpful for detecting the location and boundaries of tumour within the collapsed lung segment (Qi et al. 2009) (Fig. 7.17). In addition, preliminary experience using DW-MRI in the mediastinum has also reported a higher diagnostic accuracy (89%) for the detection of nodal metastases in patients with lung cancers compared with FDG-PET (Nomori et al. 2008).

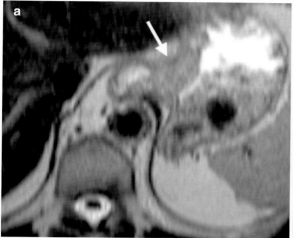
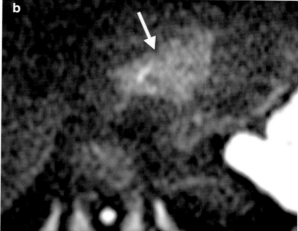

Fig. 7.16. A middle-aged man with carcinoma of the gastro-oesophageal junction (arrows). (**a**) T2-weighted imaging shows abnormal thickening of the gastro-oesophageal junction which extends into the cardia of the stomach (Type III tumour). (**b**) DW-MRI at $b = 900\,s/mm^2$ shows hyperintense impeded diffusion of the tumour and appears to demarcate the extent of disease. (With thanks to Dr. Angela Riddell, Royal Marsden Hospital, UK)

Fig. 7.17. An elderly woman with non-small cell lung cancer. (**a**) T1-weighted gradient-echo coronal imaging shows an apparent mass lesion in the left upper lobe associated with lung collapse. However, the boundaries of the tumour are not visualized. (**b**) On the $b = 800\,s/mm^2$ DW-MR image, the tumour with its hyperintense margins can be clearly distinguished from the distal collapse lung (*arrow*)

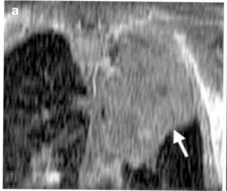
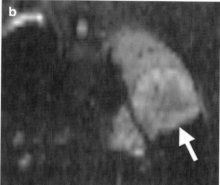

By ADC measurements, well-differentiated adenocarcinoma has been found to have higher ADC values compared with poorly differentiated adenocarcinoma and squamous cell carcinoma. However, as there is substantial overlap in the ADC values between groups of different pathologies, it would be difficult to categorize lung lesions based solely on the ADC values (MATOBA et al. 2007). Nevertheless, a relationship has been reported between tumour ADC and tumour cellularity (MATOBA et al. 2007). In another study, it was found that using the ratio of the lesion signal intensity to the signal intensity of the spinal cord on high b-value DW-MRI had a significantly higher diagnostic accuracy for diagnosing malignant lung disease compared with using ADC values (area under the curve by ROC analysis 0.91 vs. 0.60) (UTO et al. 2009).

7.3.11
Breast Tumours

DW-MRI is an attractive option for the detection of focal breast lesions as the technique is free of ionizing radiation, is quick to perform and does not require the administration of exogenous contrast material. Women with dense parenchymal tissue pose diagnostic challenges to the early detection of focal breast lesions. Free-breathing fat-suppressed echo-planar DW-MRI technique (WENKEL et al. 2007) has been shown to be of value for the detection of focal breast lesions (Fig. 7.18) at both 1.5 T (YOSHIKAWA et al. 2007) and 3 T (LO et al. 2009), although smaller cancers can be better visualized at 3 T (MATSUOKA et al. 2008).

When compared with mammography, DW-MRI showed a higher diagnostic accuracy (94 vs. 85%) for

Fig. 7.18 A 45-year-old woman with a strong family history of breast cancer. (**a**) Medial-lateral oblique digital mammogram of the right breast shows fairly dense parenchymal texture, but no definite mass lesion is identified. (**b**) DW-MRI at $b =$ 900 s/mm^2 image shows a spiculated mass in the medial right breast (*arrow*). Percutaneous biopsy of the mass confirmed invasive ductal carcinoma

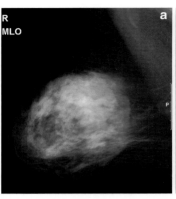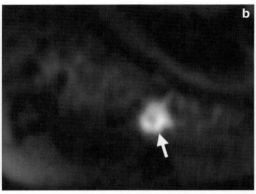

the detection of malignant breast disease, irrespective of tumour size or histology (YOSHIKAWA et al. 2007). Even without the administration of Gadolinium contrast medium, DW-MRI combined with STIR imaging was found to have a high sensitivity of 97% for the detection of breast malignancy (KUROKI-SUZUKI et al. 2007). In one study, the use of high *b*-value DW-MRI was equal to DCE-MRI (95%) but inferior to ADC maps (90%) for detecting malignant breast lesion, but the difference in diagnostic performance did not reach statistical significance (Lo et al. 2009). Interestingly, breast lesions can even be clearly visualized using the whole-body imaging DWIBS technique, thus highlighting the versatility of the DW-MRI techniques for assessing breast diseases (STADLBAUER et al. 2009).

Once a breast lesion is discovered, DW-MRI has also been applied to distinguish benign from malignant lesions. Of note is that the ADC values of breast lesions have been found to correlate with the underlying pathology but not cellularity (YOSHIKAWA et al. 2008). Generally, malignant lesions have lower ADC values compared with benign ones (WOODHAMS et al. 2005; RUBESOVA et al. 2006; PARK et al. 2007; YABUUCHI et al. 2008; Lo et al. 2009), although the cut-off value for this assessment does differ in the reported literature, varying from 0.95 to 1.6 × 10^{-3} mm^2/s. In addition, there is also significant overlap in ADC values between malignant and benign lesions. For these reasons, it is not advisable to use DW-MRI and ADC values as the sole criteria for distinguishing between benign and malignant breast diseases (KUROKI et al. 2008).

7.3.12
Head and Neck Tumours

The research application of DW-MRI in the head and neck region has largely been driven by clinical need,

focusing on the use of the technique to distinguish between benign and malignant lymphadenopathy (KING et al. 2007; VANDECAVEYE et al. 2009), the assessment of treatment response to chemoradiation (RAZEK et al. 2008; KATO et al. 2009; KIM et al. 2009) and the evaluation of post-treatment changes (VANDECAVEYE et al. 2006; ZBAREN et al. 2008). Once detected by DW-MRI, malignant nodes have been found to have lower ADC values than benign nodes. The application of DW-MRI for assessment of lymph nodes in the body will be specifically discussed in Chap. 13.

7.4
Conclusion

DW-MRI is a non-invasive imaging technique that is now being widely applied for the detection of disease in the body, with reportedly high sensitivity and diagnostic accuracy for specific tumour types and anatomical locations. However, the potential pitfalls of the technique need to be recognized, and the importance of combining DW-MRI with conventional morphological images for disease evaluation cannot be overemphasized. It is likely that DW-MRI will have a significant impact on the management of patients with cancer.

References

Abou-El-Ghar ME, El-Assmy A, Refaie HF et al (2009) Bladder cancer: diagnosis with diffusion-weighted MR imaging in patients with gross hematuria. Radiology 251: 415–421

Bruegel M, Gaa J, Waldt S et al (2008) Diagnosis of hepatic metastasis: comparison of respiration-triggered diffusion-weighted echo-planar MRI and five t2-weighted turbo spin-echo sequences. AJR Am J Roentgenol 191: 1421–1429

Coenegrachts K, Matos C, Ter Beek L et al (2008) Focal liver lesion detection and characterization: comparison of non-contrast enhanced and SPIO-enhanced diffusion-weighted single-shot spin echo echo planar and turbo spin echo T2-weighted imaging. Eur J Radiol (online)

El-Assmy A, Abou-El-Ghar ME, Mosbah A et al (2009) Bladder tumour staging: comparison of diffusion- and T(2)-weighted MR imaging. Eur Radiol 251:415–421

Filippi CG, Edgar MA, Ulug AM et al (2001) Appearance of meningiomas on diffusion-weighted images: correlating diffusion constants with histopathologic findings. AJNR Am J Neuroradiol 22: 65–72

Fujii S, Kakite S, Nishihara K et al (2008) Diagnostic accuracy of diffusion-weighted imaging in differentiating benign from malignant ovarian lesions. J Magn Reson Imaging 28: 1149–1156

Fujii S, Matsusue E, Kanasaki Y et al (2008) Detection of peritoneal dissemination in gynecological malignancy: evaluation by diffusion-weighted MR imaging. Eur Radiol 18: 18–23

Goshima S, Kanematsu M, Kondo H et al (2008) Diffusion-weighted imaging of the liver: optimizing b value for the detection and characterization of benign and malignant hepatic lesions. J Magn Reson Imaging 28: 691–697

Guo AC, Cummings TJ, Dash RC et al (2002) Lymphomas and high-grade astrocytomas: comparison of water diffusibility and histologic characteristics. Radiology 224: 177–183

Haider MA, van der Kwast TH, Tanguay J et al (2007) Combined T2-weighted and diffusion-weighted MRI for localization of prostate cancer. AJR Am J Roentgenol 189: 323–328

Ichikawa T, Erturk SM, Motosugi U et al (2006) High-B-value diffusion-weighted MRI in colorectal cancer. AJR Am J Roentgenol 187: 181–184

Ichikawa T, Erturk SM, Motosugi U et al (2007) High-b value diffusion-weighted MRI for detecting pancreatic adenocarcinoma: preliminary results. AJR Am J Roentgenol 188: 409–414

Ichikawa T, Haradome H, Hachiya J et al (1998) Diffusion-weighted MR imaging with a single-shot echoplanar sequence: detection and characterization of focal hepatic lesions. AJR Am J Roentgenol 170: 397–402

Inada Y, Matsuki M, Nakai G et al (2009) Body diffusion-weighted MR imaging of uterine endometrial cancer: is it helpful in the detection of cancer in nonenhanced MR imaging? Eur J Radiol 70: 122–127

Kato H, Kanematsu M, Tanaka O et al (2009) Head and neck squamous cell carcinoma: usefulness of diffusion-weighted MR imaging in the prediction of a neoadjuvant therapeutic effect. Eur Radiol 19: 103–109

Kim CK, Park BK, Lee HM (2009) Prediction of locally recurrent prostate cancer after radiation therapy: incremental value of 3T diffusion-weighted MRI. J Magn Reson Imaging 29: 391–397

Kim S, Jain M, Harris AB et al (2009) T1 hyperintense renal lesions: characterization with diffusion-weighted MR imaging versus contrast-enhanced MR imaging. Radiology 251: 796–807

Kim S, Loevner L, Quon H et al (2009) Diffusion-weighted magnetic resonance imaging for predicting and detecting early response to chemoradiation therapy of squamous cell carcinomas of the head and neck. Clin Cancer Res 15: 986–994

King AD, Ahuja AT, Yeung DK et al (2007) Malignant cervical lymphadenopathy: diagnostic accuracy of diffusion-weighted MR imaging. Radiology 245: 806–813

Kitajima K, Kaji Y, Kuroda K et al (2008) High b-value diffusion-weighted imaging in normal and malignant peripheral zone tissue of the prostate: effect of signal-to-noise ratio. Magn Reson Med Sci 7: 93–99

Kitazume Y, Satoh S, Taura S et al (2009) Diffusion-weighted magnetic resonance imaging detection of renal cancer presenting with diffuse peritoneal metastases in a patient with hemodialysis-associated acquired cystic disease of the kidney. J Magn Reson Imaging 29: 953–956

Koh DM, Brown G, Riddell AM et al (2008) Detection of colorectal hepatic metastases using MnDPDP MR imaging and diffusion-weighted imaging (DWI) alone and in combination. Eur Radiol 18: 903–910

Koh DM, Collins DJ (2007) Diffusion-weighted MRI in the body: applications and challenges in oncology. AJR Am J Roentgenol 188: 1622–1635

Kuroki-Suzuki S, Kuroki Y, Nasu K et al (2007) Detecting breast cancer with non-contrast MR imaging: combining diffusion-weighted and STIR imaging. Magn Reson Med Sci 6: 21–27

Kuroki Y, Nasu K (2008) Advances in breast MRI: diffusion-weighted imaging of the breast. Breast Cancer 15: 212–217

Lin G, Ng KK, Chang CJ et al (2009) Myometrial invasion in endometrial cancer: diagnostic accuracy of diffusion-weighted 3.0-T MR imaging–initial experience. Radiology 250: 784–792

Lo GG, Ai V, Chan JK et al (2009) Diffusion-weighted magnetic resonance imaging of breast lesions: first experiences at 3 T. J Comput Assist Tomogr 33: 63–69

Low RN (2007) MR imaging of the peritoneal spread of malignancy. Abdom Imaging 32: 267–283

Low RN, Barone RM, Lacey C et al (1997) Peritoneal tumor: MR imaging with dilute oral barium and intravenous gadolinium-containing contrast agents compared with unenhanced MR imaging and CT. Radiology 204: 513–520

Low RN, Gurney J (2007) Diffusion-weighted MRI (DWI) in the oncology patient: value of breathhold DWI compared to unenhanced and gadolinium-enhanced MRI. J Magn Reson Imaging 25: 848–858

Manenti G, Carlani M, Mancino S et al (2007) Diffusion tensor magnetic resonance imaging of prostate cancer. Invest Radiol 42: 412–419

Manenti G, Di Roma M, Mancino S et al (2008) Malignant renal neoplasms: correlation between ADC values and cellularity in diffusion weighted magnetic resonance imaging at 3 T. Radiol Med 113: 199–213

Matoba M, Tonami H, Kondou T et al (2007) Lung carcinoma: diffusion-weighted mr imaging–preliminary evaluation with apparent diffusion coefficient. Radiology 243: 570–577

Matsuki M, Inada Y, Tatsugami F et al (2007) Diffusion-weighted MR imaging for urinary bladder carcinoma: initial results. Eur Radiol 17: 201–204

Matsuoka A, Minato M, Harada M et al (2008) Comparison of 3.0-and 1.5-tesla diffusion-weighted imaging in the visibility of breast cancer. Radiat Med 26: 15–20

Mazaheri Y, Shukla-Dave A, Hricak H et al (2008) Prostate cancer: identification with combined diffusion-weighted MR imaging and 3D 1H MR spectroscopic imaging–correlation with pathologic findings. Radiology 246: 480–488

McVeigh PZ, Syed AM, Milosevic M et al (2008) Diffusion-weighted MRI in cervical cancer. Eur Radiol 18: 1058–1064

Morgan A, Kyriazi S, Ashley SE et al (2007) Evaluation of the potential of diffusion-weighted imaging in prostate cancer detection. Acta Radiol 48: 695–703

Naganawa S, Kawai H, Fukatsu H et al (2005) Diffusion-weighted imaging of the liver: technical challenges and prospects for the future. Magn Reson Med Sci 4: 175–186

Nagata S, Nishimura H, Uchida M et al (2008) Diffusion-weighted imaging of soft tissue tumors: usefulness of the apparent diffusion coefficient for differential diagnosis. Radiat Med 26: 287–295

Nasu K, Kuroki Y, Nawano S et al (2006) Hepatic metastases: diffusion-weighted sensitivity-encoding versus SPIO-enhanced MR imaging. Radiology 239: 122–130

Nomori H, Mori T, Ikeda K et al (2008) Diffusion-weighted magnetic resonance imaging can be used in place of positron emission tomography for N staging of non-small cell lung cancer with fewer false-positive results. J Thorac Cardiovasc Surg 135: 816–822

Ono K, Ochiai R, Yoshida T et al (2009) Comparison of diffusion-weighted MRI and 2-[fluorine-18]-fluoro-2-deoxy-D-glucose positron emission tomography (FDG-PET) for detecting primary colorectal cancer and regional lymph node metastases. J Magn Reson Imaging 29: 336–340

Parikh T, Drew SJ, Lee VS et al (2008) Focal liver lesion detection and characterization with diffusion-weighted MR imaging: comparison with standard breath-hold T2-weighted imaging. Radiology 246: 812–822

Park BK, Lee HM, Kim CK et al (2008) Lesion localization in patients with a previous negative transrectal ultrasound biopsy and persistently elevated prostate specific antigen level using diffusion-weighted imaging at three Tesla before rebiopsy. Invest Radiol 43: 789–793

Park MJ, Cha ES, Kang BJ et al (2007) The role of diffusion-weighted imaging and the apparent diffusion coefficient (ADC) values for breast tumors. Korean J Radiol 8: 390–396

Qi LP, Zhang XP, Tang L et al (2009) Using diffusion-weighted MR imaging for tumor detection in the collapsed lung: a preliminary study. Eur Radiol 19: 333–341

Razek AA, Megahed AS, Denewer A et al (2008) Role of diffusion-weighted magnetic resonance imaging in differentiation between the viable and necrotic parts of head and neck tumors. Acta Radiol 49: 364–370

Rubesova E, Grell AS, De Maertelaer V et al (2006) Quantitative diffusion imaging in breast cancer: a clinical prospective study. J Magn Reson Imaging 24: 319–324

Sakurada A, Takahara T, Kwee TC et al (2009) Diagnostic performance of diffusion-weighted magnetic resonance imaging in esophageal cancer. Eur Radiol (online)

Shinya S, Sasaki T, Nakagawa Y et al (2007) The usefulness of diffusion-weighted imaging (DWI) for the detection of gastric cancer. Hepatogastroenterology 54: 1378–1381

Shinya S, Sasaki T, Nakagawa Y et al (2008) Usefulness of diffusion-weighted imaging (DWI) for the detection of pancreatic cancer: 4 case reports. Hepatogastroenterology 55: 282–285

Stadlbauer A, Bernt R, Gruber S et al (2009) Diffusion-weighted MR imaging with background body signal suppression (DWIBS) for the diagnosis of malignant and benign breast lesions. Eur Radiol (online)

Takeuchi M, Matsuzaki K, Kubo H et al (2008) High-b-value diffusion-weighted magnetic resonance imaging of pancreatic cancer and mass-forming chronic pancreatitis: preliminary results. Acta Radiol 49: 383–386

Takeuchi M, Sasaki S, Ito M et al (2009) Urinary bladder cancer: diffusion-weighted MR imaging–accuracy for diagnosing T stage and estimating histologic grade. Radiology 251: 112–121

Tamada T, Sone T, Jo Y et al (2008) Apparent diffusion coefficient values in peripheral and transition zones of the prostate: comparison between normal and malignant prostatic tissues and correlation with histologic grade. J Magn Reson Imaging 28: 720–726

Tamai K, Koyama T, Saga T et al (2007) Diffusion-weighted MR imaging of uterine endometrial cancer. J Magn Reson Imaging 26: 682–687

Taouli B, Thakur RK, Mannelli L et al (2009) Renal lesions: characterization with diffusion-weighted imaging versus contrast-enhanced MR imaging. Radiology 251: 398–407

Thoeny HC, De Keyzer F (2007) Extracranial applications of diffusion-weighted magnetic resonance imaging. Eur Radiol 17: 1385–1393

Thomassin-Naggara I, Darai E, Cuenod CA et al (2009) Contribution of diffusion-weighted MR imaging for predicting benignity of complex adnexal masses. Eur Radiol 19: 1544–1552

Uto T, Takehara Y, Nakamura Y et al (2009) Higher sensitivity and specificity for diffusion-weighted imaging of malignant lung lesions without apparent diffusion coefficient quantification. Radiology 252: 247–254

Vandecaveye V, De Keyzer F, Nuyts S et al (2006) Detection of head and neck squamous cell carcinoma with diffusion weighted mri after (chemo)radiotherapy: correlation between radiologic and histopathologic findings. Int J Radiat Oncol Biol Phys 67: 960–971

Vandecaveye V, De Keyzer F, Vander Poorten V et al (2009) Head and neck squamous cell carcinoma: value of diffusion-weighted MR imaging for nodal staging. Radiology 251: 134–146

Wenkel E, Geppert C, Schulz-Wendtland R et al (2007) Diffusion weighted imaging in breast MRI: comparison of two different pulse sequences. Acad Radiol 14: 1077–1083

Woodhams R, Matsunaga K, Iwabuchi K et al (2005) Diffusion-weighted imaging of malignant breast tumors: the usefulness of apparent diffusion coefficient (ADC) value and ADC map for the detection of malignant breast tumors and evaluation of cancer extension. J Comput Assist Tomogr 29: 644–649

Xu J, Humphrey PA, Kibel AS et al (2009) Magnetic resonance diffusion characteristics of histologically defined prostate cancer in humans. Magn Reson Med 61: 842–850

Xu PJ, Yan FH, Wang JH et al (2009) Added value of breathhold diffusion-weighted MRI in detection of small hepatocellular carcinoma lesions compared with dynamic contrast-enhanced MRI alone using receiver operating characteristic curve analysis. J Magn Reson Imaging 29: 341–349

Yabuuchi H, Matsuo Y, Okafuji T et al (2008) Enhanced mass on contrast-enhanced breast MR imaging: lesion characterization using combination of dynamic contrast-enhanced and diffusion-weighted MR images. J Magn Reson Imaging 28: 1157–1165

Yoshida S, Fujii Y, Yokoyama M et al (2008) Female urethral diverticular abscess clearly depicted by diffusion-weighted magnetic resonance imaging. Int J Urol 15: 460–461

Yoshikawa MI, Ohsumi S, Sugata S et al (2007) Comparison of breast cancer detection by diffusion-weighted magnetic resonance imaging and mammography. Radiat Med 25:218–223

Yoshikawa MI, Ohsumi S, Sugata S et al (2008) Relation between cancer cellularity and apparent diffusion coefficient values using diffusion-weighted magnetic resonance imaging in breast cancer. Radiat Med 26: 222–226

Yoshizako T, Wada A, Hayashi T et al (2008) Usefulness of diffusion-weighted imaging and dynamic contrast-enhanced magnetic resonance imaging in the diagnosis of prostate transition-zone cancer. Acta Radiol 49: 1207–1213

Zbaren P, Weidner S, Thoeny HC (2008) Laryngeal and hypopharyngeal carcinomas after (chemo)radiotherapy: a diagnostic dilemma. Curr Opin Otolaryngol Head Neck Surg 16: 147–153

Zech CJ, Herrmann KA, Dietrich O et al (2008) Black-blood diffusion-weighted EPI acquisition of the liver with parallel imaging: comparison with a standard T2-weighted sequence for detection of focal liver lesions. Invest Radiol 43: 261–266

Zelhof B, Pickles M, Liney G et al (2009) Correlation of diffusion-weighted magnetic resonance data with cellularity in prostate cancer. BJU Int 103: 883–888

Zhang J, Tehrani YM, Wang L et al (2008) Renal masses: characterization with diffusion-weighted MR imaging–a preliminary experience. Radiology 247: 458–464

DW-MRI for Disease Characterization in the Abdomen

Ali Muhi and Tomoaki Ichikawa

CONTENTS

Ali Muhi, MD
Tomoaki Ichikawa, MD, PhD
Department of Radiology, Yamanashi University, Shimokato, Japan

SUMMARY

DW-MRI has been widely applied for the evaluation of abdominal malignancies. In the liver, the use of DW-MRI is increasing, both for lesion detection as well as for lesion characterization. However, the potential for using DW-MRI to characterize tumours of the bile duct, pancreas, kidneys and other abdominal organs continues to evolve. Disease characterization relies on comparing the relative signal attenuation of tissues on images obtained at different b-values and also on the quantitative apparent diffusion coefficient of the tissue of interest. In this chapter, we summarize the application of DW-MRI for the purpose of tumour characterization in the abdomen, enabling the differentiation of benign from malignant disease, and providing novel information which may be of diagnostic or prognostic value.

8.1

Introduction

Abdominal malignancies, such as colorectal, gastric or pancreatic cancer, are important causes of cancer-related deaths worldwide (Acs 2009). Despite advances in the multidisciplinary treatment of cancers, complete surgical removal in the early stages of disease remains the only potential curative treatment for the majority of the abdominal malignancies. Therefore, early detection and characterization of cancers, ideally before the onset of symptoms, are important to decrease cancer mortality. Although improvements in diagnostic technologies, such as multi-detector CT and fast MR imaging techniques, have changed the landscape of oncological imaging, there is still a compelling need for new imaging techniques that will improve disease characterization.

As discussed in the previous chapter, high b-value DW-MR images (e.g. >500 s/mm^2) are valuable for detecting tumours in a variety of anatomical sites in the body. For disease characterization using DW-MRI, tissue evaluation is reliant on the differential attenuation of the signal intensity between pathological and normal tissues on the high b-value images, as well as by applying the quantitative ADC values. In this chapter, we will discuss the use of high b-value DW-MR images and quantitative ADCs to distinguish tumour tissues from non-tumour tissues, and to distinguish between different pathological entities in the abdomen.

8.2
Liver Diseases

Focal liver lesions are common in patients with cancer. As such, accurate characterization of these is important to enable the right management strategy to be adopted. High b-value DW-MRI can help to distinguish solid from cystic focal liver lesions, since the signal arising from cystic lesions is usually attenuated at higher b-values. However, both benign and malignant solid hepatic lesions can demonstrate high signal intensity impeded diffusion on the high b-value images and may be thus indistinguishable on DW-MR images alone. For this reason, quantitative ADC values have been applied to aid lesion characterization. Not surprisingly, it has been found that the ADC values of benign lesions are significantly higher than those of malignant lesions, with variable degrees of overlap between the pathological entities (NAMIMOTO et al. 1997a, b; ICHIKAWA et al. 1998; KIM et al. 1999a, b; YAMADA et al. 1999; CHAN et al. 2001a, b; TAOULI et al. 2003; KOINUMA et al. 2005; BRUEGEL et al. 2008; PARIKH et al. 2008). Hence, when ADC thresholds are applied for tissue characterization, image interpretation is best made with all the available imaging sequences. In addition, since the calculated ADC can vary significantly depending on the choice of b-values, it is best to adopt ADC values and thresholds that were derived using similar imaging techniques and b-values from the reported literature for each prospective application. The application of parallel imaging to the DW-MRI acquisition does not appear to significantly influence the ADC values recorded in the liver (ONER et al. 2006). The ADC values of various liver lesions observed when using EPI DW-MRI are

summarized in Table 8.1. Note that varying threshold ADC values have been applied to distinguish benign from malignant hepatic lesions with varying diagnostic accuracies (sensitivity 74–100%, specificity 77–100%). Using these threshold values, lesions showing an ADC value below this threshold would be considered to be malignant (Table 8.1).

8.2.1
Hepatic Cyst

Simple hepatic cysts are benign developmental lesions that do not communicate with the biliary tree. They are usually discovered incidentally during routine liver examinations. The prevalence is between 2 and 7% and increases with age, with women affected more than men. Hepatic cysts generally are asymptomatic but may produce dull right upper abdominal pain if they are large in size. Rarely, they may present as an acute abdomen pain due to complications such as haemorrhage or rupture. Hepatic cysts can be solitary or multiple, with a size varying from few millimetres to several centimetres.

On low and sometimes high-b-value DW-MRI, simple hepatic cysts show high signal intensity due to T2 shine-through, and thus may mimic a haemangioma or metastasis. However, on high b-value DW-MR imaging (e.g. >750 s/mm^2), cysts are usually isointense compared to the liver parenchyma (Fig. 8.1) owing to the content of serous fluid which shows unimpeded water diffusion. Hepatic cysts, therefore, have higher ADC values compared with haemangiomas and other solid liver lesions (NAMIMOTO et al. 1997a, b; ICHIKAWA et al. 1998; MOTEKI et al. 2002; TAOULI et al. 2003; MOTEKI et al. 2006). In our experience, the ADC value of cyst is usually very high and typically >2.00 × 10^{-3} mm^2/s (e.g. 3.63 × 10^{-3} mm^2/s). However, one of the pitfalls of imaging characterization is cystic or mucinous metastases to the liver, which may mimic the appearances of cysts on the b-value DW-MRI and ADC maps.

8.2.2
Hepatic Abscess

An abscess can be a solitary collection or multiple collections of pus within the liver as a result of infection by bacteria, protozoa or fungi. Pyogenic liver abscess is the most common, which may result from biliary disease (e.g. ascending infection from obstructive biliary

Table 8.1. ADC values of normal liver and focal liver lesions reported in the published literature

	Mean ADC values (in ×10⁻³ mm²/s ± standard deviation) of focal liver lesions						
	(Namimoto et al. 1997a, b)	(Ichikawa et al. 1998)	(Kim et al. 1999a, b)	(Taouli et al. 2003)	(Bruegel et al. 2008)	(Gourtsoyianni et al. 2008)	(Parikh et al. 2008)
DW-MRI technique	Breath-hold	Breath-hold	Breath-hold	Respiratory triggered	Respiratory triggered	Respiratory triggered	Respiratory triggered
b-Values (s/mm²)	30, 1,200	1.6, 16, 55	≤850	0–500	50, 300, 600	0, 50, 500, 1,000	0, 50, 500
Normal liver	0.69 ± 0.31	2.28 ± 1.23	1.02 ± 0.25	1.83	1.24 ± 0.15	1.25–1.31	
Metastases	1.15	2.85 ± 0.59	1.06 ± 0.50	0.94 ± 0.60	1.22 ± 0.31	0.99 ± 0.07	1.50 ± 0.42
HCC	0.99	3.84 ± 0.92	0.97 ± 0.31	1.33 ± 0.13	1.05 ± 0.09	1.38 ± 0.59	1.31 ± 0.33
Cholangio-carcinoma			1.51				
Cyst	3.05		2.91 ± 1.51	3.63 ± 0.56	3.02 ± 0.31	2.55 ± 0.14	2.54 ± 0.67
Haemangioma	1.95	5.39 ± 1.23	2.04 ± 1.01	2.95 ± 0.67	1.92 ± 0.34	1.90 ± 0.19	2.04 ± 0.42
FNH and/or adenoma				1.75 ± 0.46	1.40 ± 0.15		1.49 ± 0.49
Angiomyolipoma			0.77				
Liver abscess							1.64 ± 0.05
ADC cut-off for malignant lesions			1.60	1.50	1.63	1.47	1.60

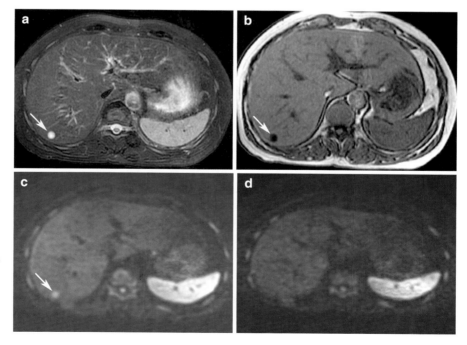

Fig. 8.1. A 63-year-old woman with hepatic cyst (*arrows*). (**a**) Axial fat-saturated T2-weighted imaging shows high signal intensity lesion in the right lobe of liver. (**b**) The lesion shows low signal intensity on opposed-phase T1-weighted imaging. (**c**) The lesion appears hyperintense on $b = 500$ s/mm² DW-MRI but becomes (**d**) isointense to the liver on $b = 1,000$ s/mm² DW-MRI

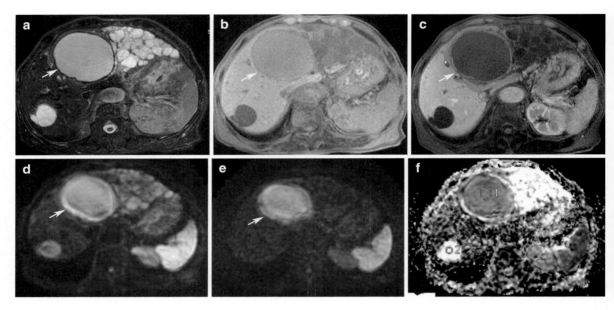

Fig. 8.2. A 76-year-old woman with a hepatic abscess (*arrows*). (**a**) Axial fat-saturated T2-weighted imaging shows a large high signal intensity abscess at the lateral segment of the left lobe (*arrow*) with distal dilatation of the intra-hepatic bile ducts. There is a simple cyst in the posterior right lobe. Note lower signal intensity of the abscess compared with the cyst and dilated ducts. (**b**) Axial fat-saturated T1-weighted imaging demonstrates low signal intensity of the abscess (*arrow*). (**c**) Gadolinium-enhanced T1-weighted imaging during portal venous phase shows a thick rim (*arrow*). (**d**) Axial DW-MRI at $b = 500\,s/mm^2$ and (**e**) axial DW-MRI at $b = 1,000\,s/mm^2$ reveal high signal intensity from the abscess but signal loss from the cyst and dilated intra-hepatic ducts. (**f**) On the ADC map, the abscess shows lower mean ADC value ($1.6 \times 10^{-3}\,mm^2/s$) than the cyst ($3.09 \times 10^{-3}\,mm^2/s$)

tract disease), portal vein infection (e.g. infective embolization or seeding of the portal vein), haematogenous spread from systemic infections, direct extension from adjacent organs (e.g. cholecystitis) or cryptogenic (up to 50% of cases). The most common pyogenic organisms are E. coli, aerobic streptococci, staphylococcus aureus and anaerobic bacteria. Symptoms of liver abscess include pyrexia, malaise, rigours, weight loss, nausea, vomiting and upper abdominal pain.

On high b-value DW-MRI, a hepatic abscess typically shows high signal intensity and low ADC value. This appearance may be explained by the dense viscous content of the abscess and the presence of cellular infiltrates within (Fig. 8.2). In one study comparing the DW-MRI appearances of hepatic abscess and cystic or necrotic tumours, it was found that abscesses showed hyperintensity on DW-MR images and low ADC values. By contrast, the cystic or necrotic portions of tumours showed hypointensity on the DW-MR b-value image and high ADC values (CHAN et al. 2001a, b). The mean ADC value was significantly lower in hepatic abscesses compared with cystic or necrotic tumours: $0.67 \pm 0.35 \times 10^{-3}\,mm^2/s$ in hepatic abscess vs. $2.65 \pm 0.49 \times 10^{-3}\,mm^2/s$ in cystic or necrotic tumour (CHAN et al. 2001a, b). It has also been suggested that early hepatic abscesses may have higher ADC values than mature hepatic abscesses (HOLZAPFEL et al. 2007). Hepatic abscesses can mimic the appearances of tumours on DW-MRI since there is overlap of their imaging appearances and ADC values. However, the clinical presentations of these conditions are often very dissimilar, which is helpful for distinguishing the two entities.

8.2.3
Hepatic Haemangioma

Haemangiomas are the most common benign tumours of the liver. They are of mesenchymal origin, composed of multiple vascular channels lined by a single endothelial cell layer and supported by thin fibrous stroma, usually solitary although multiple haemangiomas are not uncommon. The prevalence of haemangiomas ranges from 1 to 20%, and can occur at any age with women being more affected than men. These lesions

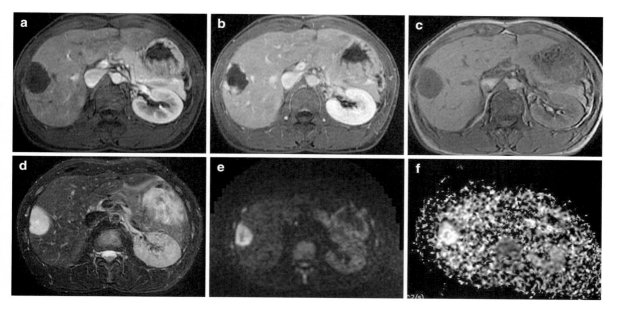

Fig. 8.3. A 41-year-old woman with hepatic haemangioma. (a) Axial contrast-enhanced MR imaging in the arterial and (b) portal venous phase show typical nodular peripheral enhancement of the haemangioma in the right lobe of liver. (c) The lesion is hypointense on unenhanced axial T1-weighted imaging and (d) is hyperintense on axial fat-suppressed T2-weighted imaging. (e) The haemangioma shows hyperintensity on axial DW-MRI imaging at $b = 1,000$ s/mm^2. (f) Note the relatively high ADC value of the haemangioma (2.7×10^{-3} mm^2/s)

are usually asymptomatic and discovered incidentally. Patients may rarely develop symptoms related to mass effect and compression of adjacent structures.

Haemangiomas display high signal intensity on low b-values DW-MR images, but usually retain their high signal intensity at high b-value ($b = 1,000$ s/mm^2) DW-MRI (Fig. 8.3). The ADC values of haemangiomas are amongst the highest of solid hepatic lesions, and are usually significantly higher than those of solid malignant tumours but lower than those of cysts (Namimoto et al. 1997a, b; Ichikawa et al. 1998; Moteki et al. 2002; Taouli et al. 2003; Moteki et al. 2006).

Although, some overlap in ADC values exist between hepatic haemangiomas and simple hepatic cysts, hepatic haemangiomas tend to retain high signal intensity on high b-value DW-MRI unlike hepatic cysts. The high ADC values of hepatic haemangiomas help to differentiate them from the most common malignant hepatic neoplasms, i.e. metastases, which show lower ADC values. Goshimai et al. (2009) using two b-values of 0 and 500 s/mm^2, found significantly higher ADC values and lower signal intensity for haemangiomas demonstrating early complete enhancement (2.18×10^{-3} mm^2/s) compared with those that showed peripheral (1.86×10^{-3} mm^2/s) and delayed

(1.71×10^{-3} mm^2/s) enhancement. Early enhancing haemangiomas have homogeneous histological architecture composed of relatively small vascular spaces (Yamashita et al. 1997), which may permit free movement of water molecules and thus show greater signal attenuation at higher b-value.

In a recent study evaluating the role of DW-MRI for characterizing hypervascular lesions in the liver (Vossen et al. 2008), it was found that the ADC value for haemangiomas (2.29×10^{-3} mm^2/s) was significantly higher than those of hepatocellular carcinoma (HCC) (1.55×10^{-3} mm^2/s), focal nodular hyperplasia (FNH) (1.65×10^{-3} mm^2/s) and metastatic neuroendocrine tumours (1.43×10^{-3} mm^2/s). The area under the receiver operating characteristic curve was 0.91 for using ADC to discriminate between haemangiomas (which included atypical lesions) and other hypervascular hepatic lesions.

8.2.4
Focal Nodular Hyperplasia

FNH is a benign tumour-like condition composed of hyperplastic hepatocytes subdivided into nodules by fibrous septa, which may form stellate scars. Vessels are present in the scars and septa, and small bile ductules are present in the lesion. Although the aetiology is unknown, congenital arteriovenous malformation may be responsible for triggering hepatocellular hyperplasia. FNH is the second most common benign tumour of the liver after hepatic haemangioma. They are well circumscribed but non-encapsulated. The tumour is usually solitary, subcapsular and smaller than 5 cm in most cases. The peak incidence is in the third to fourth decade and is more prevalent in women than men. Its association with the use of oral contraceptives is controversial. The tumour is usually discovered incidentally during imaging for other indications. Few patients show symptoms related to mass effect.

On high b-value ($b = 1,000 \, s/mm^2$) DW-MR images, FNH usually shows variable degrees of high signal intensity, while the central scar and septa, if present, usually appear of low signal intensity. Although, there is an increase in the size of hepatocytes in FNH (i.e. increase in the intracelluar space) compared to the normal hepatocyte, the increased amount of intracellular organelles and the well-developed reticulin framework supporting the cells may play a role in the impeded diffusion and increased signal intensity on DW-MR images (Fig. 8.4). The ADC value of FNH overlaps with those of malignant lesions, although many of these lesions show an ADC value which is similar or higher than normal liver parenchyma.

8.2.5
Hepatocellular Carcinoma

HCC is the most common primary malignant liver tumour accounting for 80–90% of all primary liver cancers, and is the second most common hepatic malignancy in children after hepatoblastoma. The incidence is high in certain areas of the world such as sub-Saharan Africa, Southeast Asia, Japan, Greece and Italy (5.5–20%) due to the high prevalence of hepatitis B and C infections. HCC is more frequent in men than women. The age at diagnosis varies widely according to the geographical distribution: in areas of high incidence the disease tends to affect younger populations (fourth to sixth decades), while in areas of low incidence the disease mainly affects elderly patients in their sixth to seventh decade.

The causes of HCC include: (1) chronic hepatitis C infection, (2) chronic hepatitis B infection, (3) cirrhosis, (4) alcohol, (5) carcinogens (alftatoxin, steroids, thorotrast, anabolic androgenes), and (6) metabolic diseases (haemochromatosis, alfa-1-anti-trypsin deficiency, hereditary tyrosinemia). The symptoms are insidious at onset and include malaise, fever and abdominal pain. Although jaundice is rare, the liver function test may be deranged with an elevated, alpha-fetoprotein level. Paraneoplastic syndromes may occur, including erythrocytosis, hypercalcaemia, hypoglycaemia

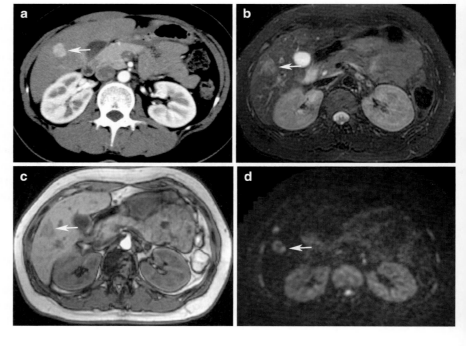

Fig. 8.4. A 29-year-old woman with focal nodular hyperplasia (FNH) (*arrows*). (**a**) Axial contrast-enhanced CT in arterial phase shows FNH in the right lobe of the liver as lesion with near uniform enhancement except for its centre. (**b**) Axial fat-suppressed T2-weighted imaging shows the lesion to be ill-defined of intermediate signal intensity. (**c**) The lesion appears hypointense on axial opposed-phase T1-weighted imaging. (**d**) The lesion is hyperintense on axial DW-MRI at $b = 1,000 \, s/mm^2$ but note low signal intensity of the central scar

and hypercholesterolaemia. By gross pathological description, HCC can be classified into expansive, infiltrative, mixed infiltrative and expansive, as well as diffuse subtypes (NAKASHIMA et al. 1987).

The signal intensity of HCC on DW-MRI is variable and appears to depend on its degree of differentiation. Based on our personal observations, about 90% of moderately to poorly differentiated HCCs show intermediate-high signal intensity on the high b-value (b = 1,000 s/mm²) DW-MR images (Fig. 8.5). While 50% of well-differentiated HCCs have isointense signal intensity on DW-MR images, 50% show intermediate signal intensity (Fig. 8.6). Furthermore, in our experience, hypovascular well-differentiated HCCs appear isointense to the liver parenchyma, but the moderately to poorly differentiated hypovascular HCCs display high signal intensity. These findings suggest that the signal intensity of HCCs on DW-MRI may not be significantly influenced by the tumour vascularity. In our experience, high b-value (b = 1,000 s/mm²) DW-MR images may sometimes be useful to differentiate between HCCs and dysplastic nodules, since dysplastic nodules are usually isointense to the liver parenchyma on DW-MRI.

In our experience, the mean ADCs of moderately ($0.71 \pm 0.26 \times 10^{-3}$ mm²/s) and poorly differentiated HCCs ($0.68 \pm 0.19 \times 10^{-3}$ mm²/s) are significantly lower than that of well-differentiated HCCs ($0.91 \pm 0.25 \times 10^{-3}$ mm²/s) and dysplastic nodules ($1.0 \pm 0.22 \times 10^{-3}$ mm²/s). Based on these observations, it is possible that tumour cellularity may be a determinant of the decreased ADC values in moderately poorly differentiated HCCs (SUGAHARA et al. 1999; LYNG et al. 2000; FILIPPI et al. 2001; GUO et al. 2002). The growth pattern (i.e. histological architecture) may also play a role in accounting for the decreased ADC value (SQUILLACI et al. 2004a, b). Tumours with compact and pseudo-glandular growth have reduced extracellular space leading to restricted diffusion in the extracellular compartment. Furthermore, the increased nuclear/cytoplasmic ratio (GUO et al. 2002) and the large number of intracellular organelles may also contribute to decreased intracellular diffusivity.

High b-value (b = 1,000 s/mm²) DW-MR images can be useful for differentiating between HCCs and benign focal liver lesions such as cysts and cavernous haemangiomas, which have higher ADC values. However, there is, unfortunately, substantial overlap in the signal intensity on DW-MRI between HCCs, metastases and intra-hepatic cholangiocarcinomas (MULLER et al. 1994; NAMIMOTO et al. 1997a, b; ICHIKAWA et al. 1998; KIM et al. 1999a, b; TAOULI et al.

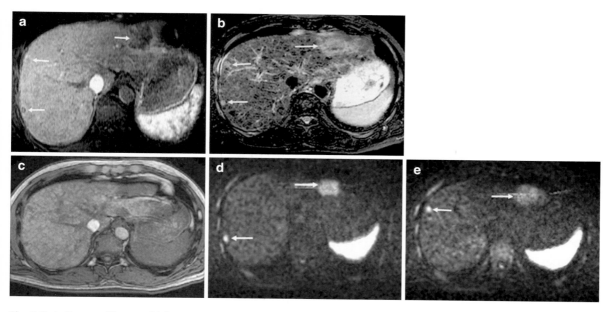

Fig. 8.5. A 45-year-old man with hypovascular poorly differentiated hepatocellular carcinomas (HCC) (*arrows*). (**a**) Axial fat-suppressed T1-weighted arterial phase Gd-EOB-DTPA enhanced imaging shows hypovascular tumours in the liver. (**b**) On unenhanced imaging, these tumours appear hyperintense to liver on axial fat-suppressed T2-weighted imaging and (**c**) hypointense on axial opposed-phase T1-weighted image. (**d**, **e**) The tumours are hyperintense relative to liver parenchyma on axial DW-MR imaging at b = 1,000 s/mm². Note signal loss from the left lobe of the liver due to cardiac motion-related artefact

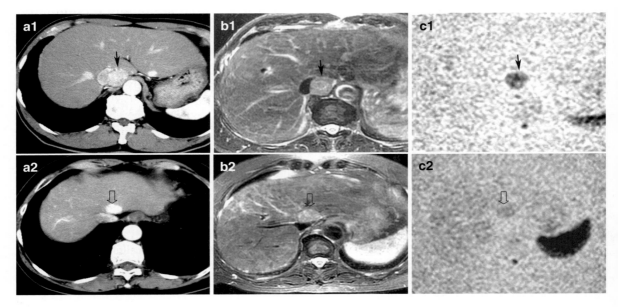

Fig. 8.6. MR imaging in two patients with moderately differentiated HCC (**a1–c1**, *arrows*) and well-differentiated HCC (**a2–c2**, *open arrows*) respectively. (**a1, a2**) Axial arterial dominant phase contrast-enhanced CT shows hypervascular tumours at similar locations in the liver. (**b1, b2**) Both tumours show high signal intensity on axial fat-suppressed T2-weighted imaging. (**c1, c2**) Axial inverted greyscale DW-MRI at $b = 1,000\,s/mm^2$. The signal is relatively suppressed from the well-differentiated tumour (*open arrow*) compared with the moderately differentiated HCC (*arrow*)

2003). TAOULI et al. reported that HCCs had lower ADC values than benign hepatic adenomas and FNHs (TAOULI et al. 2003). SUN et al. found that the ADC measurements of liver lesions could be used to differentiate HCC from hepatic metastases (SUN et al. 2005). However, in clinical practice there is often considerable overlap between HCC and metastasis making it difficult to characterize these based only on DW-MR imaging and ADC maps. For this reason, it is important to use DW-MRI in combination with conventional unenhanced and contrast-enhanced MR imaging for the best diagnosis to be made.

8.2.6
Liver Metastases

Metastases are the most common malignant tumours of the liver. The liver is the second most commonly involved organ by metastatic disease after lymph nodes. The liver may be the site of metastases from virtually any primary malignant neoplasm, but the most common primary sites include the colon, stomach, pancreas, breast and lung. Liver metastases are usually multiple involving both lobes of the liver and only 2% are solitary. Metastases vary in size, consistency, growth

pattern and vascularity. Of patients who die as a result of metastatic liver disease, only about half will have clinical signs or symptoms (HAAGA et al. 2003); the liver function tests tend to be insensitive and non-specific.

On high b-value ($b = 1,000\,s/mm^2$) DW-MR images, the non-necrotic component of metastases display high signal intensity and low ADC values, reflecting the cellularity of the solid tumour. The signal intensity of the necrotic component of metastases, however, show hypointensity on high b-value DW-MR images and high ADC values, most likely related to the increase of free water in the necrotic component (Fig. 8.7). As discussed in the previous chapter, high b-value DW-MRI shows high sensitivities and specificities for the detection of liver metastases (MOTEKI et al. 2004; NASU et al. 2006; KOH et al. 2008; PARIKH et al. 2008). Although, some metastases (e.g. from neuroendocrine tumours) appear to have the lowest ADC values among the hepatic malignant tumours, there is considerable overlap between pathological entities. Liver metastases that show a significant degree of central necrosis (e.g. colorectal liver metastases) frequently return higher mean ADC values than the normal liver (KOH et al. 2006). Interestingly, CHAN et al. reported that the mean ADC values for necrotic tumours were higher

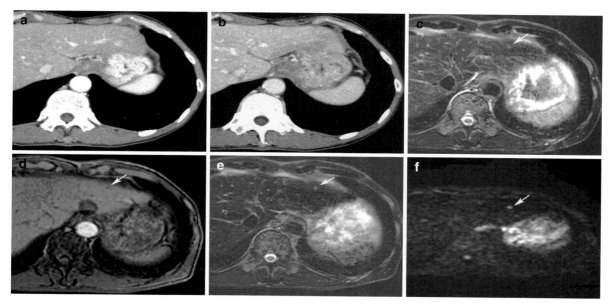

Fig. 8.7. A 58-year-old man with a small metastasis in the liver from colon cancer. (**a**) Axial CT imaging in the arterial phase and (**b**) portal venous phase of contrast enhancement. No tumour could be identified on the CT images. (**c**) Axial fat-suppressed T2-weighted imaging shows tiny hyperintense focus in the left lobe of liver (*arrow*). (**d**) The area shows subtle low signal intensity on gadolinium enhanced T1-weighted imaging (*arrow*). (**e**) The metastasis is seen as high signal intensity area (*arrow*) on axial SPIO-enhanced T2-weighted imaging. (**f**) Note the high lesion-to-background signal of the metastasis (*arrow*) on axial DW-MR imaging before SPIO at $b = 1,000\,\text{s/mm}^2$

than those of hepatic abscesses (CHAN et al. 2001a, b). SUN et al. suggested that measuring the ADC value of a lesion compared with the liver may help to differentiate HCC from hepatic metastasis because HCC usually occurs in the setting of chronic hepatitis or cirrhosis while metastases often occur in the non-cirrhotic liver (SUN et al. 2005). However, in clinical practice, it can be quite difficult to distinguish between metastases and other malignant hepatic tumours based on the signal intensity on high b-value DW-MR images or even with sophisticated calculations of the ADC value. It is thus important to interpret DW-MR images in conjunction with other MR imaging findings.

8.3

Biliary Tree and Gallbladder Tumours

8.3.1
Intra-hepatic Cholangiocarcinoma

Intra-hepatic cholangiocarcinoma is the second most common primary hepatic tumour after HCC. Intra-hepatic cholangiocarcinoma is an adenocarcinoma that originates in the small intra-hepatic bile ducts, and represents approximately 10% of all cholangiocarcinomas. These tumours are usually large, firm masses with prominent desmoplastic reaction. Mucin and calcifications are also often present. The tumour spreads by extending along intra-hepatic bile ducts or by direct infiltration into adjacent liver parenchyma. Cholangiocarcinoma usually presents in the sixth to seventh decade of life. Men are slightly more affected than women. Clinical features include abdominal pain, palpable mass, weight loss, and painless jaundice.

On DW-MRI, cholangiocarcinomas have high signal intensity on high b-value ($b = 1,000\,\text{s/mm}^2$) images and usually return low ADC values (Fig. 8.8), probably related to their high cellular density and complex histological architecture. In our opinion, it is difficult to distinguish between intra-hepatic cholangiocarcinoma, HCC and metastases based only on the ADC values and the signal intensity of the lesion on high b-value DW-MRI. Additional radiological features such as the pattern of contrast enhancement may also be helpful. However, intra-hepatic cholangiocarcinomas exhibit different enhancement patterns, depending on the histological subtype and the degree and distribution of fibrosis within the tumour (MURAKAMI et al. 1995).

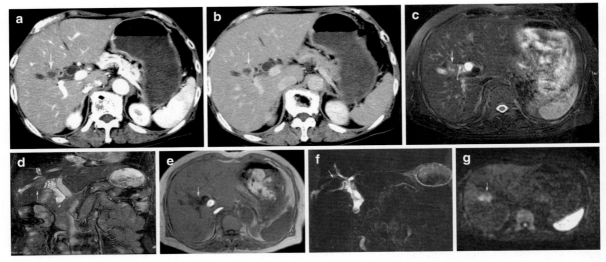

Fig. 8.8. A 76-year-old woman with an intra-hepatic cholangiocarcinoma (*open arrows*). Axial CT imaging in the (**a**) arterial dominant phase and (**b**) portal venous phase of contrast enhancement shows a heterogeneous, hypodense and ill-defined tumour in the right lobe of liver. (**c**) On MR imaging, the mass shows intermediate to high signal intensity on axial fat-suppressed T2-weighted imaging and (**d**) coronal fast T2-weighted imaging. (**e**) The tumour is hypointense on the axial T1-weighted imaging. (**f**) On coronal breath-hold single-shot fast spin-echo T2-weighted MR cholangiography, there is narrowing of the right segmental intra-hepatic bile duct (*arrow*). (**g**) Axial DW-MRI at $b = 1,000 \, \text{s/mm}^2$ shows tumour to be hyperintense to the liver parenchyma

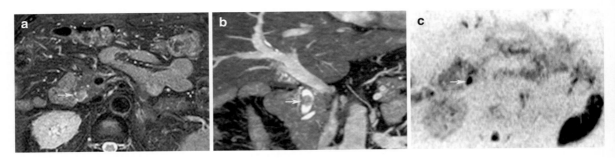

Fig. 8.9. A 67-year-old man with cholangiocarcinoma arising from the common bile duct (*arrows*). (**a**) Axial fat-suppressed fast spin-echo T2-weighted imaging shows intraductal polypoidal mass of intermediate signal intensity. (**b**) Coronal fat-suppressed T2-weighted image shows the tumour within the common bile duct. (**c**) Axial inverted *grey scale* DW-MRI at $b = 1,000 \, \text{s/mm}^2$ demonstrates tumour as focus of reduced signal intensity

8.3.2
Extra-hepatic Cholangiocarcinoma

Cancer of the bile ducts occurs most commonly at the distal common bile duct. Bile duct cancers occur less frequently at the ductal confluence, proximal duct or mid-duct. The peak age of incidence is in the sixth to seventh decade and occurs more frequently in men. The most common pattern of tumour growth is focal infiltration of the ductal wall resulting in a focal stricture. Other tumour patterns include intraluminal polypoidal mass and diffuse sclerosis. The clinical presentation includes obstructive jaundice, cholangitis, abdominal pain and weight loss.

In our experience, on high b-value ($b = 1,000 \, \text{s/mm}^2$) DW-MRI, the polypoidal or papillary type of bile duct cancer can show high signal intensity and low ADC values (Fig. 8.9). High b-value DW-MRI may thus help towards evaluating the patient with biliary obstruction and jaundice. High b-value DW-MRI may prove to be useful in differentiating between malignant obstruction (e.g. due to bile duct cancer or

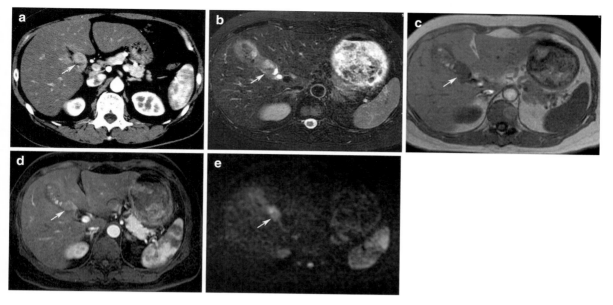

Fig. 8.10. A 53-year-old female patient with gallbladder carcinoma (*arrows*) and adenomyomatosis. (**a**) Arterial phase contrast-enhanced CT shows heterogeneous enhancing tumour at the gallbladder neck. (**b**) The tumour appears mildly hyperintense on the axial fat-suppressed T2-weighted imaging. (**c**) Axial in-phase T1-weighted imaging demonstrates low signal intensity of the tumour. The body and fundus of the gallbladder show high signal intensity (adenomyomatosis). (**d**) Gd-EOB-DTPA enhanced T1-weighted imaging during the arterial dominant phase. The tumour exhibits hypervascularity relative to the adenomyomatosis. (**e**) The tumour is hyperintense on axial DW-MRI at $b = 1,000\,\text{s/mm}^2$ while the adenomyomatosis shows subtle high signal intensity

pancreatic cancer) and benign obstruction (e.g. due to choledocholithiasis or benign stricture) and in defining the level of biliary obstruction.

8.3.3
Gallbladder Carcinoma

Gallbladder cancer is the fifth most common gastrointestinal malignancy. One hypothesis suggests chronic irritation of the gallbladder wall by gallstones as a possible aetiology and thus the vast majority of gallbladder cancers are associated with gallstones with the prevalence of disease higher in women than in men. The peak age of incidence is in the sixth to seventh decade. There is also association with porcelain gallbladder, inflammatory bowel disease and chronic cholecystitis. Gallbladder carcinoma can appear as focal or diffuse wall thickening, intra-luminal polypoidal mass or a mass that replaces the gallbladder. The clinical features include abdominal pain, malaise, vomiting, weight loss and obstructive jaundice. Up to 80% of patients present with advanced disease at the time of diagnosis and the prognosis is poor.

On high b-value ($b = 1,000\,\text{s/mm}^2$) DW-MR imaging, gallbladder carcinoma demonstrates non-specific high signal intensity and low ADC (Fig. 8.10). In clinical practice, high b-value may prove to be of value in differentiating gallbladder carcinoma from adenomyomatosis and other benign gallbladder processes.

8.4
Pancreatic Tumours

The majority (80%) of pancreatic neoplasms are ductal adenocarcinomas. Cystic tumours such as mucinous cystic tumour and serous cystic tumours are uncommon, accounting for only 5% of all pancreatic tumours.

8.4.1
Solid Pancreatic Tumours

8.4.1.1
Pancreatic Ductal Adenocarcinoma

Pancreatic ductal adenocarcinomas are the most common pancreatic malignant tumours, accounting for about 80% of all pancreatic cancers. Pancreatic ductal adenocarcinoma is the fourth leading cause of cancer-related death after lung, prostate/breast and colon cancer (Acs 2009). In terms of sites of disease, approximately 62% involve the pancreatic head while 26% occur in the pancreatic body, and 12% involve the pancreatic tail. The disease tends to affect elderly people and is more common in men than in women. The aetiology of the disease is uncertain but factors such as smoking, alcohol, diabetes, high-fat diet, hereditary pancreatitis and industrial exposures are implicated.

Clinical symptoms and signs develop late and the presentation depends on the site of the tumour. Tumours in the body and tail produce symptoms late in the course of disease, such as abdominal pain radiating to the back. Pancreatic adenocarcinoma arising in the pancreatic head is the most frequent malignant cause of obstructive jaundice. Severe pain almost invariably indicates the spread of tumour to the perivascular neural plexus. Weight loss and anorexia are common. The disease usually presents late with retroperitoneal invasion, metastases to the regional or distal lymph nodes, liver, lungs and bone. Only 14% of tumours are confined to the pancreas at the time of diagnosis.

Despite advances in imaging, the treatment and prognosis of the disease have not significantly changed due to the frequent late presentation of disease. Hence, early diagnosis and accurate staging of pancreatic cancer is crucial in improving outcomes. Even though recent advances in imaging techniques have contributed to the accurate diagnosis of pancreatic cancer, the condition is still often diagnosed late. Differentiation from pancreatitis and benign tumours is also important since the prognosis of pancreatic adenocarcinoma is very poor and is curable only by surgical resection.

High b-value ($b = 1,000$ s/mm^2) DW-MRI has evolved as an additional imaging modality, which may be helpful in distinguishing pancreatic tumour from the normal glandular tissue. Ichikawa et al. (2007) reported a sensitivity and specificity of 92 and 96% for the detection of pancreatic ducal adenocarcinoma using high b-value DW-MRI. DW-MRI can be performed as an adjunct to a conventional MR imaging study. DW-MRI has the potential to become a technique for screening patients with symptoms suggestive of pancreatic adenocarcinoma. If successful, this technique may be extended to evaluate patients who have hereditary predisposition for pancreatic cancer such as patients with hereditary pancreatitis, multiple endocrine neoplasia (MEN) type 1, and Gardner's syndrome.

Although CT and MR imaging are advantageous in providing precise anatomical delineation of pancreatic tumours, they are less specific in differentiating malignant and benign lesions (Neff et al. 1984; Lammer et al. 1985; Ho et al. 1996). Kim et al. found that intra-pancreatic fibrotic changes associated with chronic pancreatitis, as visualized on contrast-enhanced CT and MR imaging, could not be distinguished from pancreatic adenocarcinoma (Kim et al. 2001). The confirmatory feature to distinguish between the two entities was the presence of local or distant tumour spread. Despite reports describing the usefulness of high b-value DW-MRI with its high sensitivity and specificity in detecting pancreatic carcinoma, differentiation from inflammatory lesions remains challenging (Ichikawa et al. 2007; Shinya et al. 2008).

The ADC value of the normal pancreas varies within the reported literature (Ichikawa et al. 1999; Yamada et al. 1999; Chow et al. 2003; Yoshikawa et al. 2006). This variation could be accounted for by age-related changes such as glandular atrophy, fatty replacement and fibrosis (Yoshikawa et al. 2006). Clearly, the choice of b-values used for the calculation of the ADC would also influence the results. Regional variations in ADC value in the pancreas has also been reported, with the values being lower in the pancreatic tail compared with the head or the body, although the basis for this difference is uncertain (Yoshikawa et al. 2006).

There is also substantial variation in the reported value of pancreatic cancers in the literature. In one study performed using b-values of 0 and 400 s/mm^2, the ADC values of pancreatic carcinoma ranged from 0.93 to 2.42×10^{-3} mm^2/s (Niwa et al. 2009). Perhaps not surprisingly, the reported ADC values of pancreatic tumours relative to the pancreas could be influenced by the presence of necrosis or cystic change within the tumour, and also to the degree of glandular and fatty involution in the remnant pancreas. While a few studies have reported higher ADC values of pancreatic carcinoma relative to the normal pancreas (Yoshikawa et al. 2006), the majority indicate that pancreatic cancers have lower ADC values than the normal pancreas (Ichikawa et al. 1999; Lee et al. 2008; Muraoka et al. 2008; Takeuchi et al. 2008; Fattahi et al. 2009).

Using DW-MRI with two b-values (0 and 500 s/mm^2), Muraoka et al. (2008) found that the mean ADC value of tumours ($1.27 \pm 0.52 \times 10^{-3}$ mm^2/s) was significantly lower than for non-cancerous tissue ($1.90 \pm 0.41 \times 10^{-3}$ mm^2/s). Interestingly, the authors also found that the mean ADC value was significantly higher in tumours classified pathologically as showing loose fibrosis ($1.88 \pm 0.39 \times 10^{-3}$ mm^2/s) vs. those that were classified as showing dense fibrosis ($1.01 \pm 0.29 \times 10^{-3}$ mm^2/s), with a good correlation between

ADC values and the proportion of collagenous fibres within the tumours.

In our experience, when applying ADC (using b-values of 0, 500 and 1,000 s/mm^2) for the characterization of focal pancreatic mass lesions, we have found the mean ADC value of pancreatic adenocarcinomas ($1.02 \pm 0.17 \times 10^{-3}$ mm^2/s) to be significantly higher than that of the acute mass-forming pancreatitis ($0.81 \pm 0.19 \times 10^{-3}$ mm^2/s). In another study using b-values of 0 and 600 s/mm^2, it was found that the mean ADC value of pancreatic cancer ($1.46 \pm 0.18 \times 10^{-3}$ mm^2/s) was significantly lower than the remaining pancreas ($2.11 \pm 0.32 \times 10^{-3}$ mm^2/s) or mass-forming pancreatitis ($2.09 \pm 0.18 \times 10^{-3}$ mm^2/s), although it was unclear whether the ADC values for the pancreatitis were derived in the acute or chronic phases of inflammation (FATTAHI et al. 2009). In an earlier study, little difference was observed in the ADC values of acute and chronic pancreatitis (YOSHIKAWA et al. 2006). Clearly,

there appears to be significant variations in the ADC values recorded of acute and chronic pancreatitis, and the temporal evolution of the ADC values in inflammation of the pancreas warrants further evaluation.

Despite the reported variations in ADC values of focal pancreatic mass lesions, our experience suggests that it may be possible to distinguish pancreatic adenocarcinomas and acute mass-forming pancreatitis from the mass-forming pancreatitis during the chronic phase by visual assessment of the high b-value DW-MRI, the former often showing high signal intensity on high b-value DW-MRI, whereas the latter displaying slight hyperintensity to isointensity relative to the pancreatic parenchyma (Fig. 8.11). The merits of using visual assessment of high b-value DW-MR images for distinguishing between pancreatic adenocarcinoma and mass-forming pancreatitis has been corroborated by other authors (TAKEUCHI et al. 2008; FATTAHI et al. 2009). Thus, high b-value

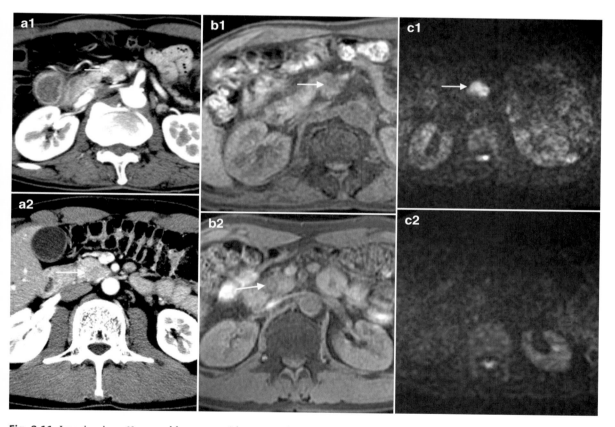

Fig. 8.11. Imaging in a 63-year-old woman with pancreatic adenocarcinoma (**a1–c1**) and a 47-year-old man with mass-forming pancreatitis in chronic phase (**a2-c2**). (**a1, a2**) Axial contrast-enhanced CT in arterial phase shows both tumours and pancreatitis as hypovascular masses (*arrows*). (**b1, b2**) Axial fat-saturated T1-weighted imaging. Pancreatic adenocarci- noma shows low signal intensity relative to pancreatic paren- chyma (**b**, *arrow*), but mass-forming pancreatitis is less well seen (**b2**). (**c1, c2**) Axial DW-MRI at $b = 1,000$ s/mm^2. Pancreatic adenocarcinoma shows hyperintensity relative to the pancreatic parenchyma (**c**, *arrow*), but the mass-forming pancreatitis appears isointense and is not identified

DW-MRI appears to be a promising technique for differentiating between these conditions.

8.4.1.2
Neuroendocrine Tumours

Neuroendocrine tumours of the pancreas, formerly called islet cell tumours, arise from the islets of Langerhans. Neuroendocrine tumours may be functioning or non-functioning, benign or malignant. They include insulinoma which arise from B cell, gastrinoma from P cell, glucagonoma from A cell, somatostatinoma from D1 cells, vipoma (secretes vasoactive intestinal polypeptide) from EC cells and PPoma from PP cells. The clinical symptoms are either related to hormone secretion, to invasion of adjacent structures or distant metastases by malignant tumours. Neuroendocrine tumours can occur in isolation or be associated with MEN syndrome type 1, and they could be single or multiple.

Insulinoma is the most common type of neuroendocrine neoplasms accounting for 70–75% of all tumours. They are usually small (<2 cm), solitary and 90% are benign. The symptoms associated with insulinoma are related to insulin secretion and include Whipple's triad (hypoglycaemia, low fasting-glucose and relief of symptoms by administration of glucose), palpitations, sweating, tremor, headache, confusion and coma. The tumour usually affects patients in their fourth to sixth decade and men are affected less than women. Insulinoma have a predilection for the head of the pancreas.

Gastrinoma accounts for about 20% of neuroendocrine tumours. Unlike insulinoma, most gastrinoma are malignant with up to 40% of patients having metastases at the time of diagnosis. Gastrinoma tends to affect younger individuals in their fourth to fifth decade, with men affected more often than women. Patients present with symptoms related to excessive production of gastrin, which include severe peptic ulcers refractory to traditional treatment and diarrhoea. Gastrinomas tend to be multiple, and may be associated with Type 1 MEN syndrome.

Non-functioning neuroendocrine tumours are the third most common tumour in the pancreas, accounting for 15–45% of all tumours. They present as large masses, usually with evidence of metastases at the time of diagnosis.

The diagnosis of functioning neuroendocrine tumours is usually made clinically. The role of imaging is to determine the location, size and number of tumours. Based on our experience so far, neuroendocrine tumours show high signal intensity on the high b-value DW-MRI (Fig. 8.12), probably related to their cellularity and have a mean ADC value ($0.56 \pm 0.29 \times 10^{-3}$ mm^2/s) which is lower than that of pancreatic ductal adenocarcinoma (Ichikawa et al., unpublished data). Bakir et al reported that DWI is equally sensitive to the conventional MRI for the detection of islet cell tumors, and the mean ADC values of islet cell tumour were significantly higher than that of the normal pancreas (Bakir et al. 2009). Variations in the ADC value of neuroendocrine pancreatic tumours may be related to underlying tissue necrosis or cystic change, perfusion characteristics and choice of b-values. However, it appears that high b-value DW-MRI has the potential to be used for the preoperative localization of functioning neuroendocrine tumours and could be used as an adjunct for the diagnosis of non-functioning neuroendocrine tumours. However, further research into this area is needed.

8.4.2
Cystic Pancreatic Tumours

Cystic pancreatic tumours include pseudocysts, serous cystic tumours, mucinous cystic tumours, intra-ductal papillary mucinous neoplasms, solid and papillary epithelial neoplasms, as well as cystic islet cell tumours. Mucinous cystic tumours are premalignant, while serous cystic tumour and pseudocysts are usually benign. In cystic fluid, molecular diffusion is correlated with the viscosity of the fluid. Hence, characterization of the nature of pancreatic cysts may be possible using DW-MRI.

8.4.2.1
Intra-ductal Papillary Mucinous Neoplasm (IPMN)

Intra-ductal papillary mucinous neoplasms are characterized by excessive secretion of mucin, resulting in progressive ductal dilatation or cyst formation. These tumours have a primarily intra-ductal papillomatous growth pattern and involvement of the pancreatic duct may take one of three forms: segmental involvement of the main pancreatic duct, diffuse involvement of the main pancreatic duct and cystic involvement of a branch duct. IPMN tends to affect elderly people in the sixth and seventh decade, and both men and women are equally affected. The clinical symptoms include recurrent episodes of pancreatitis, dull abdominal pain, pancreatic insufficiency and not

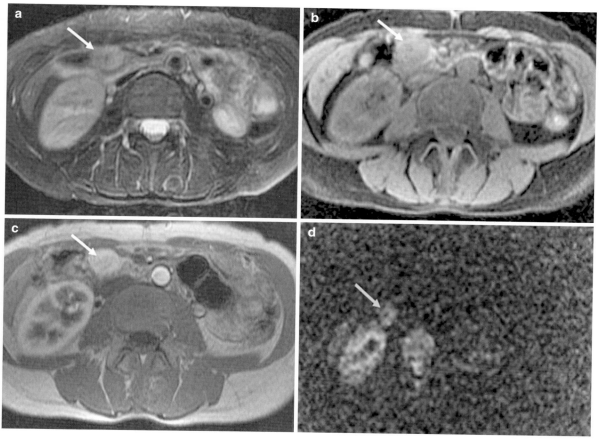

Fig. 8.12. A 38-year-old woman with neuroendocrine tumour of the pancreas (*arrows*). (**a**) Axial fat-suppressed T2-weighted imaging shows heterogeneous intermediate signal-intensity mass at the pancreatic head. (**b**) The mass appears isointense on fat-suppressed T1-weighted imaging. (**c**) The tumour shows avid enhancement on the axial arterial phase gadolinium contrast-enhanced fat-suppressed T1-weighted imaging. (**d**) The tumour is hyperintense on axial DW-MRI at $b = 1,000\,\text{s/mm}^2$

unusually, the disease may be discovered incidentally during imaging for other abdominal conditions. As IPMN is a pre-malignant condition, accurate pre-operative diagnosis is important because the disease has excellent prognosis after surgical treatment.

Yamashita et al. has reported that IPMN shows high signal intensity on DW-MRI, and the ADC (2.7×10^{-3} $\pm\ 0.9 \times 10^{-3}\,\text{mm}^2/\text{s}$) is lower than that of serous fluid ($5.8 \pm 2.0 \times 10^{-3}\,\text{mm}^2/\text{s}$) (YAMASHITA et al. 1998). The high signal intensity reported by Yamashita et al. may be related to the use of relatively low b-values (30 and 300 s/mm²) that were used in the study. From our own unpublished data from a series of 15 patients with IPMNs, all tumours displayed isointensity-hypointensity relative to the pancreatic parenchyma at a high b-value of 1,000 s/mm² and returned a mean ADC value of ($2.9 \pm 0.36 \times 10^{-3}\,\text{mm}^2/\text{s}$) (Fig. 8.13). Furthermore, the high b-value DW-MRI proved useful

in detecting the solid component in two tumours, which showed high signal intensity on DW-MRI and returned a low ADC value ($0.7 \pm 0.17 \times 10^{-3}\,\text{mm}^2/\text{s}$) (Fig. 8.14). Thus, the high b-value DW-MRI was helpful in differentiating intra-ductal papillary mucinous component from the solid carcinoma. However, we could not reliably differentiate IPMN from other cystic neoplasm on the basis of the DW-MRI signal intensity and ADC values. Irie et al. (2002) also found ADC values to be unhelpful in distinguishing between mucinous and serous cystic tumours of the pancreas.

8.4.2.2
Mucinous Cystic Neoplasm

Mucinous cystic neoplasms are rare cystic tumours of the pancreas. The tumour is lined by columnar,

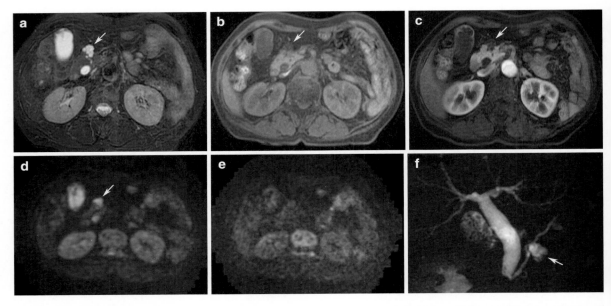

Fig. 8.13. A 70-year-old woman with branch duct type of intra-ductal papillary mucinous neoplasm (IPMN) (*arrow*). (**a**) Axial fat-suppressed T2-weighted imaging shows high signal intensity lobulated cystic mass at the pancreatic head, which appears (**b**) hypointense on the axial fat-suppressed T1-weighted imaging. (**c**) Axial gadolinium contrast-enhanced fat-suppressed T1-weighted imaging shows no significant en-hancing component. (**d**) On axial DW-MRI at $b = 500\,s/mm^2$, the tumour is hyperintense to the pancreatic parenchyma. (**e**) However, on axial DW-MRI at $b = 1,000\,s/mm^2$, the tumour becomes isointense to the surrounding pancreas. (**f**) Maximum intensity projection of T2-weighted MR cholangiopancreaticography shows tumour mass in communication with the main pancreatic duct

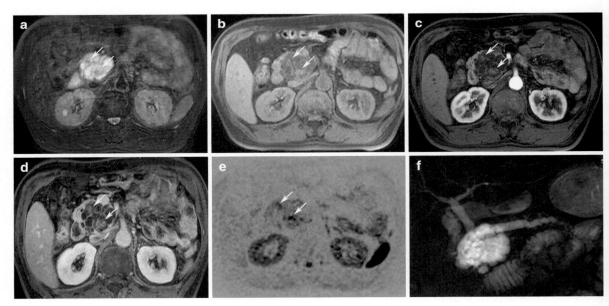

Fig. 8.14. A 59-year-old man with intra-ductal papillary mucinous carcinoma. (**a**) Axial T2-weighted imaging shows lobulated high signal intensity mass at the pancreatic head with two intermediate signal intensity mural nodules (*arrows*). (**b**) Axial fat-suppressed T1-weighted imaging demonstrates the mass as area of low signal intensity with mural nodules (*arrows*) of intermediate signal intensity. (**c**) Axial arterial phase and (**d**) delayed phase gadolinium contrast-enhanced fat-suppressed T1-weighted imaging shows enhancement of mural nodules and thick septal enhancement. (**e**) Axial DW-MRI at $b = 1,000\,s/mm^2$ shows mural nodules of high signal intensity relative to the cystic component of the tumour. (**f**) Coronal single-shot T2-weighted imaging demonstrates communication of the mass with the main pancreatic duct

mucin-producing epithelium. Mucinous cystic neoplasms may be unilocular or mutilocular. Secondary cysts along the internal wall are common. Solid papillary excrescences sometimes protrude from the wall into the interior of these tumours. Mucinous cystic neoplasms are pre-malignant or malignant tumours. The tumour tends to affect young patients in their fourth to fifth decade and is more common in women. The clinical symptoms are non-specific and include epigastric pain, which may radiate to the back, anorexia, weakness and weight loss.

On high b-value ($b = 1{,}000\,\text{s/mm}^2$) DW-MRI, mucinous cystic tumours display isointensity to intermediate signal intensity, which may be related to the higher viscosity of the mucin content of the tumour. We found mucinous cystic tumours to have lower ADC values than serous fluid and cerebrospinal fluid ($2.4 \pm 0.28 \times 10^{-3}\,\text{mm}^2/\text{s}$) (Fig. 8.15). As with IPMN,

high b-value DW-MRI may help to demonstrate the solid component of the tumours as high signal intensity foci on DW-MRI and lower ADC values. Due to their malignant potential all cystic mucinous tumours should always be surgically resected where possible.

8.4.2.3
Serous Cystadenoma

Serous cystadenoma are also called microcystic cystadenoma. The condition is more common in elderly patients in the sixth to seventh decade. Men and women are equally affected. Clinical symptoms are variable and include non-specific abdominal pain or weight loss, more commonly as an incidental finding. Typical serous cystadenomas are composed of multiple small cysts which do not contain mucin. The cysts vary in size

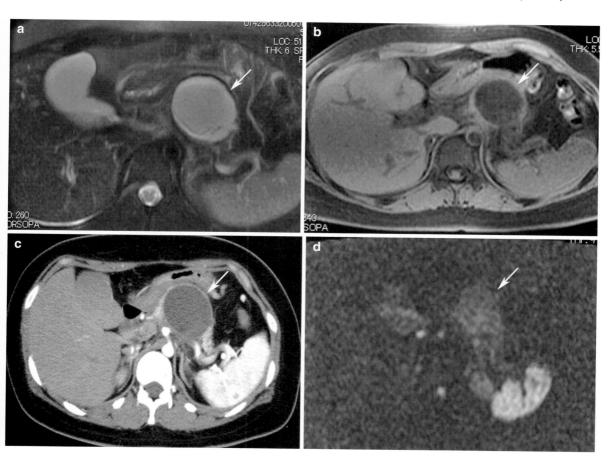

Fig. 8.15. A 22-year-old woman with mucinous cystic tumour (*arrows*) in the distal body of pancreas. (**a**) Axial fat-suppressed T2-weighted imaging shows ovoid high signal intensity cystic tumour in the pancreatic body. (**b**) Axial fat-suppressed T1-weighted imaging demonstrates low signal intensity of the tumour relative to the pancreatic parenchyma. (**c**) Axial arterial phase contrast-enhanced CT shows cystic tumour with no appreciable enhancement or solid component. (**d**) Axial DW-MRI at $b = 1{,}000\,\text{s/mm}^2$ shows tumour to be slightly hyperintense to the pancreatic parenchyma

from 0.2 to 2.0 cm and the size of the tumours ranges from 1.4 to 27 cm, with a mean diameter of 10.8 cm and occur most commonly at the head of pancreas.

On high b-value (b = 1,000 s/mm^2) DW-MRI, a serous cystadenoma is typically isointense to the pancreatic parenchyma due to the relatively free diffusion of water protons in the serous fluid. Yamashita et al. reported a mean ADC value of ($5.8 \pm 2.0 \times 10^{-3}$ mm^2/s) (YAMASHITA et al. 1998) in these tumours, but in our experience, serous cystadenoma have a mean ADC value of (2.6×10^{-3} mm^2/s). This discrepancy is probably related to the use of low b-value by Yamashita et al., with contamination by perfusion effects resulting in higher ADC values observed in their series. Asymptomatic serous cystadenomas do not require surgical excision because they are rarely malignant.

8.4.2.4
Solid and Papillary Epithelial Neoplasms

Solid and papillary epithelial neoplasms of the pancreas are rare, non-functioning low-grade malignant tumours. These affect mainly young women. The tumour is usually large with a mean diameter of 10 cm at time of diagnosis, well-encapsulated, and often demonstrates haemorrhage and necrosis. Solid and papillary epithelial neoplasm usually arises from the tail of the pancreas. The tumour could be solid, cystic or partly solid and partly cystic. Solid and papillary epithelial neoplasm is potentially curable by surgical resection.

The solid component of solid and papillary neoplasm has high signal intensity on high b-value DW-MRI, again reflecting the lower diffusivity of the solid component. The cystic component usually shows isointensity to hypointensity reflecting mobility of free water (Fig. 8.16). Based on our unpublished data, we found the mean ADC of the solid component to be $1.3 \pm 0.47 \times 10^{-3}$ mm^2/s, while the mean ADC of the cystic component was $2.6 \pm 0.24 \times 10^{-3}$ mm^2/s.

8.4.2.5
Pseudocyst

A pseudocyst is a fluid collection consisting of necrotic material, proteinaceous debris and enzymatic material that is confined by a fibrous capsule. Most cystic masses of the pancreas encountered in clinical practice are pseudocysts. Pancreatic pseudocysts are not lined by epithelium, are usually unilocular, and can have a thin or a thick wall of uniform thickness. They develop most often as a complication of acute or chronic pancreatitis. Pancreatic pseudocyst may also develop secondary to pancreatic trauma or surgery.

In one study evaluating DW-MRI in cystic lesions of the pancreas, abscesses, hydatid and neoplastic cysts appeared hyperintense on the b = 1,000 s/mm^2 images, whereas most of the simple and pseudocysts were isointense (INAN et al. 2008). In our experience, pseudocysts display isointensity to hypointensity on high b-value DW-MRI and high return ADC values ($3.08 \pm 0.35 \times 10^{-3}$ mm^2/s) (Fig. 8.17), although the ADC value of the cyst fluid was observed to be lower than that of cerebrospinal fluid. This is perhaps to be expected since the necrotic content of pseudocyst may increase its viscosity, thereby limiting water mobility. The reported ADC values of the various focal pancreatic lesions are summarized in Table 8.2.

8.5
Colorectal Carcinoma

In the Western world, colorectal carcinoma is second in incidence after lung cancer in men and breast carcinoma in women. There is association with high-fat low-fibre diet, streptococcus infection, alcohol and tobacco. Familial adenomatous polyposis and hereditary non-polyposis colorectal cancer have an increased risk of colorectal cancer. There is also increase in the incidence of the disease in patients with inflammatory bowel diseases. Approximately 75% of the cases are sporadic with no predisposing factors. The disease tends to affect elderly people with a peak incidence in the seventh decade, with men more frequently affected than women. The symptoms may include rectal bleeding, change in bowel habit, weakness, malaise, weight loss and abdominal or pelvic pain. On high b-value DW images (b = 1,000 s/mm^2) colorectal cancers are usually hyperintense compared with the normal bowel wall and faecal material, which are hypointense (Fig. 8.18) (NASU et al. 2004; ICHIKAWA et al. 2006; SHINYA et al. 2009).

8.6
Renal Tumours

Renal cysts display low signal intensity on the high b-value DW-MR images and higher ADC values than that of renal parenchyma. However, complicated renal

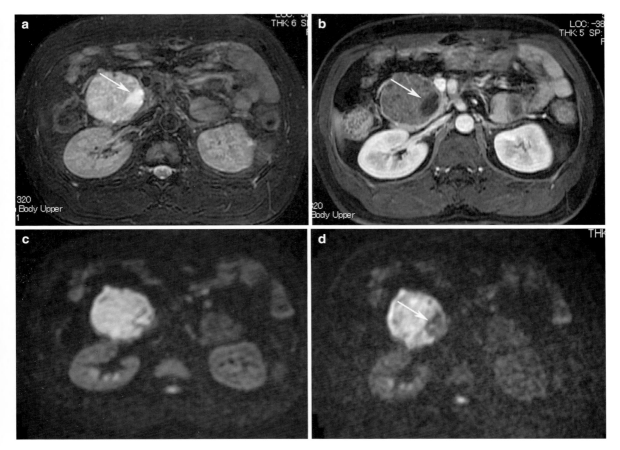

Fig. 8.16. A 35-year-old man with solid and pseudopapillary tumour of the pancreas. (**a**) Axial fat-suppressed T2-weighted imaging shows heterogeneous high signal intensity lesion at the pancreatic head. The medial portion of the tumour shows higher signal intensity relative to the rest of the tumour (*arrow*). (**b**) Axial gadolinium contrast-enhanced fat-suppressed T1-weighted imaging shows heterogeneous tumour enhancement. The medial portion does not enhance after contrast administration suggesting its cystic nature (*arrow*). (**c**) Axial DW-MRI image at $b = 500$ s/mm^2. The tumour is hyperintense relative to the adjacent pancreatic parenchyma. (**d**) Axial DW-MRI at $b = 1,000$ s/mm^2. The tumour is hyperintense but the medial cystic portion now shows signal loss (*arrow*)

cysts tend to show lower ADC values than simple renal cysts, which are probably related to the higher viscosity within the complicated cyst as a result of haemorrhage or proteinaceous content (Fig. 8.19).

In our experience, hydronephrosis and simple renal cysts show overlapping ADC values. However, pyonephrosis return very high signal intensity on high b-value DW-MRI and have measurably lower ADC than hydronephrosis. The thick fluid in the collecting system of the pyonephrotic kidneys has very high viscosity and cellularity, thus resulting in impeded diffusion and the low ADC value. High b-value DW-MRI and ADC can aid differentiation between pyonephrosis and hydronephrosis (Chan et al. 2001a, b; Cova et al. 2004). The application of

DW-MRI for the assessment of renal function and obstructive uropathy is discussed in detail in Chap. 5.

Renal tumours typically show high signal intensity on DW-MRI and low ADC values, which is related to cellular density and complex histological architecture (Cova et al. 2004; Squillaci et al. 2004a, b; Manenti et al. 2008; Zhang et al. 2008; Kim et al. 2009; Taouli et al. 2009). Solid tumour tissues show lower ADCs compared with necrotic or cystic tumour tissue (Kim et al. 2009). Although the ADC of cystic tumour tissue has been reported to be lower than that of uncomplicated renal cysts (Zhang et al. 2008), the experience is not universal (Taouli et al. 2009). Zhang et al. reported that benign cysts and necrotic or cystic tumour areas have significantly different ADCs, even though they

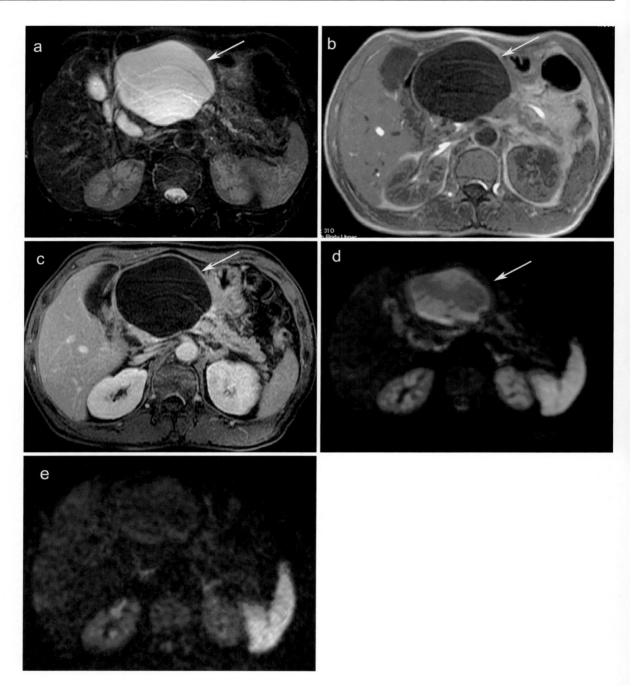

Fig. 8.17. A 58-year-old man with large pseudocyst of the pancreas (*arrow*). (**a**) Axial fat-suppressed T2-weighted imaging shows large cystic mass at the pancreatic body associated with dilatation of the main pancreatic duct. (**b**) The cyst returns low signal intensity on axial T1-weighted imaging (**c**) Axial gadolinium contrast-enhanced fat-suppressed T1-weighted imaging shows no enhancement of the cyst. (**d**) Axial DW-MRI at $b = 500\,\mathrm{s/mm^2}$ shows mild hyperintensity of the cyst. (**e**) However, the cyst becomes isointense to the rest of the pancreas on the axial DW-MRI image at $b = 1{,}000\,\mathrm{s/mm^2}$. Note hypointensity of the main pancreatic duct on both b-value images (**d**) and (**e**)

Table 8.2. Reported ADC values of focal pancreatic lesions

Studies	Mean ADC values (in $\times 10^{-3}$ mm^2/s $\pm$ standard deviations) of focal pancreatic lesions					
	(Ichikawa et al. unpublished)	(Niwa et al. 2009)	(Fattahi et al. 2009)	(Takeuchi et al. 2008)	(Lee et al. 2008)	(Irie et al. 2002)
b-Values (s/mm^2)	0, 500, 1,000	0, 1,000	0, 6,000	0, 800	0, 1,000	30, 300, 900
Pancreatic adenocarcinoma	1.02 ± 0.17	0.72−1.88	1.46 ± 0.18	1.38 ± 0.32+	1.23 ± 0.18	
Acute mass-forming pancreatitis	0.81 ± 0.19					
Chronic mass-forming pancreatitis				1.00 ± 0.18		
Mass-forming pancreatitis (not specified)			2.09 ± 0.18		1.04 ± 0.18	
Neuroendocrine tumour	0.56 ± 0.29				1.30 ± 0.41	
IPMN	2.9 ± 0.36					
Mucinous cystadenoma	2.4 ± 0.28					2.8 ± 1.0
Serous cystadenoma	2.6 ± 0.28					2.9
Solid pseudopapillary tumour (solid component)	1.3 ± 0.47				1.16 ± 0.36	
Solid pseudopapillary tumour cystic component	2.6 ± 0.24					
Pseudocyst	3.08 ± 0.35					2.9 ± 1.2

IPMN intra-ductal papillary mucinous neoplasm

may have a similar appearance on conventional (i.e. T1-weighted, T2-weighted and contrast-enhanced) MR images (Zhang et al. 2008). However, the value of DW-MRI for the characterization of the indeterminate renal cystic lesion needs to be further assessed in larger prospective series.

For solid renal lesions, it has been found that the fat-containing angiomyolipoma have significantly lower ADC values compared with renal cell carcinoma and the normal renal parenchyma (Yoshikawa et al. 2006; Taouli et al. 2009). Among renal cancers, one study performed using a 3 T MR system found no significant difference in the ADC value between different histological tumour subtypes (Manenti et al. 2008). However, in another study performed at 1.5 T, papillary renal cell tumours were reported to have lower ADC values than non-papillary tumours, which could be attributed to the architectural organization of papillary cancers (Taouli et al. 2009). In the same study, it was also found that oncocytomas have significantly

higher ADC values compared with solid renal cell carcinoma (Taouli et al. 2009). It has also been observed that solid renal cell carcinomas which demonstrate high T1 signal intensity have lower ADC values compared with other renal cell carcinomas which show T1 hypointensity (Zhang et al. 2008). Interestingly, although DW-MRI can be applied for the characterization of renal masses, it has been found to be less accurate compared with dynamic contrast-enhanced MR imaging (Taouli et al. 2009).

8.7

DW-MRI for Nodal Characterization in the Abdomen

High b-value DW-MRI is a sensitive technique for detecting lymph nodes throughout the body. In our experience, lymph node metastases can show high

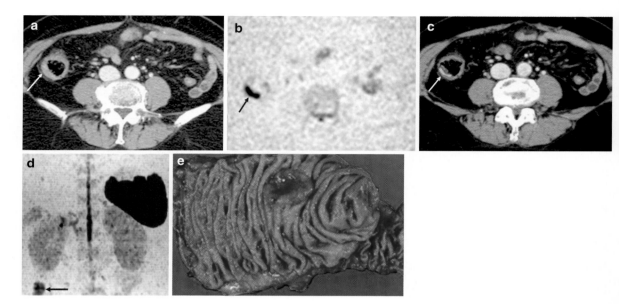

Fig. 8.18. A 55-year-old man with carcinoma of the ascending colon. (**a**) Axial contrast-enhanced CT shows eccentric wall thickening in the ascending colon (*arrow*). (**b**) Axial DW-MRI at $b = 1,000\,\text{s/mm}^2$. The tumour appears darker compared to the rest of colonic wall on the inverted *grey scale* image (*arrow*). (**c**) Axial fusion of $b = 1,000\,\text{s/mm}^2$ and CT image local- izes the tumour in the colonic wall. (**d**) Inverted *grey scale* coronal maximum intensity projection of $b = 1,000\,\text{s/mm}^2$ DW-MRI shows the tumour as a low signal intensity focus (*arrow*). (**e**) Gross pathology of the surgical resection shows the polypoidal morphology of tumour

signal intensity on the high b-value (b=1000,2000 s/mm(2)) image and return a lower mean ADC value 0.63 +/- 0.22 x 10(-3) mm(2)/s than benign lymph nodes 0.83 +/- 0.28 x 10(-3) mm(2)/s (unpublished data). However, the positive predictive value is not as high because both normal and reactive lymph nodes also demonstrate high signal intensity on the high b-value DW-MRI. There is also the practical issue of trying to accurately measure the ADC values of lymph nodes which are normal in size or minimally enlarged. The combination of signal intensity on high b-value DW-MRI, ADC value, and lymph node size may help to improve the positive predictive value/specificity of nodal assessment. It is likely that the use of DW-MRI for nodal characterization will continue to evolve as more experience in this area is accrued. A further discussion of this subject is presented in Chap. 13.

8.8
Peritoneal Metastases

Many primary tumours can metastasize to the peritoneum, omentum and mesentery. The most common are from the ovaries, stomach, pancreas and colon. The mode of spread is by direct invasion, lymphatic permeation, peritoneal seeding or haematogenous. The imaging patterns include mesenteric stranding, nodules, plaques, masses, omental caking and ascites. The clinical features include abdominal pain, abdominal distension and weight loss. High b-value DW-MRI shows high signal intensity for the metastatic peritoneal tumours. Mimics of peritoneal metastasis are rare, and include tuberculous peritonitis, mesenteric panniculitis, leiomyomatosis peritonealis disseminata, extramedullary haematopoiesis, and chronic leak from an ovarian dermoid cyst with granulomatous peritonitis. The DW-MRI appearances of these conditions have not been fully established.

8.9
Conclusions

In this chapter, we have demonstrated how DW-MRI may be applied for lesion characterization in the abdomen. Both qualitative evaluation of high b-value DW-MR images and quantitative evaluation of ADC maps are employed for lesion characterization. The

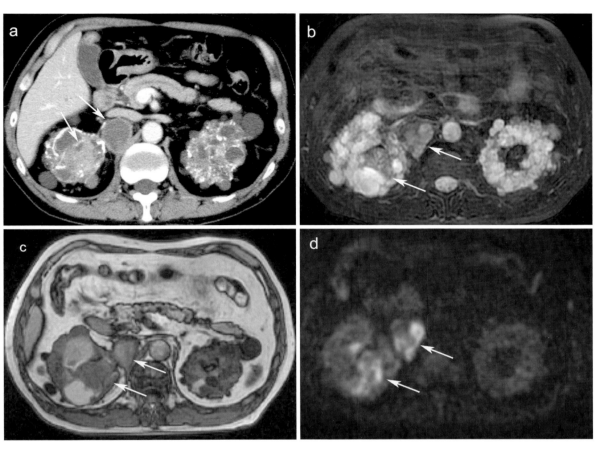

Fig. 8.19. A 58-year-old man with adult polycystic kidney disease and renal cell carcinoma. (**a**) Axial arterial phase contrast-enhanced CT shows a poorly defined hypervascular tumour (*arrow*) at upper pole of right kidney. There is an additional mass behind the inferior vena cava with peripheral rim enhancement in keeping with a lymph node metastasis (*arrowhead*). (**b**) Axial fat-suppressed T2-weighted imaging shows tumour to be lower in signal intensity compared with the renal cysts (*arrow*). The lymph node metastasis is isointense to the renal tumour. (**c**) Axial opposed-phase T1-weighted imaging. The tumour (*arrow*) and lymph node (*arrowhead*) are hypointense. (**d**) Axial DW-MRI at $b = 1,000\,s/mm^2$. The tumour (*arrow*) and nodal metastasis (*arrowhead*) are hyperintense

usage of DW-MRI is now more established in the liver, but experience is building for its application to other abdominal sites. DW-MRI has been found to add value to the evaluation of focal pancreatic and renal disease.

References

ACS (2009) Cancer Facts and Figures 2009, American Cancer Society, Atlanta

Bakir B, Salmaslioglu A et al (2009) Diffusion weighted MR imaging of pancreatic islet cell tumors. Eur J Radiol

Bruegel M, Holzapfel K et al (2008) Characterization of focal liver lesions by ADC measurements using a respiratory triggered diffusion-weighted single-shot echo-planar MR imaging technique. Eur Radiol 18:477–485

Chan JH, Tsui EY et al (2001a) Diffusion-weighted MR imaging of the liver: distinguishing hepatic abscess from cystic or necrotic tumor. Abdom Imaging 26:161–165

Chan JH, Tsui EY et al (2001b) MR diffusion-weighted imaging of kidney: differentiation between hydronephrosis and pyonephrosis. Clin Imaging 25:110–113

Chow LC, Bammer R et al (2003) Single breath-hold diffusion-weighted imaging of the abdomen. J Magn Reson Imaging 18:377–382

Cova M, Squillaci E et al (2004) Diffusion-weighted MRI in the evaluation of renal lesions: preliminary results. Br J Radiol 77:851–857

Fattahi R, Balci NC et al (2009) Pancreatic diffusion-weighted imaging (DWI): comparison between mass-forming focal pancreatitis (FP), pancreatic cancer (PC), and normal pancreas. J Magn Reson Imaging 29:350–356

Filippi CG, Edgar MA et al (2001) Appearance of meningiomas on diffusion-weighted images: correlating diffusion constants with histopathologic findings. AJNR Am J Neuroradiol 22:65–72

Goshima S, Kanematsu M et al (2009) Hepatic hemangioma: correlation of enhancement types with diffusion-weighted MR findings and apparent diffusion coefficients. Eur J Radiol 70:325–330

Gourtsoyianni S, Papanikolaou N et al (2008) Respiratory gated diffusion-weighted imaging of the liver: value of apparent diffusion coefficient measurements in the differentiation between most commonly encountered benign and malignant focal liver lesions. Eur Radiol 18:486–492

Guo AC, Cummings TJ et al (2002) Lymphomas and high-grade astrocytomas: comparison of water diffusibility and histologic characteristics. Radiology 224:177–183

Haaga JR, Lanzieri CF et al (2003) MR imaging of the whole body. Mosby, St.Louis, MO

Ho CL, Dehdashti F et al (1996) FDG-PET evaluation of indeterminate pancreatic masses. J Comput Assist Tomogr 20: 363–369

Holzapfel K, Rummeny E et al (2007) Diffusion-weighted MR imaging of hepatic abscesses: possibility of different apparent diffusion coefficient (ADC)-values in early and mature abscess formation. Abdom Imaging 32:538–539

Ichikawa T, Erturk SM et al (2006) High-B-value diffusion-weighted MRI in colorectal cancer. AJR Am J Roentgenol 187:181–184

Ichikawa T, Erturk SM et al (2007) High-b value diffusion-weighted MRI for detecting pancreatic adenocarcinoma: preliminary results. AJR Am J Roentgenol 188:409–414

Ichikawa T, Haradome H et al (1998) Diffusion-weighted MR imaging with a single-shot echoplanar sequence: detection and characterization of focal hepatic lesions. AJR Am J Roentgenol 170:397–402

Ichikawa T, Haradome H et al (1999) Diffusion-weighted MR imaging with single-shot echo-planar imaging in the upper abdomen: preliminary clinical experience in 61 patients. Abdom Imaging 24:456–461

Inan N, Arslan A et al (2008) Diffusion-weighted imaging in the differential diagnosis of cystic lesions of the pancreas. AJR Am J Roentgenol 191:1115–1121

Irie H, Honda H et al (2002) Measurement of the apparent diffusion coefficient in intraductal mucin-producing tumor of the pancreas by diffusion-weighted echo-planar MR imaging. Abdom Imaging 27:82–87

Kim S, Jain M et al (2009) T1 Hyperintense renal lesions: characterization with diffusion-weighted MR imaging versus contrast-enhanced MR imaging. Radiology 251:796–807

Kim T, Murakami T et al (1999) Diffusion-weighted single-shot echoplanar MR imaging for liver disease. AJR Am J Roentgenol 173:393–398

Kim T, Murakami T et al (2001) Pancreatic mass due to chronic pancreatitis: correlation of CT and MR imaging features with pathologic findings. AJR Am J Roentgenol 177: 367–371

Koh DM, Brown G et al (2008) Detection of colorectal hepatic metastases using MnDPDP MR imaging and diffusion-weighted imaging (DWI) alone and in combination. Eur Radiol 18:903–910

Koh DM, Scurr E et al (2006) Colorectal hepatic metastases: quantitative measurements using single-shot echo-planar diffusion-weighted MR imaging. Eur Radiol 16: 1898–1905

Koinuma M, Ohashi I et al (2005) Apparent diffusion coefficient measurements with diffusion-weighted magnetic reso-nance imaging for evaluation of hepatic fibrosis. J Magn Reson Imaging 22:80–85

Lammer J, Herlinger H et al (1985) Pseudotumorous pancreatitis. Gastrointest Radiol 10:59–67

Lee SS, Byun JH et al (2008) Quantitative analysis of diffusion-weighted magnetic resonance imaging of the pancreas: usefulness in characterizing solid pancreatic masses. J Magn Reson Imaging 28:928–936

Lyng H, Haraldseth O et al (2000) Measurement of cell density and necrotic fraction in human melanoma xenografts by diffusion weighted magnetic resonance imaging. Magn Reson Med 43:828–836

Manenti G, Di Roma M et al (2008) Malignant renal neoplasms: correlation between ADC values and cellularity in diffusion weighted magnetic resonance imaging at 3 T. Radiol Med 113:199–213

Moteki T, Horikoshi H (2006) Evaluation of hepatic lesions and hepatic parenchyma using diffusion-weighted echo-planar MR with three values of gradient b-factor. J Magn Reson Imaging 24:637–645

Moteki T, Horikoshi H et al (2002) Evaluation of hepatic lesions and hepatic parenchyma using diffusion-weighted reordered turboFLASH magnetic resonance images. J Magn Reson Imaging 15:564–572

Moteki T, Sekine T (2004) Echo planar MR imaging of the liver: comparison of images with and without motion probing gradients. J Magn Reson Imaging 19:82–90

Muller MF, Prasad P et al (1994) Abdominal diffusion mapping with use of a whole-body echo-planar system. Radiology 190:475–478

Murakami T, Nakamura H et al (1995) Contrast-enhanced MR imaging of intrahepatic cholangiocarcinoma: pathologic correlation study. J Magn Reson Imaging 5:165–170

Muraoka N, Uematsu H et al (2008) Apparent diffusion coefficient in pancreatic cancer: characterization and histopathological correlations. J Magn Reson Imaging 27: 1302–1308

Nakashima O, Kojiro M (1987) Hepatocellular carcinoma: an atlas of its pathology. Springer, Tokyo

Namimoto T, Yamashita Y et al (1997) Focal liver masses: characterization with diffusion-weighted echo-planar MR imaging. Radiology 204:739–744

Nasu K, Kuroki Y et al (2004) Diffusion-weighted single shot echo planar imaging of colorectal cancer using a sensitivity-encoding technique. Jpn J Clin Oncol 34:620–626

Nasu K, Kuroki Y et al (2006) Hepatic metastases: diffusion-weighted sensitivity-encoding versus SPIO-enhanced MR imaging. Radiology 239:122–130

Neff CC, Simeone JF et al (1984) Inflammatory pancreatic masses. Problems in differentiating focal pancreatitis from carcinoma. Radiology 150:35–38

Niwa T, Ueno M et al (2009) Advanced pancreatic cancer: the use of the apparent diffusion coefficient to predict response to chemotherapy. Br J Radiol 82:28–34

Oner AY, Celik H et al (2006) Single breath-hold diffusion-weighted MRI of the liver with parallel imaging: initial experience. Clin Radiol 61:959–965

Parikh T, Drew SJ et al (2008) Focal liver lesion detection and characterization with diffusion-weighted MR imaging: comparison with standard breath-hold T2-weighted imaging. Radiology 246:812–822

Shinya S, Sasaki T et al (2008) Usefulness of diffusion-weighted imaging (DWI) for the detection of pancreatic cancer: 4 case reports. Hepatogastroenterology 55:282–285

Shinya S, Sasaki T et al (2009) The efficacy of diffusion-weighted imaging for the detection of colorectal cancer. Hepatogastroenterology 56:128–132

Squillaci E, Manenti G et al (2004a) Correlation of diffusion-weighted MR imaging with cellularity of renal tumours. Anticancer Res 24:4175–4179

Squillaci E, Manenti G et al (2004b) Diffusion-weighted MR imaging in the evaluation of renal tumours. J Exp Clin Cancer Res 23:39–45

Sugahara T, Korogi Y et al (1999) Usefulness of diffusion-weighted MRI with echo-planar technique in the evaluation of cellularity in gliomas. J Magn Reson Imaging 9: 53–60

Sun XJ, Quan XY et al (2005) Quantitative evaluation of diffusion-weighted magnetic resonance imaging of focal hepatic lesions. World J Gastroenterol 11:6535–6537

Takeuchi M, Matsuzaki K et al (2008) High-b-value diffusion-weighted magnetic resonance imaging of pancreatic cancer and mass-forming chronic pancreatitis: preliminary results. Acta Radiol 49:383–386

Taouli B, Thakur RK et al (2009) Renal lesions: characterization with diffusion-weighted imaging versus contrast-enhanced MR imaging. Radiology 251:398–407

Taouli B, Vilgrain V et al (2003) Evaluation of liver diffusion isotropy and characterization of focal hepatic lesions with two single-shot echo-planar MR imaging sequences: prospective study in 66 patients. Radiology 226:71–78

Vossen JA, Buijs M et al (2008) Receiver operating characteristic analysis of diffusion-weighted magnetic resonance imaging in differentiating hepatic hemangioma from other hypervascular liver lesions. J Comput Assist Tomogr 32: 750–756

Yamada I, Aung W et al (1999) Diffusion coefficients in abdominal organs and hepatic lesions: evaluation with intravoxel incoherent motion echo-planar MR imaging. Radiology 210: 617–623

Yamashita Y, Namimoto T et al (1998) Mucin-producing tumor of the pancreas: diagnostic value of diffusion-weighted echo-planar MR imaging. Radiology 208:605–609

Yamashita Y, Ogata I et al (1997) Cavernous hemangioma of the liver: pathologic correlation with dynamic CT findings. Radiology 203:121–125

Yoshikawa T, Kawamitsu H et al (2006) ADC measurement of abdominal organs and lesions using parallel imaging technique. AJR Am J Roentgenol 187:1521–1530

Zhang J, Tehrani YM et al (2008) Renal masses: characterization with diffusion-weighted MR imaging–a preliminary experience. Radiology 247:458–464

DW-MRI for Disease Characterization in the Pelvis

9

Masoom A. Haider, Yasaman Amoozadeh, and Kartik S. Jhaveri

CONTENTS

Masoom A. Haider, MD, FRCPC
Yasaman Amoozadeh, MD
Kartik S. Jhaveri, MD
Joint Department of Medical Imaging, University Health Network,
Princess Margaret Hospital, University of Toronto, Toronto, ON
M5G 2M9, Canada

SUMMARY

The tissue diffusivity of pelvic cancers is usually lower than most benign processes and is reflected by a lower ADC value. When performing DW-MRI in the pelvis, avoidance of air in the bowel or rectum, together with the optimization of imaging pulse sequences are important to achieve optimal image quality. In the pelvis, DW-MRI using b-values of 800–1,000 s/mm^2 with the application of parallel imaging can be recommended to achieve sufficient suppression of the background signal. DW-MRI is showing added value for the detection and characterization of cancers, particularly in the prostate and in gynaecological malignancies. DW-MRI may also play a role in lymph node characterization, disease prognostication and tumour response assessment in a variety of pelvic malignancies such as prostate and rectal cancer. The application of pelvic DW-MRI continues to evolve and further studies will help to establish its role in clinical practice.

9.1

Introduction

As in other regions of the body, pelvic cancers often have lower tissue diffusivity, which is observed as hyperintense signal intensity on the high b-value DW-MR image, and a lower ADC than normal tissues. As a result, there is the potential for DW-MRI to deliver additional diagnostic value when it is added to the standard pelvic MR imaging by improving lesion conspicuity for disease detection and in the characterization of pelvic malignancies. Although studies evaluating DW-MRI in inflammatory pelvic disease are being undertaken, such data are still limited. In this chapter, we will explore and review the current state-of-the-art DW-MRI for the characterization of pelvic malignancies.

9.2
Prostate Cancer

9.2.1
Background

As many as one in six men in developed countries such as the United States will be diagnosed with prostate cancer (AMERICAN CANCER SOCIETY 2008). As ultrasound is only able to visualize a small percentage of prostate cancers, the primary method of diagnosing prostate cancer is by systematic transrectal ultrasound (TRUS) guided biopsy. In a patient presenting with a raised serum prostate-specific antigen (PSA) level and suspected of underlying prostate cancer, an initial negative prostate biopsy may prompt repeat biopsy with 12 or more cores taken from the prostate gland. However, should this also remain negative for prostate cancer, then repeated extended biopsies may be necessary (DJAVAN et al. 2001). Thus, if MR imaging is able to localize primary prostate cancer accurately, then MR imaging could be used as a roadmap for targeted biopsy to facilitate a quicker diagnosis, thus avoiding the risks and discomfort of repeated prostate biopsies with multiple needle passes.

Studies have shown the added value of T2-weighted MR imaging combined with proton spectroscopy (MRS) for localizing prostate cancer. T2-weighted imaging has been shown to provide limited localization information with sensitivity and specificity of 67–81 and 46–69%, respectively. MRS has shown promise in prostate cancer localization with sensitivities of 73% and specificities of 80%; however, in these studies, up to 26% of the sextants were inadequately evaluated and eliminated from the analysis (SCHEIDLER et al. 1999; WEFER et al. 2000; MULLERAD et al. 2005). Interestingly, in a multi-institutional study (ACRIN), the accuracy of combining 1.5 T endorectal MR imaging with MR spectroscopic imaging for the sextant localization of prostate cancer in the peripheral zone (PZ) was found to be equal to that of T2-weighted MR imaging alone (WEINREB et al. 2009). This has motivated investigation into other MR imaging methods such as DW-MRI for prostate cancer detection and characterization.

9.2.2
Technical Considerations

DW-MRI is commonly performed using echo planar imaging (EPI)-based pulse sequences. Typically a single-shot acquisition is performed with a high number of signal averages. At image acquisition, b-values of 800–1,000 s/mm^2 are widely used. The choice of b-values may be in part limited by the measurement signal-to-noise, which can vary according to the vendor platform. On some imaging systems, higher b-values of 1,000–1,500 s/mm^2 can be achieved without sacrificing signal-to-noise.

Image interpretation can be performed by reviewing the DW-MR images or the ADC maps, although ADC maps may be more useful in prostate cancers due to variable degrees of T2 shine-through from the normal PZ. Prostate cancers typically exhibit high signal intensity restricted diffusion on the high b-value image and return a low ADC value. On source DW-MR images, tumour conspicuity is lost at b-values of 600 s/mm^2 or less (Fig. 9.1). However, a b-value of 2,000 s/mm^2 may also not add value with current imaging systems (KITAJIMA et al. 2008), especially if they are noise-limited.

Magnetic susceptibility artefact principally caused by rectal gas or air in the endorectal coil should be minimized to avoid spatial distortion. Methods to overcome this include reduction of the echo time by using parallel imaging, filling the endorectal coil with various substances which bring the susceptibility to a similar value to human tissue or the use of non-EPI-based DW-MRI methods such as line scan diffusion (CHAN et al. 2003) or fast spin-echo (KOZLOWSKI et al. 2008). Fluids which have been used in the endorectal coil include perfluorocarbon (FC-77 Fluorinert, 3M, St. Paul, MN) (CHOI et al. 2008) and barium (ROSEN et al. 2007) while ultrasound gel can be considered in the rectum in cases where no endorectal coil is used. Placing fluids in the endorectal coil balloon represents an off-label use of the device and has not as yet been approved by the regulatory authorities or manufacturer but is being more commonly used in clinical practice. Susceptibility artefacts from hip prostheses may be particularly problematic and EPI-based DW-MRI may have limited application in these patients. The administration of anti-peristaltic drugs such as Buscopan (hyoscine-N-butyl bromide) or glucagon also helps to reduce motion and susceptibility artefacts arising within the pelvis.

Once the DW-MR images are acquired, the ADC is usually calculated by mono-exponential fitting to the data. However, there is interest in applying more

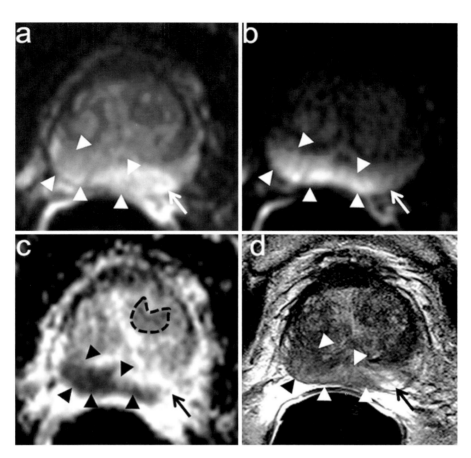

Fig. 9.1. DW-MRI of prostate cancer. A 65-year-old male with right peripheral zone (PZ) cancer extending across the midline (*black* and *white arrowheads*); Gleason score 7 (4 + 3). Images were obtained at the same location using a 1.5 T MRI with an endorectal coil filled with perfluorocarbon (FC-77). (**a**) Axial DW-MRI with *b*-value of 400 s/mm². Tumour (*white arrowheads*) is not defined because of T2 shine-through in the PZ (*white arrow*). (**b**) DW-MRI with *b*-value = 1,000 s/mm² allows visualization of bright tumour (*white arrowheads*). The higher sensitivity to water diffusion at this *b*-value results in more suppression of normal PZ signal (*white arrow*). (**c**) ADC map clearly shows dark tumour (*black arrowheads*) reflecting low ADC (0.666 × 10⁻³ mm²/s). The effect of near field signal increase deep the endorectal coil is eliminated allowing maximal tumour conspicuity. PZ (*black arrow*) exhibits the highest ADC (1.452 × 10⁻³ mm²/s). The transition zone exhibits intermediate ADC and a heterogeneous architecture. A central gland nodule (*dotted line*) has an ADC as low as 0.983 × 10⁻³ mm²/s. (**d**) T2-weighted image showing tumour (*arrowheads*) and normal PZ (*black arrow*)

sophisticated data fitting models, such as the use of bi-exponential fitting (RICHES et al. 2009; SHINMOTO et al. 2009) or fractional ADC calculation (RICHES et al. 2009), with the aim of improving the discriminatory value of these tests.

9.2.3
DW-MRI Properties of Prostatic Tissues

The use of different *b*-values, field strengths, acquisition protocols and manufacturer systems has resulted in a wide reported range of mean ADC. However, for a given protocol and hardware platform the results are consistent, showing the highest mean ADC is in the PZ (1.54–2.99 × 10⁻³ mm²/s) followed by the central gland (CG) (0.9–2.14 × 10⁻³ mm²/s) and then cancers (0.8–1.66 × 10⁻³ mm²/s) (GIBBS et al. 2001, 2007; KUMAR et al. 2006; MANENTI et al. 2007; REN et al. 2008; TAMADA et al. 2008; VAN AS et al. 2008; XU et al. 2009; ZELHOF et al. 2009) (Fig. 9.1). Prostate cancers exhibit lower ADC than normal prostatic tissue but with a degree of overlap. The lower ADC values in prostate cancers have been shown to correlate with a higher cellularity determined by histology (XU et al. 2009; ZELHOF et al. 2009). A correlation between tumour ADC and the degree of tumour differentiation (Gleeson score) has also been suggested (YOSHIMITSU et al. 2008).

Using DTI, fractional anisotropy (FA) has been demonstrated within the prostate gland. FA has been shown to be higher in the normal prostate than in cancers, reflecting the relative lack of structural organization in cancers, but with a wide range of reported values between studies (0.155–0.47 for PZ, 0.249–0.41 for CG, 0.27 for cancer) (SINHA et al. 2004; GIBBS et al. 2007; MANENTI et al. 2007; GURSES et al. 2008).

9.2.4
Tissue Characterization for Diagnosis and Staging

Multi-parametric studies which add DW-MRI have shown improved diagnostic performance compared to T2-weighted imaging alone (area under the ROC curve [A_z], A_z = 0.81–0.96 for ADC + T2 compared to A_z = 0.81–0.85 for T2 alone) (CHAN et al. 2003; SHIMOFUSA et al. 2005; HAIDER et al. 2007; KIM et al. 2007a; MAZAHERI et al. 2008; REN et al. 2008; YOSHIMITSU et al. 2008; LIM et al. 2009). The ability of DW-MRI to detect and characterize cancer is dependent on the size and composition of the tumour as well as its location. Tumours less than 4–5 mm in diameter are more difficult to detect. Benign nodules in the CG also exhibit low ADC and this can make the detection of cancer more difficult in this region. Despite this limitation, in some series ADC improved the detection of CG tumours (YOSHIMITSU et al. 2008), although confident diagnosis of tumours arising in the transitional zone or CG using DW-MRI remains challenging due to the overlap in ADC values between cancers and benign prostatic hypertrophy.

Using FA maps derived from DTI may provide additional characterization of benign vs. malignant tissue but further studies are required (SINHA et al. 2004; MANENTI et al. 2007; GURSES et al. 2008). Nevertheless, DTI appears promising for further characterization of changes in the CG and transitional zone. In a recent study, Xu et al. (2009) found that non-fibromuscular tissues (such as prostate cancers, the normal prostate and epithelial benign prostatic hypertrophy) showed no significant FA. Interestingly, no significant diffusion anisotropy differential was found in the PZ between cancerous and non-cancerous PZ tissues (Xu et al. 2009). However, in areas where there was bundling of fibromuscular structures, such as in stromal benign prostatic hypertrophy, diffusion anisotropy could be observed and distinguished from glandular epithelial benign prostatic hypertrophy (Xu et al. 2009). Thus,

combining the use of ADC and FA values may help to further improve our ability to distinguish cancers from benign changes in the prostate gland.

A list of published ADC values for benign and malignant prostatic tissue is presented in Table 9.1. It should be kept in mind that inflammatory processes within the prostate can also have lower ADC values. Prostatitis can reduce the ADC value and produce a false positive appearance of cancer (Fig. 9.2). Not surprisingly, there is an overlap in the ADC values between prostatitis and prostate cancer, and more research is needed to determine how these two entities may be confidently distinguished.

DW-MRI is generally of lower spatial resolution than T2 images and as a result may not provide added value for the detection of extracapsular tumour extension for staging unless a significant increase in spatial resolution can be obtained. DW-MRI may be of added value in detecting nodal and bone metastases but definitive data is not yet available. Early report of combining DW-MRI with USPIO-enhanced MR imaging has shown the potential of such an approach to improve nodal staging accuracy in patients with genitourinary malignancies (THOENY et al. 2009).

9.2.5
Characterizing Tumours for Disease Prognostication and Response Assessment

Quantitative assessment of ADC might have prognostic value. Preliminary studies have shown a difference in ADC between patients with low risk and intermediate risk of disease suggesting further prospective studies of DW-MRI as an outcome predictor may be warranted (DESOUZA et al. 2008; YOSHIMITSU et al. 2008). However, issues of repeatability of ADC measurements will need to be addressed (GIBBS et al. 2007). In one study of patients on active surveillance for early stage organ-confined prostate cancer, the baseline ADC measurement was found to be a significant independent predictor for both adverse repeat biopsy findings ($p < 0.0001$; hazard ratio: 1.3; 95%, confidence interval: 1.1–1.6), and time to radical treatment ($p < 0.0001$; hazard ratio: 1.5; 95%, confidence interval: 1.2–1.8) (VAN As et al. 2008).

Other than prostatectomy, prostate cancer can be treated using radiation, anti-androgen drugs, and focal treatments such as microwave, cryotherapy, photodynamic therapy and high intensity focused ultrasound. There is generally a decrease in ADC immediately after thermal therapy and within a few days of photodynamic therapy (HUANG et al. 2006; CHEN et al. 2008; CHENG et al. 2008) which may help in monitoring outcomes and the need for retreatment (Fig. 9.3), although, experience in the application of DW-MRI to assess tumour response in humans using such techniques, is still accumulating. In one study evaluating ADC changes in response to carbon-ion radiotherapy, the ADC value was found to increase in tumour areas after treatment but not in the normal prostate gland (TAKAYAMA et al. 2008). The application of DW-MRI to evaluate treatment response of cancers will be discussed in detail in Chaps. 10 and 11.

9.3
Rectal Cancer

9.3.1
Background

Colorectal cancer detection is principally performed with clinical examination, endoscopy or CT colonography. MR imaging is being used more frequently for local staging of rectal cancer as part of a patient-tailored treatment approach based on the risk of local recurrence. Patients with disease that has spread beyond the rectum into the mesorectal fat (T3) may be considered for neoadjuvant chemo-radiation therapy, particularly if the cancer has extended close to the rectal fascia, which represents the line for mesorectal surgical dissection. In the MERCURY study (MERCURY STUDY GROUP 2007), T2-weighted MR imaging was shown to be accurate to 0.5 mm for assessment of depth of tumour extension into the mesorectal fat and is now routinely being used in many clinical centres to help decide if neoadjuvant therapy is required. Despite these strong results, T2-weighted MR imaging has its limitations in assessing nodal status, treatment response and local recurrence. DW-MRI has shown promise in these areas.

9.3.2
DW-MRI Characteristics of Rectal Cancer

MR imaging is not used as a screening test for rectal cancer. Rectal cancer has a low ADC compared to normal surrounding tissues. At b-values of 800–1,000 s/mm^2 rectal cancers are conspicuous on the source high b-value DW-MR images as bright regions (Fig. 9.4) (NASU et al. 2004). Hosonuma et al. reported

ADC values of 1.374×10^{-3} mm^2/s in rectal cancers at a b-value of 800 s/mm^2. The diagnostic sensitivity was high in detecting all 15 rectal cancers but specificity was intermediate at 65% (13/20) (HOSONUMA et al. 2006). The utility of DW-MRI in the context of evaluating rectal cancers on a background of inflammatory bowel disease has not been established.

9.3.3
Characterization of Lymph Nodes

In addition to the depth of extramural tumour invasion and distant metastases, nodal status is an independent adverse prognostic factor in rectal cancer with the risk of local recurrence increasing with the number of positive nodes (STEINBERG et al. 1986; MORAN et al. 1992; PARK et al. 1999). Size criteria perform poorly in discriminating between benign and malignant lymph nodes. In pathological series, cancer is reported in 15–32% of nodes ≤5 mm in diameter in patients with rectal cancer (DWORAK 1989; BROWN et al. 2003). FDG-PET has not been particularly useful for local node assessment in rectal cancer with sensitivities in the order of 50% (TSUNODA et al. 2008). This may be related to the proximity of malignant nodes in the mesorectal fat to the primary tumour, making them difficult to resolve on imaging. Internal signal characteristics and irregularity of nodal margins can be helpful in distinguishing benign from malignant nodes using high resolution T2-weighted MR imaging reaching sensitivities of 85% (BROWN et al. 2003). It is possible that DW-MRI can improve the diagnostic accuracy. Preliminary reports have suggested lower ADCs in metastatic lymph nodes than benign nodes in rectal cancer. There is added diagnostic value seen in particular with nodes between 5 and 10 mm in size, the area under the ROC curve increasing from 0.78 with T2-weighted imaging to 0.90 when combined with DW-MRI (KIM et al. 2007b) (Fig. 9.5), but further work is required to determine the optimal nodal assessment criteria.

9.4
Transitional Cell Carcinoma of the Urinary Bladder

9.4.1
Background

Cystoscopy is the primary diagnostic modality for definitive assessment of benign and malignant bladder

Table 9.1. Reported ADC values of prostatic tissues and cancer

Authors	Year	Tissue	Subjects	b-Values (s/mm^2)	ADC (mm^2/s × 10^{-3})
REN et al.	2008	Cancer	21	0, 500	0.93 ± 0.16
		Benign peripheral zone	16		1.82 ± 0.07
		Benign central gland	16		1.35 ± 0.05
DESOUZA et al.	2008	*Low risk group*		0,100, 300, 500, 800	
		Cancer	26		1.65 ± 0.33
		Benign peripheral zone	26		2.19 ± 0.24
		Benign central gland	26		1.77 ± 0.18
		Intermediate/high risk group			
		Cancer	18		1.50 ± 0.25
		Benign peripheral zone	18		2.04 ± 0.30
		Benign central gland	18		1.74 ± 0.15
TAMADA et al.	2008	Benign peripheral zone	125	0, 800	1.80 ± 0.27
		Benign central gland	125		1.34 ± 0.14
		Cancer peripheral zone	90		1.02 ± 0.25
		Cancer central gland	90		0.94 ± 0.21
MAZAHERI et al.	2008	Cancer peripheral zone	38	0, 800	1.39 ± 0.23
		Benign peripheral zone	38		1.69 ± 0.24
YOSHIMITSU et al.	2008	Well-differentiated cancer	37	0, 500, 1,000	1.19 ± 0.15
		Moderately differentiated cancer	37		1.10 ± 0.24
		Poorly differentiated cancer	37		0.93 ± 0.20
KOZLOWSKI et al.	2008	*FSE*		0, 600	
		Cancer	14		0.99 ± 0.16
		Benign peripheral zone	14		1.57 ± 0.28
		Benign central gland	14		1.37 ± 0.18
		EPI			
		Cancer	15		1.21 ± 0.25
		Benign peripheral zone	15		1.99 ± 0.20
		Benign central gland	15		1.51 ± 0.12
KIM et al.[a]	2007	Cancer peripheral zone	37	0, 1,000	1.30 ± 0.26
		Cancer central gland	37		1.35 ± 0.24
		Benign peripheral zone	37		1.96 ± 0.20
		Benign central gland	37		1.75 ± 0.23
MANENTI et al. [a]	2007	Cancer peripheral zone	30	0, 1,000	1.06 ± 0.37
		Benign peripheral zone	30		1.95 ± 0.38
		Benign central gland	30		1.59 ± 0.40
DESOUZA ET AL.	2007	Cancer peripheral zone	33	0, 300, 500, 800	1.30 ± 0.30
		Benign peripheral zone	33		1.71 ± 0.16
		Benign central gland	33		1.46 ± 0.14
TANIMOTO et al.	2007	Cancer	9	0, 1,000	0.93 ± 0.11
		Benign peripheral zone	9		1.72 ± 0.35
		Benign central gland	9		1.46 ± 0.16
REINSBERG et al.	2007	Cancer ≥30% of voxel	42	0, 300, 500,800	1.19 ± 0.24
		Cancer ≥70% of voxel	42		1.03 ± 0.18
		Benign peripheral zone	42		1.51 ± 0.27
		Benign central gland	42		1.31 ± 0.20
KUMAR et al.	2006	Benign peripheral zone	7	0, 250, 500, 750, 1,000	1.5 ± 0.2
		Benign central gland	7		0.9 ± 0.1
		Cancer peripheral zone (metabolite ratio <1.4, PSA > 20)	13		0.8 ± 0.1
		Cancer peripheral zone (metabolite ratio <1.4, PSA 4–20)	20		1.0 ± 0.2

Table 9.1. (Continued)

Authors	Year	Tissue	Subjects	b-Values (s/mm²)	ADC (mm²/s × 10⁻³)
Pⁱᶜᵏˡᵉˢ et al. [a]	2006	Cancer	49	0, 500	1.38 ± 0.32
		Benign peripheral zone	9		1.60 ± 0.25
		Benign central gland	9		1.27 ± 0.14
Sᴀᴛᴏ et al.	2005	Cancer peripheral zone	23	0, 300, 600	1.08 ± 0.39
		Cancer central gland	23		1.13 ± 0.42
		Benign peripheral zone	23		1.80 ± 0.41
		Benign central gland	23		1.58 ± 0.37
Hᴏssᴇɪɴᴢᴀᴅᴇʜ et al.	2004	Cancer peripheral zone	10	0, 1,000	1.27 ± 0.37
		Benign peripheral zone	10		1.61 ± 0.26
Issᴀ	2002	Cancer peripheral zone	19	64–786	1.38 ± 0.52
		Benign peripheral zone	7		1.91 ± 0.46
		Benign central gland	7		1.63 ± 0.30
Gɪʙʙs et al.	2001	Benign peripheral zone	8	0–720	1.25 ± 0.23
		Benign central gland	8		1.17 ± 0.18
		Cancer	12		2.73 ± 0.70

FSE fast spin echo; *EPI* echo planar imaging
[a]Indicates DWI carried out at 3 T

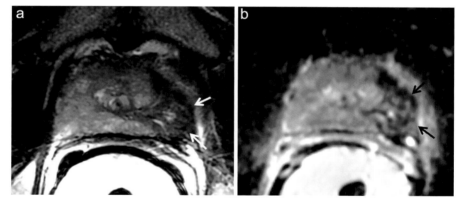

Fig. 9.2. Granulomatous prostatitis. A 51-year-old male with elevated PSA. (**a**) Axial T2-weighted image showing a low signal intensity region in the left peripheral zone (PZ) (*arrows*). (**b**) ADC map calculated from *b*-value 0 s/mm² and *b*-value 600 s/mm² acquisitions shows a region of relatively low ADC (*black arrows*) in the left PZ, shown at biopsy to be extensive granulomatous inflammation. No cancer was found

mucosal diseases. Thus, the role of MR imaging in the assessment of bladder diseases has been limited to suspected large, locally invasive tumours being assessed for exenterative procedures or radiation planning.

The commonest type of bladder cancer is transitional cell carcinoma. Approximately 70–80% of patients will present with superficial tumours which do not extend deeper than the subepithelial connective tissue (TNM stage, ≤T1, N0, M0). These patients are highly curable and are treated with transurethral resection (TUR) and fulguration, with or without

intravesical therapies. Following such procedures, these patients will undergo routine surveillance as the risk of long-term recurrence is up to 80%.

Patients with muscle-invasive disease or extension beyond the bladder may undergo cystectomy or combinations of radiation and chemotherapy. Cystoscopy and TUR can significantly underestimate the local disease extent in the bladder. For example, in a study of 58 patients with stage T1 disease in whom a second TUR was performed 2–6 weeks later, 28% of patients were found to have T2 disease and 24% had residual disease

Fig. 9.3. Decrease in ADC in regions of necrosis following focal ablative therapy. A 65-year-old man was treated with photodynamic therapy for recurrent prostate cancer after radiation therapy. This produces vascular occlusion and tissue necrosis. Contrast-enhanced axial T1-weighted images (*left column*); ADC maps (*right column*). The baseline appearance of the prostate is shown in the *top row* and the appearance at 7 days post-treatment in the *bottom row*. Note focal areas of low ADC scattered within the treated regions on the ADC maps within the devascularized tissue (*dotted lines*)

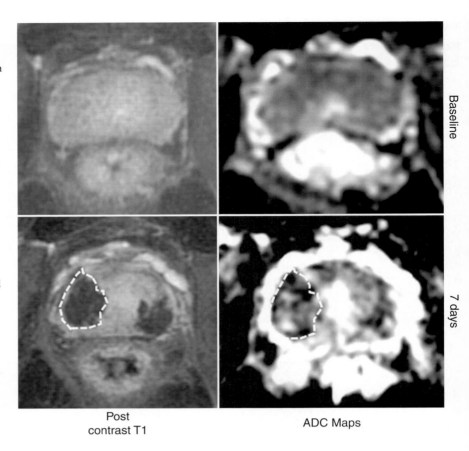

Post contrast T1   ADC Maps

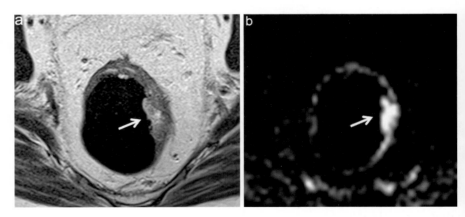

Fig. 9.4. Rectal cancer. A 78-year-old male with rectal cancer. (a) Axial T2-weighted image obtained with rectal barium shows a sessile mass on the left rectal wall (*arrow*). (b) DW-MRI obtained with a *b*-value of 1,000 s/mm² shows suppression of almost all background signal but retention of high signal intensity in the rectal carcinoma (*arrow*) allowing for high contrast between the tumour and background tissues

(HERR 1999) following resection. Hence, if DW-MRI could help distinguish post-TUR healing from residual tumour and also provide an assessment of the depth of tumour invasion into muscle, this would be of great value. In addition, the potential role of using DW-MRI for the detection of recurrent tumours reliably without the need for repeated cystoscopy is also worth investigating. These areas of DW-MRI research

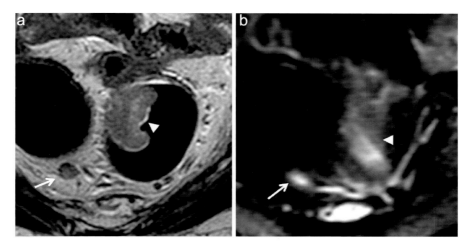

Fig. 9.5. Metastatic node from rectal cancer. A 65-year-old female with rectal cancer and a 6 mm metastatic node. (**a**) Axial T2-weighted image shows a node in the left mesorectal fat (*arrow*) and the primary cancer (*arrowhead*). (**b**) DW-MRI obtained with a *b*-value of 1,000 s/mm² shows retained high signal intensity in this node (*arrow*) with a low ADC (not shown). Note distortion of the rectal tumour (*arrowhead*) by susceptibility artefact

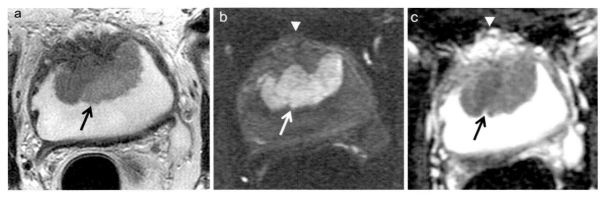

Fig. 9.6. Large polypoid transitional cell carcinoma. A 61-year-old male with a large anterior transitional cell carcinoma of the urinary bladder invading the outer half of muscularis propria (stage T2b). (**a**) Axial T2-weighted image shows a lobulated tumour attached to the anterior bladder wall (*arrow*). (**b**) DW-MRI obtained with a *b*-value of 600 s/mm² shows a bright cap (*arrow*) and a lower signal base (*arrowhead*). (**c**) ADC map shows low ADC of the bulk of the tumour and cap (*arrow*) but high ADC at the base of the tumour and in the muscularis propria, possibly related to the fibrovascular core and/or oedema

in bladder cancer are currently unfulfilled although some early data have become available.

9.4.2
DW-MRI of Bladder Carcinoma

Transitional cell carcinoma has a low ADC value. Bladder carcinomas can be seen against the low signal intensity of the muscular bladder wall and the low signal of urine on the high *b*-value DW-MR images (Matsuki et al. 2007; El-Assmy et al. 2008) (Fig. 9.6). For some tumours, the stalk or base may exhibit a higher ADC than the cellular cap of the tumour. However, data is lacking on the ability of DW-MRI to distinguish malignant from inflammatory tissue or post-TUR healing from residual or recurrent tumour. Recently, the combination of DW-MRI with T2-weighted imaging has been shown to be more accurate than T2-weighted imaging and contrast-enhanced T1-weighted imaging for the assessment of the depth of tumour invasion in the bladder wall (El-Assmy et al. 2009; Takeuchi et al. 2009). The potential value of DW-MRI for assessing pelvic sidewall nodal disease is also being investigated (Thoeny et al. 2009).

Uterine Malignancy

9.5.1
Tissue Characterization for Diagnosis

Small endometrial abnormalities on endovaginal ultrasound can be assessed using MR imaging. Submucosal fibroids can be distinguished from endometrial polyps using T2-weighted and T1-weighted gadolinium contrast-enhanced imaging. Initial experience using DW-MRI suggests that the technique may further improve the diagnostic accuracy in distinguishing benign from malignant pathologies.

The ADC value of endometrial cancer is lower (0.864–0.88×10^{-3} mm²/s) than that of benign lesions such as small submucosal leiomyomas and endometrial polyps or normal endometrium (1.277–1.53×10^{-3} mm²/s) (Fujii et al. 2008b). A summary of published ADC values for uterine pathologies is shown in Table 9.2. Differentiation of degenerated leiomyomas from leiomyosarcomas of the uterus with standard MR imaging is difficult. However, it has been shown that the mean ADC value of leiomyosarcomas is lower than that of degenerated leiomyomas and normal myometrium but overlaps with cellular and ordinary leiomyoma (Tamai et al. 2008). As with other pelvic cancers b-values of 800–1,000 s/mm² appear to yield good results.

9.5.2
Tumour Staging

In clinical practice, endometrial cancer is staged surgically by hysterectomy and bilateral salpingo-oophorectomy, thus the role of MR imaging has been limited. The incidence of cancer spread beyond the uterus in low-grade endometrial cancer confined to the endometrium is extremely low. In patients with low-grade tumours, if imaging could reliably determine the depth of myometrial invasion, a simple hysterectomy might be considered in patients with superficial disease without the need for subspecialty surgical oncology expertise for more radical surgery including pelvic sidewall nodal dissection, thus reducing the health care costs and saving a premenopausal patient an unnecessary oophorectomy and increasing morbidity. In centres where surgical nodal dissections are routinely performed, the prevalence of such surgery could also be reduced.

Currently, the combination of T2-weighted MR imaging and contrast-enhanced MR imaging has an accuracy of 77–89% and a negative predictive value as high as 91% in the assessment of myometrial invasion (Manfredi et al. 2004; Ortashi et al. 2008; Savelli et al. 2008). However, the negative predictive value has been reported to be as low as 42% if only T2-weighted sequences are used (Nakao et al. 2006). Shen et al. have shown DW-MRI alone to have a

Table 9.2. ADC values of normal uterine cervix and pathologies

Authors	Year	Tissue	Subjects	b-values (s/mm²)	ADC (mm²/s × 10⁻³)
McVeigh et al.	2008	Cervical cancer	47	0, 600	1.09 ± 0.20
		Normal cervix	26		2.09 ± 0.46
Tamai et al.	2008	Uterine sarcoma	7	0, 500, 1,000	1.17 ± 0.15
		Ordinary leiomyoma	43		0.88 ± 0.27
		Degenerated leiomyoma	6		1.70 ± 0.11
		Cellular leiomyoma	2		1.19 ± 0.18
		Normal myometrium	20		1.62 ± 0.11
Shen et al.	2008	Endometrial cancer	21	0, 1,000	0.86 ± 0.31
		Benign endometrial lesions (hyperplasia/polyp)	7		1.27 ± 0.21
Fujii et al.	2008	Endometrial cancer	11	0, 1,000	0.98 ± 0.21
		Carcinosarcoma	2		0.97 ± 0.02
		Submucosal leiomyoma	8		1.37 ± 0.28
		Endometrial polyp	4		1.58 ± 0.45
Tamai et al.	2007	Endometrial cancer	18	0, 500, 1,000	0.88 ± 0.16
		Normal endometrium	12		1.53 ± 0.10
Naganawa et al.	2005	Cervical cancer	12	0, 300, 600	1.09 ± 0.20
		Normal cervix	10		1.79 ± 0.24

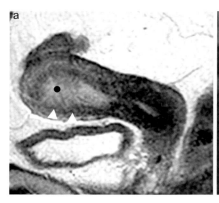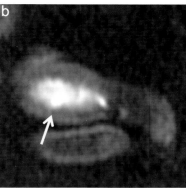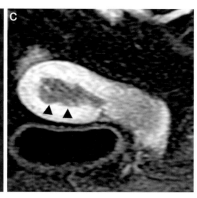

Fig. 9.7. TNM stage T1b endometrial cancer. DW-MRI of a 65-year-old female patient with pathologically proven endometrial carcinoma with myometrial invasion of less than one-third of the myometrial thickness. Fusion of T2 and DW-MR images may add further accuracy to assessment. (**a**) Sagittal T2-weighted MRI shows thickening of the endometrium (*black dot*), and possible irregularity of the myometrial/endometrial interface (*white arrowheads*) but definitive endometrial invasion is difficult to diagnose. (**b**) DW-MRI obtained with a *b*-value of 600 s/mm² shows a clear nodular area of invasion (*arrow*) into the inferior myometrium. (**c**) Post-contrast fat-suppressed T1-weighted spoiled gradient-echo image shows some irregularity of the endometrial–myometrial interface (*black arrowheads*) but invasion is not as clearly demonstrated as with DW-MRI

limited accuracy of 62%; however, they suggest when combined with contrast-enhanced MR imaging, DW-MRI may be of added value (Fig. 9.7) (SHEN et al. 2008). LIN et al. (2009) recently demonstrated that for evaluating myometrial involvement, the addition of fused T2-weighted and DW-MRI to dynamic contrast-enhanced or dynamic contrast-enhanced and T2-weighted imaging was significantly better compared with dynamic contrast-enhanced imaging alone ($p < 0.001$) or dynamic contrast-enhanced and T2-weighted ($p = 0.001$) imaging. T2-weighted imaging combined with fused T2-weighted and DW-MRI was also better than dynamic contrast-enhanced and T2-weighted imaging ($p = 0.001$). The highest diagnostic accuracy was achieved by using dynamic contrast-enhanced MR imaging with fused T2-weighted and DW-MR images (Az = 0.91) (LIN et al. 2009).

9.6
Cervical Cancer

9.6.1
DW-MRI Characteristics of Primary Tumour

The ADC of cervical cancer (1.09×10^{-3} mm²/s) is substantially lower than normal cervical stroma (1.79–2.09×10^{-3} mm²/s) which aides disease detection using DW-MRI (NAGANAWA et al. 2005; MCVEIGH

et al. 2008). There are a number of prognostic indicators for patient outcome in cervical cancer, including the clinical stage and the tumour size (STEHMAN et al. 1991). Nodal status is also a strong prognostic indicator but it is not optimally predicted with current imaging methods (SELMAN et al. 2008).

It would be of value if ADC of the tumour could provide an independent prognostic measure or a measure that was predictive of node positivity. For patients with advanced disease undergoing chemo-radiation therapy MCVEIGH et al. (2008) showed that the average median ADC (mADC) of cervical carcinomas ($1.09 \pm 0.20 \times 10^{-3}$ mm²/s) was significantly lower than that of the normal cervix ($2.09 \pm 0.46 \times 10^{-3}$ mm²/s) ($p < 0.001$). In addition, the median ADC values of tumours were lower in FIGO stages T1b/T2a (0.986×10^{-3} mm²/s) compared to T2b (1.21×10^{-3} mm²/s) and T3/T4 (1.10×10^{-3} mm²/s) ($p < 0.001$). This suggests that the ADC value may be related to tumour aggressiveness. In the same study it was found that ADC was not predictive of relapse-free survival although those patients who had a complete response to chemo-radiation therapy had a lower ADC at baseline (MCVEIGH et al. 2008).

9.6.2
Characterizing Lymph Nodes

As with rectal cancer, the ADC of metastatic nodes in cervix and uterine cancers has been shown to be lower than in benign nodes. Lin et al. showed an increase in the sensitivity for nodal metastases from 25 to 83% while maintaining specificity of 98–99% by comparing the ADC value of lymph nodes to that of the primary tumour (LIN et al. 2008). Whether DW-MRI technique is sufficient to supplant FDG-PET for nodal assessment requires further explorations but initial results are promising (BOUGHANIM et al. 2008).

9.7
Ovarian Cancer

Although US and MR imaging characterize many adnexal cysts as benign or malignant, a large proportion of cases remain equivocal requiring surgery or continued follow-up. Keratin containing areas of cystic teratomas have shown low ADC (NAKAYAMA et al. 2005) but this is usually not a diagnostic dilemma as fat can easily be detected in such lesions using other pulse sequences. In a study of 77 women with complex adnexal masses prior to surgery, the following features on $b = 1,000$ s/mm^2 DW-MRI and conventional imaging were found to be the most important predictors of benignity: low b_{1000} signal intensity within the solid component (positive likelihood ratio (PLR) = 10.9), low T2 signal intensity within the solid component (PLR = 5.7), absence of solid portion (PLR = 3.1), absence of ascites or peritoneal implants (PLR = 2.3) and absence of papillary projections (PLR = 2.3). Interestingly, the ADC measurements were not helpful in distinguishing between benign and malignant adnexal masses (THOMASSIN-NAGGARA et al. 2009). DW-MRI has also been shown to be useful in demonstrating the subtle signs of peritoneal carcinomatosis indicative of malignancy (FUJII et al. 2008a).

9.8
Inflammatory Disease

DW-MRI can depict inflammatory processes in the bowel and other pelvic organs. Few studies have been published on the added value of DW-MRI for inflammatory bowel disease. The best assessment of bowel inflammation is typically done with the use of intravenous Gadolinium (Gd)-based contrast agents. With the growing concern regarding the use of Gd-based contrast agents because of the risk of nephrogenic systemic fibrosis, a pulse sequence that could provide added value for the assessment of fistulae and avoid contrast administration would be valuable. Preliminary data has suggested little added value in the assessment of perianal fistulae in Crohn's disease compared to contrast-enhanced and T2-weighted MR imaging combined (BOURIKAS et al. 2008), but further work is necessary on a larger series of patients to see if performance is comparable to existing sequences. There are a host of other inflammatory processes within the pelvis from appendicitis to pelvic inflammatory disease where the role of DW-MRI currently remains undefined. The ability of DW-MRI to discriminate between inflammatory vs. malignant conditions in the pelvis is also yet to be established.

9.9
Conclusions

DW-MRI is being applied to characterize diseases in the prostate, bladder and gynaecological system, and the results based on published series are encouraging. There is also promise for the use of DW-MRI for the characterization of nodal diseases in the pelvis. DW-MRI may increase confidence in the diagnosis of malignant disease, and provide additional information to guide tumour therapy.

References

American Cancer Society (2008) Cancer facts and figures 2008 ACS, Atlanta, GA

Boughanim M, Leboulleux S, Rey A et al (2008) Histologic results of para-aortic lymphadenectomy in patients treated for stage IB2/II cervical cancer with negative [18F]fluorodeoxyglucose positron emission tomography scans in the para-aortic area. J Clin Oncol 26: 2558–2561

Bourikas L, Xyda A, Koutroubakis I et al (2008) The impact of diffusion-weighted-MR imaging in detecting and staging anorectal Crohn's fistulas: comparison with conventional MRI. In: Third Congress of the European Crohn's and Colitis Organisation (Inflammatory Bowel Diseases), Lyon Convention Centre, Lyon, France

Brown G, Richards CJ, Bourne MW et al (2003) Morphologic predictors of lymph node status in rectal cancer with use of high-spatial-resolution MR imaging with histopathologic comparison. Radiology 227: 371–377

Chan I, Wells W III, RV Mulkern et al (2003) Detection of prostate cancer by integration of line-scan diffusion, T2-mapping and T2-weighted magnetic resonance imaging; a multi-channel statistical classifier. Med Phys 30: 2390–2398

Chen J, Daniel BL, Diederich CJ et al (2008) Monitoring prostate thermal therapy with diffusion-weighted MRI. Magn Reson Med 59: 1365–1372

Cheng HL, Haider MA, Dill-Macky MJ et al (2008) MRI and contrast-enhanced ultrasound monitoring of prostate microwave focal thermal therapy: an in vivo canine study. J Magn Reson Imaging 28: 136–143

Choi H, Ma J (2008) Use of perfluorocarbon compound in the endorectal coil to improve MR spectroscopy of the prostate. AJR Am J Roentgenol 190: 1055–1059

Desouza NM, Riches SF, Vanas NJ et al (2008) Diffusion-weighted magnetic resonance imaging: a potential non-invasive marker of tumour aggressiveness in localized prostate cancer. Clin Radiol 63: 774–782

Djavan B, Ravery V, Zlotta A et al (2001) Prospective evaluation of prostate cancer detected on biopsies 1, 2, 3 and 4: when should we stop? J Urol 166: 1679–1683

Dworak O (1989) Number and size of lymph nodes and node metastases in rectal carcinomas. Surg Endosc 3: 96–99

El-Assmy A, Abou-El-Ghar ME, Mosbah A et al (2009) Bladder tumour staging: comparison of diffusion- and T(2)-weighted MR imaging. Eur Radiol 19: 1575–1581

El-Assmy A, Abou-El-Ghar ME, Refaie HF et al (2008) Diffusion-weighted MR imaging in diagnosis of superficial and invasive urinary bladder carcinoma: a preliminary prospective study. ScientificWorldJournal 8: 364–370

Fujii S, Matsusue E, Kanasaki Y et al (2008a) Detection of peritoneal dissemination in gynecological malignancy: evaluation by diffusion-weighted MR imaging. Eur Radiol 18: 18–23

Fujii S, Matsusue E, Kigawa J et al (2008b) Diagnostic accuracy of the apparent diffusion coefficient in differentiating benign from malignant uterine endometrial cavity lesions: initial results. Eur Radiol 18: 384–389

Gibbs P, Pickles MD, Turnbull LW (2007) Repeatability of echo-planar-based diffusion measurements of the human prostate at 3 T. Magn Reson Imaging 25: 1423–1429

Gibbs P, Tozer DJ, Liney GP et al (2001) Comparison of quantitative T2 mapping and diffusion-weighted imaging in the normal and pathologic prostate. Magn Reson Med 46: 1054–1058

Gurses B, Kabakci N, Kovanlikaya A et al (2008) Diffusion tensor imaging of the normal prostate at 3 Tesla. Eur Radiol 18: 716–721

Haider MA, van der Kwast TH, Tanguay J et al (2007) Combined T2-weighted and diffusion-weighted MRI for localization of prostate cancer. AJR Am J Roentgenol 189: 323–328

Herr HW (1999) The value of a second transurethral resection in evaluating patients with bladder tumors. J Urol 162: 74–76

Hosonuma T, Tozaki M, Ichiba N et al (2006) Clinical usefulness of diffusion-weighted imaging using low and high b-values to detect rectal cancer. Magn Reson Med Sci 5: 173–177

Hosseinzadeh K, Schwarz SD (2004) Endorectal diffusion-weighted imaging in prostate cancer to differentiate malignant and benign peripheral zone tissue. J Magn Reson Imaging 20: 654–661

Huang Z, Haider MA, Kraft S et al (2006) Magnetic resonance imaging correlated with the histopathological effect of Pd-bacteriopheophorbide (Tookad) photodynamic therapy on the normal canine prostate gland. Lasers Surg Med 38: 672–681

Issa B (2002) In vivo measurement of the apparent diffusion-coefficient in normal and malignant prostatic tissues using echo-planar imaging. J Magn Reson Imaging 16: 196–200

Kim CK, Park BK, Lee HM et al (2007a) Value of diffusion-weighted imaging for the prediction of prostate cancer location at 3T using a phased-array coil: preliminary results. Invest Radiol 42: 842–847

Kim MY, Kim AY, Ha HK et al (2007b) MRI in rectal cancer: added value of diffusion-weighted Imaging (DWI) for discrimination of metastatic lymph nodes. In: 93rd Scientific Assembly and Annual Meeting of the Radiological Society of North America (RSNA 2007), Chicago, IL, USA

Kitajima K, Kaji Y, Kuroda K et al (2008) High b-value diffusion-weighted Imaging in normal and malignant peripheral zone tissue of the prostate: effect of signal-to-noise ratio. Magn Reson Med Sci 7: 93–99

Kozlowski P, Chang SD, Goldenberg SL (2008) Diffusion-weighted MRI in prostate cancer – comparison between single-shot fast spin echo and echo planar imaging sequences. Magn Reson Imaging 26: 72–76

Kumar V, Jagannathan NR, Kumar R et al (2006) Correlation between metabolite ratios and ADC values of prostate in men with increased PSA level. Magn Reson Imaging 24: 541–548

Lim HK, Kim JK, Kim KA et al (2009) Prostate cancer: apparent diffusion coefficient map with T2-weighted images for detection–a multireader study. Radiology 250: 145–151

Lin G, Ho KC, Wang JJ et al (2008) Detection of lymph node metastasis in cervical and uterine cancers by diffusion-weighted magnetic resonance imaging at 3T. J Magn Reson Imaging 28: 128–135

Lin G, Ng KK, Chang CJ et al (2009) Myometrial invasion in endometrial cancer: diagnostic accuracy of diffusion-weighted 3.0-T MR imaging–initial experience. Radiology 250: 784–792

Manenti G, Carlani M, Mancino S et al (2007) Diffusion tensor magnetic resonance imaging of prostate cancer. Invest Radiol 42: 412–419

Manfredi R, Mirk P, Maresca G et al (2004) Local-regional staging of endometrial carcinoma: role of MR imaging in surgical planning. Radiology 231: 372–378

Matsuki M, Inada Y, Tatsugami F et al (2007) Diffusion-weighted MR imaging for urinary bladder carcinoma: initial results. Eur Radiol 17: 201–204

Mazaheri Y, Shukla-Dave A, Hricak H et al (2008) Prostate cancer: identification with combined diffusion-weighted MR imaging and 3D 1H MR spectroscopic imaging–correlation with pathologic findings. Radiology 246: 480–488

McVeigh PZ, Syed AM, Milosevic M et al (2008) Diffusion-weighted MRI in cervical cancer. Eur Radiol 18: 1058–1064

MERCURY Study Group (2007) Extramural depth of tumor invasion at thin-section MR in patients with rectal cancer: results of the MERCURY study. Radiology 243: 132–139

Moran MR, James EC, Rothenberger DA et al (1992) Prognostic value of positive lymph nodes in rectal cancer. Dis Colon Rectum 35: 579–581

Mullerad M, Hricak H, Kuroiwa K et al (2005) Comparison of endorectal magnetic resonance imaging, guided prostate biopsy and digital rectal examination in the preoperative anatomical localization of prostate cancer. J Urol 174: 2158–2163

Naganawa S, Sato C, Kumada H et al (2005) Apparent diffusion coefficient in cervical cancer of the uterus: comparison with the normal uterine cervix. Eur Radiol 15: 71–78

Nakao Y, Yokoyama M, Hara K et al (2006) MR imaging in endometrial carcinoma as a diagnostic tool for the absence of myometrial invasion. Gynecol Oncol 102: 343–347

Nakayama T, Yoshimitsu K, Irie H et al (2005) Diffusion-weighted echo-planar MR imaging and ADC mapping in the differential diagnosis of ovarian cystic masses: usefulness of detecting keratinoid substances in mature cystic teratomas. J Magn Reson Imaging 22: 271–278

Nasu K, Kuroki Y, Kuroki S et al (2004) Diffusion-weighted single shot echo planar imaging of colorectal cancer using a sensitivity-encoding technique. Jpn J Clin Oncol 34: 620–626

Ortashi O, Jain S, Emannuel O et al (2008) Evaluation of the sensitivity, specificity, positive and negative predictive values of preoperative magnetic resonance imaging for staging endometrial cancer. A prospective study of 100 cases at the Dorset Cancer Centre. Eur J Obstet Gynecol Reprod Biol 137: 232–235

Park YJ, Park KJ, Park JG et al (1999) Prognostic factors in 2230 Korean colorectal cancer patients: analysis of consecutively operated cases. World J Surg 23: 721–726

Pickles MD, Gibbs P, Sreenivas M et al (2006) Diffusion-weighted imaging of normal and malignant prostate tissue at 3.0T. J Magn Reson Imaging 23: 130–134

Reinsberg SA, Payne GS, Riches SF et al (2007) Combined use of diffusion-weighted MRI and 1H MR spectroscopy to increase accuracy in prostate cancer detection. AJR Am J Roentgenol 188: 91–98

Ren J, Huan Y, Wang H et al (2008) Diffusion-weighted imaging in normal prostate and differential diagnosis of prostate diseases. Abdom Imaging 33: 724–728

Riches SF, Hawtin K, Charles-Edwards EM et al (2009) Diffusion-weighted imaging of the prostate and rectal wall: comparison of biexponential and monoexponential modelled diffusion and associated perfusion coefficients. NMR Biomed 22: 318–325

Rosen Y, Bloch BN, Lenkinski RE et al (2007) 3T MR of the prostate: reducing susceptibility gradients by inflating the endorectal coil with a barium sulfate suspension. Magn Reson Med 57: 898–904

Savelli L, Ceccarini M, Ludovisi M et al (2008) Preoperative local staging of endometrial cancer: transvaginal sonography vs. magnetic resonance imaging. Ultrasound Obstet Gynecol 31: 560–566

Scheidler J, Hricak H, Vigneron DB et al (1999) Prostate cancer: localization with three-dimensional proton MR spectroscopic imaging–clinicopathologic study. Radiology 213: 473–480

Selman TJ, Mann C, Zamora J et al (2008) Diagnostic accuracy of tests for lymph node status in primary cervical cancer: a systematic review and meta-analysis. CMAJ 178: 855–862

Shen SH, Chiou YY, Wang JH et al (2008) Diffusion-weighted single-shot echo-planar imaging with parallel technique in assessment of endometrial cancer. AJR Am J Roentgenol 190: 481–488

Shimofusa R, Fujimoto H, Akamata H et al (2005) Diffusion-weighted imaging of prostate cancer. J Comput Assist Tomogr 29: 149–153

Shinmoto H, Oshio K, Tanimoto A et al (2009) Biexponential apparent diffusion coefficients in prostate cancer. Magn Reson Imaging 27: 355–359

Sinha S, Sinha U (2004) In vivo diffusion tensor imaging of the human prostate. Magn Reson Med 52: 530–537

Stehman FB, Bundy BN, DiSaia PJ et al (1991) Carcinoma of the cervix treated with radiation therapy. I. A multi-variate analysis of prognostic variables in the Gynecologic Oncology Group. Cancer 67: 2776–2785

Steinberg SM, Barkin JS, Kaplan RS et al (1986) Prognostic indicators of colon tumors. The Gastrointestinal Tumor Study Group experience. Cancer 57: 1866–1870

Takayama Y, Kishimoto R, Hanaoka S et al (2008) ADC value and diffusion tensor imaging of prostate cancer: changes in carbon-ion radiotherapy. J Magn Reson Imaging 27: 1331–1335

Takeuchi M, Sasaki S, Ito M et al (2009) Urinary bladder cancer: diffusion-weighted MR imaging–accuracy for diagnosing T stage and estimating histologic grade. Radiology 251: 112–121

Tamada T, Sone T, Toshimitsu S et al (2008) Age-related and zonal anatomical changes of apparent diffusion coefficient values in normal human prostatic tissues. J Magn Reson Imaging 27: 552–556

Tamai K, Koyama T, Saga T et al (2008) The utility of diffusion-weighted MR imaging for differentiating uterine sarcomas from benign leiomyomas. Eur Radiol 18: 723–730

Tanimoto A, Nakashima J, Kohno H et al (2007) Prostate cancer screening: the clinical value of diffusion-weighted imaging and dynamic MR imaging in combination with T2-weighted imaging. J Magn Reson Imaging 25: 146–152

Thoeny HC, Triantafyllou M, Birkhaeuser FD et al (2009) Combined ultrasmall superparamagnetic particles of iron oxide-enhanced and diffusion-weighted magnetic resonance imaging reliably detect pelvic lymph node metastases in normal-sized nodes of bladder and prostate cancer patients. Eur Urol. 55:761–769

Thomassin-Naggara I, Darai E, Cuenod CA et al (2009) Contribution of diffusion-weighted MR imaging for predicting benignity of complex adnexal masses. Eur Radiol 19: 1544–1552

Tsunoda Y, Ito M, Fujii H et al (2008) Preoperative diagnosis of lymph node metastases of colorectal cancer by FDG-PET/CT. Jpn J Clin Oncol 38: 347–353

Van As N, Charles-Edwards E, Jackson A et al (2008) Correlation of diffusion-weighted MRI with whole mount radical prostatectomy specimens. Br J Radiol 81: 456–462

van As NJ, de Souza NM, Riches SF et al (2008) A study of diffusion-weighted magnetic resonance imaging in men with untreated localised prostate cancer on active surveillance. Eur Urol

Wefer AE, Hricak H, Vigneron DB et al (2000) Sextant localization of prostate cancer: comparison of sextant biopsy, magnetic resonance imaging and magnetic resonance spectroscopic imaging with step section histology. J Urol 164: 400–404

Weinreb JC, Blume JD, Coakley FV et al (2009) Prostate cancer: sextant localization at MR imaging and MR spectroscopic imaging before prostatectomy–results of ACRIN prospective multi-institutional clinicopathologic study. Radiology 251: 122–133

Xu J, Humphrey PA, Kibel AS et al (2009) Magnetic resonance diffusion characteristics of histologically defined prostate cancer in humans. Magn Reson Med 61: 842–850

Yoshimitsu K, Kiyoshima K, Irie H et al (2008) Usefulness of apparent diffusion coefficient map in diagnosing prostate carcinoma: correlation with stepwise histopathology. J Magn Reson Imaging 27: 132–139

Zelhof B, Pickles M, Liney G et al (2009) Correlation of diffusion-weighted magnetic resonance data with cellularity in prostate cancer. BJU Int 103: 883–888

DW-MRI Assessment of Cancer Response to Chemoradiation

Brian D. Ross, Craig J. Galbán, and Alnawaz Rehemtulla

SUMMARY

MR imaging is widely used in the radiological diagnosis of oncology patients as it provides excellent soft tissue differentiation using routine anatomical MR imaging. A variety of MR acquisition sequences are available which can yield images of biophysical, physiological, metabolic, or functional properties of tissues. Imaging of response to oncological treatments has traditionally used single or multidirectional measurements of tumour dimensions following completion of therapy. Development of an MR imaging biomarker that would allow for early prediction of tumour response to therapeutic intervention would be a significant achievement as it could individualize clinical management of cancer patients in a timely fashion and improve outcome. This goal is very important as standard risk factors currently used in patient assessment cannot account for the variable and unpredictable treatment responses encountered by patients with similar risk profiles. This chapter will overview the use of diffusion-weighted MR imaging (DW-MRI) as a method of providing a potentially early surrogate marker of response to therapy in oncological imaging.

10.1

Overview of Current Cancer Treatment Response Assessment

Management of patients with solid malignancies involves the diagnosis, treatment planning, and assessment of treatment response or recurrence. MR imaging plays a key role in patient management, as it is able to provide cross-sectional images and three-dimensional acquisition of anatomical regions, thus

Brian D. Ross, PhD
Craig J. Galbán, PhD
Alnawaz Rehemtulla, PhD
Department of Radiology, Center for Molecular Imaging, 109 Zina Pitcher Place , Ann Arbor, MI 48109-2200, USA

allowing precise radiographic measurements of tumour location and size. However, reaching a consensus on how tumour boundaries should be optimally defined or how tumour response/progression should be scored is still a subject of debate. While a single method to determine tumour response has not been developed, solid tumour response based on a single linear summation of selected target lesions, termed "response evaluation criteria in solid tumours" (RECIST) (THERASSE et al. 2000), has been widely adopted for clinical protocols. This method of linear summation has gained acceptance as it provides for a relatively rapid and reproducible approach, thus facilitating its use in clinical trials. The standardized RECIST criteria also take into account differences in slice thickness, minimum tumour sizes, and frequency of evaluations. However, there is a growing concern that response measurements may not be adequately addressed by RECIST when tumours are treated with conventional cytotoxic therapy (JAFFE 2006), as well as more recently developed molecularly targeted agents which can provide therapeutic benefit without significantly reducing the tumour volume (CHOI et al. 2004; STRUMBERG et al. 2005). These current issues reveal an urgent need to develop more reliable response measures which are linked to clinical outcome and that can evaluate response to treatment sooner than current imaging methodologies.

Introduction of DW-MRI for Cancer Treatment Response Assessment

The development of functional imaging techniques such as DW-MRI has created new opportunities but also the need to carefully evaluate this imaging biomarker for its ability to accurately measure tumour response across organ sites and tumour types. In brief, the concept of using DW-MRI for cancer treatment response assessment is that, since molecular diffusion is a thermally driven random translational motion of water molecules within tumour tissue (also referred to as Brownian motion), treatment-induced alterations of the cellular density of a tumour would be reflected as a change in its MR imaging quantified diffusion value. This is possible due to the fact that the diffusion coefficient of pure water at body temperature is approximately $3 \times 10^{-3}\,mm^2/s$; therefore, free water molecules have a displacement distance of 0.03 mm, or 30 μm in 50 ms, which is in the order of the typical diffusion time interval used clinically. As the diameter of a tumour cell is on the order of, and other cellular structures (i.e. micrometres membranes, organelles and macromolecules) span even smaller dimensions, a water molecule will encounter many interactions with cellular or subcellular entities over the diffusion measurement interval. Therefore, in general, the more slow-moving macromolecules, cell membranes and other structures in the microenvironment, will result in a reduction of water mobility within that spatial region under measurement. The more dense the structures within tumour tissue are, the more impeded the water mobility will be, which is quantified as an apparent diffusion coefficient (ADC) value (see Chap. 1).

ADC values have been shown to correlate inversely with cell density in a variety of tumour types providing evidence for its use as a non-invasive imaging biomarker of cell density (HUMPHRIES et al. 2007; KINOSHITA et al. 2008; ZELHOF et al. 2008). However, caution must be exercised in the interpretation of the ADC value as a lower ADC value for a tumour may not necessarily reflect an underlying larger number of cells per unit volume, as other factors such as cell size, relative extracellular vs. intracellular volume, and membrane permeability can also affect water mobility and thus the ADC value. Some studies have revealed no regional correlation between ADC and the cell density in heterogeneous gliomas (SADEGHI et al. 2008). Thus, even within a given tissue or cell type, ADC may not be a reliable indicator of the relative cellularity but monitoring changes over time during treatment of an individual tumour may yield useful information related to treatment outcome, as changes from baseline measurements provide an opportunity to quantify changes within the same tumour.

For DW-MRI to be widely adopted as an imaging biomarker, the technique should provide quantifiable data, be reproducible between instruments and manufacturers, and be consistent between different clinical sites. The intra-observer and inter-observer variability in ADC measurements also need to be quantified. Although the biophysical interactions of water with tissue structures are complex and acquisition techniques are not precisely consistent between institutions, the measured ADC values of normal tissues appear to be remarkably consistent across investigators, MR hardware platforms, and operating field strengths as long as comparable acquisition techniques are used (SASAKI et al. 2008).

The application of DW-MRI for measurement of response to cancer treatment involves an

Fig. 10.1. Overview of quantifying diffusion changes using whole tumour statistic histogram-based approach. An ADC map of an invasive ductal breast carcinoma obtained prior to treatment is generated from the patient's DW-MRI scans. This is repeated at an early time point following treatment induction. Tumour margins are delineated and the distribution of tumour ADC values are plotted in a histogram format for each time interval. Histogram analysis yields whole-tumour statistical metrics such as the mean or percentage change in tumour ADC as a quantitative assessment of treatment response

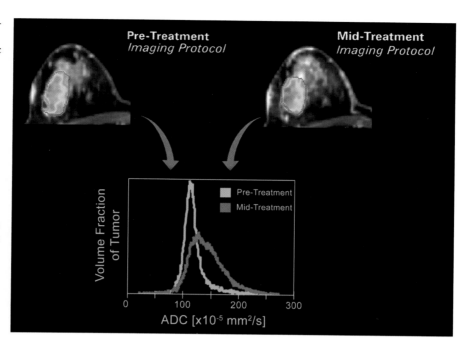

understanding of the key MR acquisition parameter defining the degree of sensitivity to diffusion, namely the *b*-value (LE BIHAN et al. 1988, 1991). The *b*-value increases with magnetic gradient strength, duration, and the temporal separation of gradient pulses used to encode and decode molecular positions, thus higher *b*-values yield higher diffusion weighting in the resultant MR image. Two or more *b*-values are typically acquired to separate diffusion effects from other MR imaging contrasts. For most cancer applications, one low ($b = 0$ s/mm^2) and one high ($b = 800–1,000$ s/mm^2) value are used although much higher *b*-values of up to 4,000 s/mm^2 are also being actively investigated to provide for additional sensitivity to tissue alterations such as the loss of cells during cancer treatment. DW-MR images acquired with a high *b*-value will exhibit high mobility environments (e.g. necrotic cyst and cerebrospinal fluid) as low intensity regions, whereas environments that impede molecular mobility, such as cellular-dense tissues, will appear relatively bright. Typically, the high *b*-value DW-MRI will have contrast that appears reversed to the corresponding ADC map because ADC displays intensity in proportion to mobility.

The application of DW-MRI as an early treatment response biomarker requires quantification of changes in tumour ADC values in an individual patient prior to and during therapy, with the goal of using the quanti-

fied parameter as a surrogate for clinical efficacy in a manner that conventional anatomical imaging cannot. There are two commonly used summary statistics for quantification and reporting of tumour treatment response using ADC values: (1) the change in the mean ADC value and (2) the voxel-by-voxel change.

The use of DW-MRI for monitoring treatment response requires a baseline or pretreatment diffusion study followed by an additional scan soon after commencement of therapy (i.e. after a few days or up to several weeks into treatment). However, the timing of the posttreatment imaging would depend on the drug or therapy being administered. As shown in Fig. 10.1, quantitative ADC maps are initially generated for each of the interval scans. Delineation of the ROI/VOI defining the tumour margins is then accomplished by the radiologist, from which all of the ADC values from the individual voxels comprising the tumour mass can be obtained to generate a histogram plot for each measurement time point. The mean ADC value for the ADC histogram distribution can then be determined and a change from baseline to treatment can be reported as the difference or a percentage change. The advantage of this approach is that it is a relatively simple procedure assuming that the quality of the data was reasonable and the tumour margins could be adequately delineated. However, the sensitivity of detecting changes in treatment-associated ADC values

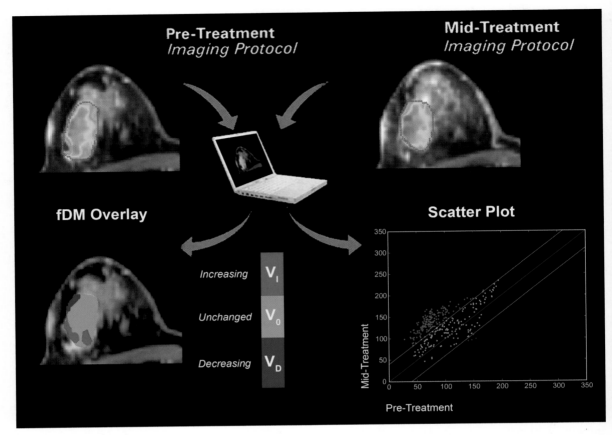

Fig. 10.2. Overview of voxel-by voxel analysis (fDM). The analytical approach uses two interval DW-MRI examinations of a breast cancer patient to generate pre- and posttreatment initiation ADC maps. The ADC maps are spatially registered using a computer algorithm. Once aligned, a voxel-by-voxel analysis is accomplished to identify and colour encode voxels which have either increased (*red*), decreased (*blue*), or remained unchanged (*green*) as a colour overlay on the corresponding anatomical image. Quantification of these changes using a scatter plot analysis provides for a reporting metric of response given in terms of a percentage of total tumour volume with increased ADC. (Adapted from MOFFAT et al. 2005)

may be attenuated in situations where there is significant heterogeneity of response (i.e. diffusion values increased and decreased in voxels within the tumour after treatment) or when there is significant heterogeneity in ADC values pre-therapy.

In order to compensate for the potential for treatment-associated heterogeneity in ADC values, an alternative approach was developed and evaluated. This analytical method uses a voxel-by-voxel comparison of tumour changes over time and is known as the functional diffusion map (fDM) (MOFFAT et al. 2005). This approach initially mirrors the same data collection, generation of ADC maps and ROI/VOI contouring procedures as described above for generation of mean ADC values. However, the fDM approach requires that the pretreatment ADC map is spatially registered with a posttreatment interval ADC map from the same patient using a computer registration algorithm as shown in Fig. 10.2. Thus, a map of voxel-by-voxel differences can be generated using a predetermined threshold of statistically significant change, allowing quantification of the relative area or percent of tumour volume which demonstrated a significant change (increase or decrease) in ADC values. The ADC changes can be encoded as a colour map and overlaid on the anatomical MR image to obtain spatial correlation and localization of the ADC changes within the tumour. The fDM approach provides an opportunity to follow spatial heterogeneity of treatment response within the tumour, which can in principle provide an opportunity to adapt therapy in "real-time" during treatment for any individual patient. The fDM approach is currently being evaluated in clinical trials for validation, and has been applied to the study of brain, bone, as well as head and neck tumours. One of the requirements for using the fDM approach is good image registration between imaging studies, which can be challenging in the body. Sophisticated registration algorithms need to be implemented to deal with the effects of motion in the body, and also to account for possible change in tumour size between studies.

It may be worth mentioning that when calculating the ADC value, a mono-exponential fitting is usually applied across a range of b-values. However, using a bi-exponential model can allow for the estimation of tissue diffusivity (D) and the perfusion fraction (F_p). Fractionated calculation of ADCs using low or high b-values can also be performed. These techniques can provide information that reflect changes in tissue diffusivity and tissue perfusion, and may be worth investigating in treatments that affect tumour vasculature (THOENY et al. 2005; LE BIHAN 2008).

Although this review focuses on DW-MRI in tumour response evaluation, it should be added that there will certainly be instances when other functional imaging techniques will furnish unique or complementary information, which could enhance the interpretation of the treatment response.

10.3

DW-MRI as a Clinical Biomarker of Cancer Treatment Response

DW-MRI is a non-invasive technique that can be used to quantify the thermal motion of water molecules in tumour tissue. This measurement is sensitive to the underlying tumour microenvironment and as this can change following therapy, diffusion has the potential to provide feedback related to the treatment effects over time. Changes in tumour ADC values during treatment have been shown to correlate with outcome, suggesting a role for DW-MRI as a predictive imaging biomarker of early response (HAMSTRA et al. 2008). The rapidly increasing pace and cost associated with drug development provides strong impetus to identify biomarkers that can be used to assess tumour biology and to monitor the effects of therapy. The motivation for developing a validated imaging biomarker of treatment response is in part due to its potential to non-invasively and repeatedly interrogate the entire tumour mass over time (or in the case of metastatic disease,

multiple tumours at once). An additional advantage of imaging over histological assessment of biopsy samples is that it allows for evaluating the heterogeneity of both the tumour and its response to therapy. DW-MRI is particularly attractive as it provides a quantitative biophysical diffusion value for each tumour voxel thus providing its spatial distribution, the ADC value generated is largely independent of instrument manufacturer and magnetic field strength, the measurements can be obtained without the need for contrast agents (except if it is needed to define the tumour extent) and finally, DW-MRI can be acquired in a relatively short period of time. Overall, these features provide DW-MRI with the potential to provide for a standardized imaging measurement of tumour treatment response. This was recently highlighted by a National Cancer Institute-sponsored open consensus conference resulting in a consensus on the use of DW-MRI as a cancer imaging biomarker where it was stated that "there is an extraordinary opportunity for DW-MRI to evolve into a clinically valuable imaging tool, potentially important for drug development" (PADHANI et al. 2009).

In recent years, clinical studies investigating the use of DW-MRI as a prognostic imaging biomarker of response have been reported in a wide variety of cancer types, including liver, breast, bone, soft tissue (sarcoma), central nervous system (CNS), head and neck, lymph node and rectum (Table 10.1) (CHENEVERT et al. 2000; SHARMA et al. 2009). Most of the studies have been single institution studies with small sample sizes although there are four specific studies to date that have reported results from relatively large patient populations (N ≥ 34) (HAMSTRA et al. 2005, 2008; KAMEL et al. 2006; SHARMA et al. 2009).

10.4

Assessment of Tumour Response Using DW-MRI

10.4.1
Liver Tumours

The optimal treatment for patients with hepatic malignancies is liver resection; however, the majority of patients are not suitable for primary surgery. Therefore, chemotherapy is often administered to downstage and downsize the tumours. DW-MRI studies following systemic chemotherapy of liver metastases from colorectal, gastric and breast cancer have reported good correlation of response with

Table 10.1. Clinical DW-MRI Studies

Site	Number	Treatment[a]	Timing[b]	Reference
Bone	24	RT	1–6 months	BYUN et al. (2002)
Bone	1	Hormone	2 & 8 weeks	LEE et al. (2007)
Breast	10	Chemotherapy	3 weeks	PICKLES et al. (2006)
Breast	11	Chemotherapy	15–18 weeks	YANKEELOV et al. (2007)
Breast	56	Neoadjuvant chemotherapy	After each cycle	SHARMA et al. (2009)
Cervical	20	Chemotherapy/RT	2 weeks	HARRY et al. (2008)
CNS	2	Chemotherapy/RT	Serial	CHENEVERT et al. (2000)
CNS	3	CED	Serial	MARDOR et al. (2001)
CNS	8	RT	3–10 days	MARDOR et al. (2003)
CNS	20	Stereotactic RT	2–4 weeks	TOMURA et al. (2006)
CNS	20	Chemotherapy/RT	3 weeks	MOFFAT et al. (2005)
CNS	34	RT ± Chemotherapy	3 weeks	HAMSTRA et al. (2005)
CNS	60	RT ± Chemotherapy	1 & 3 weeks	HAMSTRA et al. (2008)
CNS	21	Stereotactic radiosurgery	1 week, 1 & 3 months	HUANG et al. (2008)
CNS	3	Chemotherapy	23–41 days	SCHUBERT et al. (2006)
CNS	1	Chemotherapy	Fourth cycle	JAGER et al. (2005)
CNS	15	CED	Daily	LIDAR et al. (2004)
Liver	13	Chemotherapy	4 & 11 days	THEILMANN et al. (2004)
Liver	23	Chemotherapy	3, 7 & 42 days	CUI et al. (2008)
Liver	20	Chemotherapy	12 weeks	KOH et al. (2007)
Lymph node	1	Chemotherapy	Four courses	NAKAYAMA et al. (2008)
Rectum	14	Chemotherapy then RT	NA	DZIK-JURASZ et al. (2002)
Rectum	8	Chemotherapy/RT	1 week	KREMSER et al. (2003)
Rectum	9	Chemotherapy/RT	2, 3 & 4 week	HEIN et al. (2003)
Sarcoma	18	Chemotherapy	NA	HAYASHIDA et al. (2006)
Sarcoma	8	Chemotherapy	NA	UHL et al. (2006)
Sarcoma	23	Chemotherapy	57 days	DUDECK et al. (2008)
Sarcoma	29	Radiation	11–31 days	EINARSDOTTIR et al. (2004)

[a]*RT* radiation therapy; *CED* convection-enhanced delivery of chemotherapy
[b]Timing of response evaluation relative from start of treatment. *NA* Not available in text

increased tumour ADC values following treatment (KOH et al. 2007; CUI et al. 2008; THEILMANN et al. 2004).

The ability of DW-MRI to predict response to chemotherapy in patients with colorectal and gastric hepatic metastases was reported in a clinical study involving imaging of 87 hepatic metastases in 23 colorectal and gastric cancer patients before and at 3, 7, and 42 days after initiating chemotherapy (CUI et al. 2008). In this study, clinical outcome was assigned using changes in tumour size following completion of treatment and tumours were identified as either responding or non-responding accordingly. While 38 metastases were found to be responding, 49 metastases were identified as being non-responding. It was found that tumour ADC values increased early on days 3 or 7 for responding lesions but not in non-responding lesions ($p = 0.002$). A correlation was found between final tumour size reduction and early ADC changes (day 3, $p = 0.004$; day 7, $p < 0.001$) in this patient population (Cui et al. 2008). Overall, ADC was found to have significant promise for detecting early response to chemotherapy of hepatic metastases from colorectal and gastric carcinomas. Similar results were observed in 40 metastatic lesions of colorectal cancer undergoing chemotherapy with high pretreatment ADC values correlating with poor response to treatment. A significant increase in mean ADC was observed in metastatic lesions that responded to therapy at completion of chemotherapy (Koh et al. 2007).

In another study involving 13 patients with 60 measurable metastatic liver lesions from breast cancer, DW-MRI was used to follow changes after initiation of chemotherapy (Theilmann et al. 2004). Baseline DW-MR images were obtained and repeated at intervals corresponding to 4, 11, and 39 days following start of therapy. This study showed that early increase in ADC values could be observed using DW-MRI, which could predict response by 4 or 11 days after treatment initiation, with the best correlation of ADC changes in tumour lesions with volumes less than $8\,cm^3$ prior to therapy.

These results revealed that ADC measurements could be successfully obtained in liver lesions and that ADC values were promising for quantifying and predicting response of liver metastases to effective chemotherapy.

10.4.2
Nodal Disease

DW-MRI was evaluated in a case report for its potential to detect treatment response in a patient with para-aortic lymph node metastases from bladder cancer (Nakayama et al. 2008). Prior to treatment, the lymph node showed high signal intensity on DW-MRI indicating a cellular dense lesion with low ADC values. Following four cycles of a combination of gemcitabine and cisplatin chemotherapy, the lesion showed reduction of signal intensity on DW-MRI corresponding to an increase in ADC which was correlated with the morphological response of the lesion. Although this was a limited study in a single patient, it nevertheless illustrates the potential value of DW-MRI to quantify treatment response in metastatic lymph nodes.

10.4.3
Breast Cancer

Treatment of primary breast cancer using systemic chemotherapy significantly reduces the risk of disease recurrence and death (Buzdar et al. 2005; Romond et al. 2005; Slamon et al. 2006). Recently, the use of neoadjuvant therapy vs. adjuvant therapy has been investigated in several clinical trials (Mauriac et al. 1999; Wolmark et al. 2001; Gianni et al. 2005). The conceptual advantage of neoadjuvant therapy is that it provides for early intervention of potential systemic disease, may reduce the dissemination of loose cells after surgical resection and can decrease tumour size prior to surgery, subsequently reducing the extent of surgery. While some studies have shown little evidence to support enhanced survival benefits using neoadjuvant chemotherapy (NACT) as compared with adjuvant regimens, preoperative therapy is still preferentially administered as it can potentially downstage the primary tumour in the majority of women resulting in improved rates for breast-conserving surgery (Scholl et al. 1994; Makris et al. 1998; Broet et al. 1999).

DW-MRI lends itself to the evaluation of preoperative therapy regimens as it may provide tumour response assessment to drugs prior to invasive perturbation of the mass. This may prove to be an exceptional opportunity for evaluation of imaging biomarkers as studies have shown that the ability of chemotherapy regimens to elicit a pathologic complete response (CR) correlates with enhanced long-term disease survival (Robertson et al. 1994; Sataloff et al. 1995; Chang et al. 1999; Kuerer et al. 1999). Evaluation of the effectiveness of systemic preoperative therapy relies on post-surgical assessment of the excised tumour tissue, which is too late to allow for tailoring and optimization of therapy. Since pathological CR correlates with long-term disease-free survival, the ability to assess CR by non-invasively using DW-MRI in a timely fashion, would allow for customization of NACT regimens to optimize tumour response prior to surgery.

Several studies have reported the ability of ADC measurements to detect treatment-induced changes in primary breast cancer (Pickles et al. 2006; Yankeelov et al. 2007; Sharma et al. 2009). A common finding between these studies was that increased ADC values were detected in responding tumours. In one study of 56 patients with locally advanced breast cancer (SHARMA et al. 2009), the tumour ADC values, tumour volume and tumour diameter were measured to determine whether these variables could predict response to NACT. The percentage change in the mean ADC values, tumour volume and tumour diameter measurements after each cycle of NACT were determined, which showed that there was a statistically significant difference in the ADC value between clinical responders and non-responders after the first cycle of treatment, but not when the tumour volume or diameter were evaluated. The results suggest that DW-MRI may be a valuable early predictor of response to NACT and thus has the potential to inform effective treatment management. This data provides encouraging evidence for continuing to investigate DW-MRI as a marker for early tumour response in NACT-treatment patients.

Figure 10.3 illustrates DW-MRI for quantification of breast cancer response to NACT with T2-weighted MR imaging of a breast tumour. VOI definition of tumour boundaries was accomplished and DW-MRI colour overlays are shown for pretreatment imaging and at 10 days' post-initiation of NACT. ADC histograms are provided for each VOI corresponding to the pretreatment (blue) and posttreatment (red) measurements. A significant shift to higher diffusion values was observed 10 days following therapy. An alternative analytical approach was also accomplished on the same patient data using the fDM or voxel-by-voxel approach. The colour fDM overlay is shown alongside the corresponding scatter plot analysis revealing those tumour voxels which had shown a significant increase in ADC values (red). Heterogeneity of treatment response is visible in both types of analyses. This patient was later, following surgical resection, determined to have a clinical response to therapy. Figure 10.3 demonstrates that DW-MRI data may be acquired in primary breast cancers and different analytical approaches can be applied to quantify the treatment-associated changes in the ADC values in these patients.

10.4.4
Tumours of the Central Nervous System

Although the CNS is the domain of the neuroradiologist rather than body imaging specialists, DW-MRI has been used in the brain for a considerably longer

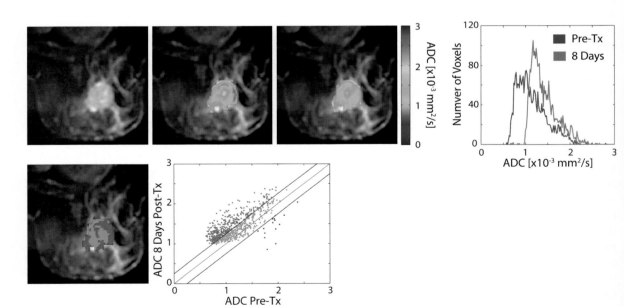

Fig. 10.3. MR imaging corresponding to pretreatment T2-weighted image (*top left*), pretreatment ADC map (*top middle*) and mid-treatment ADC map (*top right*) overlaid on pretreatment T2-weighted images in a patient with breast cancer. ADC histograms are also provided showing change in the overall ADC distribution within the tumour mass. Functional diffusion map overlaid on pretreatment T2-weighted image (*bottom left*) and corresponding scatter plot (*bottom right*) is shown. This representative patient was diagnosed as a responder by radiological response and had significant increases in ADC values by both metrics. (Data kindly provided by Pickles and Turnbull)

period of time and it is valuable to learn how ADC value changes in relation to therapy in cranial tumours, with a view to applying this experience elsewhere in the body.

Preliminary data reported in two patients with high-grade primary brain tumours that changes in ADC could be detected weeks before tumour response was observable using standard clinical volumetric measurements (CHENEVERT et al. 2000). In another study, convection-enhanced delivery of chemotherapy (CED) directly into the tumour was accomplished and changes in ADC could be detected 1 day following treatment (MARDOR et al. 2001). In a follow-up study by the same investigators evaluating ten metastatic or primary brain tumours treated with radiotherapy, six treated tumours regressed by 35–89% (partial response) and in all six tumours, a significant increase in diffusion as early as 3 days after treatment was detected (MARDOR et al. 2003). Tissue diffusivity was either unchanged or decreased in four lesions found to be stable or progressive after treatment. The early increases in mean ADC values were correlated with subsequent tumour response ($p < 0.006$) (MARDOR et al. 2003). Other studies of CNS tumours have also reported the predictive value of ADC values changes in relation to response after chemotherapy or radiotherapy (LIDAR et al. 2004; JAGER et al. 2005; SCHUBERT et al. 2006; TOMURA et al. 2006; HUANG et al. 2008).

In an effort to develop an analytical approach which would help to improve the ability to use ADC measurements as a prognostic imaging biomarker of response, fDM was developed and evaluated in three different studies (HAMSTRA et al. 2005, 2008; MOFFAT et al. 2005). In these prospective trials of DW-MRI, patients with primary brain tumours underwent a baseline scan within 1 week prior to treatment, followed by the first intra-treatment scan at 1 or 3 weeks. Patients were treated with 6 weeks of fractionated radiation. In an initial report, the mean ADC was weakly correlated with subsequent radiological response by size measurement criteria. However, fDM analysis was able to discriminate between patients who had progressive disease (PD), stable disease, or a partial response (MOFFAT et al. 2005). In a companion study, 34 patients with World Health Organization (WHO) grade 3/4 gliomas were evaluated by fDM at 3 weeks into fractionated radiation therapy (RT) (HAMSTRA et al. 2005). The fDM measurement determined from the 3-week interval scan from baseline correlated with radiological response as well as progression-free and overall survival (OS) (HAMSTRA et al. 2005). Patients in which fDM stratified as having

PD had an OS of 8.2 months whereas patients stratified by fDM as having a favorable response to therapy had an improved OS of 18.2 months ($p < 0.008$). These results were validated in a recent study in which 60 patients with high-grade glioma were evaluated using fDM (HAMSTRA et al. 2008). In this study, receiver operating characteristic curve analysis was used to evaluate fDM as a function of patient survival at 1 year. Cox and log-rank proportional hazards models were utilized to assess the OS. It was found that patients alive at 1 year compared with those who died as a result of disease had a significantly larger increase in their diffusion values in response to therapy. Representative examples of a responding and a non-responding patient by fDM analysis are shown in Fig. 10.4. Overall, it was shown that the volume of tumour with increased diffusion by fDM criteria at 3 weeks was the strongest predictor of patient survival at 1 year, with a larger fDM change predicting for longer median survival (52.6 vs. 10.9 months; log-rank, $p < 0.003$). Radiological response measured at 10 weeks was determined to have a similar prognostic value for outcomes (median survival, 31.6 vs. 10.9 months). However, the outcome stratification by radiological response and fDM was found to differ in 25% of cases, and a composite index including fDM and radiological response was found to be a more robust predictor of overall patient survival. Hence, combining fDM and radiological response criteria was proposed as a possible method to identify patients in whom the radiological response may not correlate with the clinical outcome. These studies have shown that compared with conventional imaging, fDM can provide an earlier assessment of equal predictive value, but the combination of fDM and standard radiological response criteria resulted in a more accurate prediction of patient survival than either metric alone.

10.4.5
Bone Malignancies

An interesting opportunity for investigating DW-MRI as an imaging biomarker of cancer treatment response assessment is for the evaluation of osseous lesions. In this regard, there are currently no accepted methods for quantifying response of primary or metastatic cancers within skeletal sites and in fact response is not considered measurable by RECIST (THERASSE et al. 2000). The ability to determine response of osseous lesions to therapy would provide a major breakthrough for imaging and have a major impact in

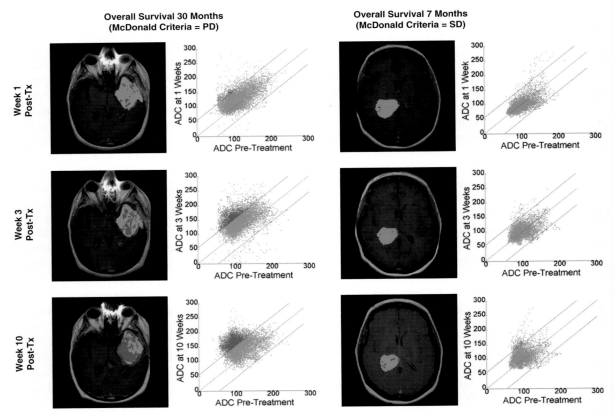

Fig. 10.4. Representative fDM analysis for two patients with glioblastoma treated with fractionated radiation therapy (RT) and concurrent temozolamide, and followed with serial DW-MRI. The patient on the left was scored as progressive disease (PD) by McDonald criteria at week 10 and had overall survival (OS) of 30 months. The patient on the right was scored as stable disease and had OS of 7 months. Depicted anatomical images are single slices of the T1 post-contrast images at each time point (1, 3, and 10 weeks post the start of RT from *top* to *bottom*) with a pseudo-colour overlay of the fDM. *Red voxels* indicate regions that underwent a sig-nificant rise in apparent diffusion coefficient at each time point as compared to pretreatment whereas *green* regions had unchanged ADC. The *scatter plots* depict data for the entire tumour volume and not just for the displayed slice at each scan interval and present the pretreatment ADC on the *x*-axis and posttreatment ADC for the indicated time-point on the *y*-axis. The *central red line* represents unity while the flanking *blue lines* represent the 95% confidence intervals with those voxels that increased above the 95% confidence interval coded in *red* (Hamstra et al. 2008)

this clinical population which includes a large population of patients with metastatic breast and prostate cancer to the bone.

10.4.5.1
Primary Bone Tumours

In a recent study, quantitative DW-MRI was evaluated for monitoring the therapeutic response of primary bone tumours including osteogenic and Ewing sarcomas (Hayashida et al. 2006). DW-MRI examination was performed before and after therapy, and ADC changes were compared with bone tumour volume before and after treatment. Patients were grouped according to whether their tumours showed less than 90% or more than 90% necrosis after treatment. Changes in ADC value and tumour volume were compared between these groups where it was found that the change in ADC values were statistically greater in the group with >90% necrosis than in the <90% necrosis group ($p = 0.003$). Furthermore, it was observed that there was no significant difference in the changes in tumour volume ($p = 0.065$), thus monitoring of ADC values by DW-MRI was determined to be promising for monitoring the therapeutic response of primary bone sarcomas.

In a different study, correlation between the ADC values obtained from osteosarcomas following chemotherapy with the corresponding regions on pathological analysis was accomplished to relate the histology to the diffusion measurements (Uhl et al. 2006). In this study, necrotic areas, confirmed by macroscopic and histological examination, revealed ADC values up to 2.7 (mean, 2.3 ± 0.2); whereas areas of viable tumour were found to have significantly lower ADC values (mean, 0.8 ± 0.3; $p = 0.01$).

10.4.5.2
Metastatic Cancers

In a recent study, the feasibility of clinically translating the functional diffusion map (fDM) imaging biomarker for quantifying the spatiotemporal effects of bone tumour response in a patient treated for metastatic prostate cancer with bone metastases was reported (Lee et al. 2007). In this study, a patient was evaluated by DW-MRI prior to treatment and at 2 and 8 weeks after commencement of treatment to quantify changes in the tumour diffusion values. Figure 10.5 illustrates three metastatic lesions identified for fDM analysis, all of which demonstrated early changes in diffusion values at 2 weeks, which increased further at 8 weeks posttreatment initiation. Evident in the fDM colour overlays are significant regions of increased (red) and decreased (blue) diffusion values within each of the monitored tumours. A comparison of the mean ADC changes using whole tumour volume statistic (i.e. histogram analysis) with increased ADC changes quantified using voxel-by-voxel analysis (i.e. fDM) revealed improved sensitivity of fDM over mean ADC value in lesions showing heterogeneous changes over time. The fDM changes showed correlation with a decrease in the patient's prostate-specific antigen (PSA) levels suggesting treatment response. It was also reported in this study that the CT, radionuclide bone scans, and anatomical MR images obtained posttreatment were not useful for the assessment of treatment effectiveness. This study presents the feasibility of applying the fDM approach in osseous lesions following treatment and provides intriguing data which warrant further investigation of fDM as a quantitative imaging biomarker.

Another important area in which DW-MRI may prove useful for monitoring treatment response is in metastatic disease to the spine. Currently, monitoring the response to therapy using plain radiography, radionuclide bone scan, and conventional spin-echo sequence MR imaging has not proven satisfactory. A recent study investigated signal intensity changes of bone marrow following RT using DW-MRI to evaluate if this visual approach could detect response to therapy in metastatic disease of the spine (Byun et al. 2002). Images were obtained in 24 patients prior to and following RT. A comparison was made of the signal intensity changes of the metastatic disease of the vertebral bone marrow before and following treatment between conventional spin-echo and diffusion-weighted MR images. In 23 patients with metastatic disease to the spine which showed clinical improvement following therapy, the signal intensity decreased on the highest acquired b-value images during follow-up. The T1-weighted/ T2-weighted imaging findings and volume of abnormality did not correlate with clinical improvement. In contrast, in the one patient who had increasing symptoms after RT, the mean ADC decreased, whereas in the remaining 23 patients who experienced clinical improvement, mean ADC increased by 56%. Furthermore, persistent hyperintense bone marrow on the high b-value images was observed in this non-responding patient. This study concluded that decreased signal intensity of metastatic disease on DW-MRI correlated with successful therapy in metastatic disease of the vertebral bone marrow (Byun et al. 2002).

10.4.6
Soft Tissue Sarcomas

Musculoskeletal soft-tissue masses are frequently imaged using magnetic resonance because of the superior soft tissue contrast to define tumour location and extent. Such anatomical images are also used to follow treatment response by comparing tumour dimensions prior to and following completion of treatment (Kransdorf et al. 2000). In tumours that are not being treated by primary surgical resection, DW-MRI could be used to determine early treatment response to fractionated radiotherapy schedules. To date, two studies have evaluated the ability of DW-MRI to quantify response in soft tissue sarcomas (Einarsdottir et al. 2004; Dudeck et al. 2008).

Fig. 10.5. Functional diffusion map analysis of treatment response in a patient with three distinct metastatic lesions to the bone from prostate cancer. Regional changes of ADC are plotted on anatomical images to provide a visual representation and quantification of treatment-induced changes in ADC values. fDM analysis of the femoral head lesion at (**a**) 2 and (**b**) 8 weeks after treatment initiation revealed distinct regions of red voxels signifying areas with significant increases in ADC ($>26 \times 10^{-6}$ mm^2/s). fDM analysis of the sacral lesion at (**c**) 2 and (**d**) 8 weeks after treatment revealed significant regions of increased ADC (red voxels). fDM analysis of the ilium lesion at (**e**) 2 and (**f**) 8 weeks after treatment also show large regions of increased ADC values (red voxels). (Bar graph) Comparison of mean ADC changes using histogram analysis with respect to baseline reveals that no statistically significant change could be detected. A comparison of fDM values with histogram analysis at 2 weeks post-therapy revealed that a decrease of 0.7 ± 4.8% was detectable using mean ADC values whereas fDM demonstrated a 24 ± 1.6% increase in ADC. Furthermore, at 8 weeks, mean ADC values increased by 8.3 ± 4.3% whereas fDM demonstrated a 38 ± 5.2% increase in ADC (LEE et al. 2007)

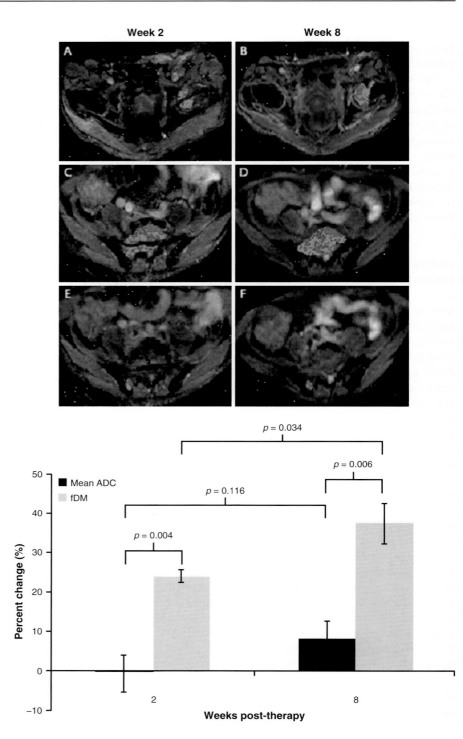

In an initial study, 29 patients were evaluated in which 16 patients had benign lesions and 13 patients were diagnosed with sarcomas (EINARSDOTTIR et al. 2004). Four of the sarcoma patients were examined both before and following RT using DW-MRI. The mean ADC values were obtained from a large VOI circumscribing each lesion. The baseline comparison of the ADC values of the benign lesions with those of non-treated sarcomas revealed no significant difference between the groups suggesting that the ADC value may not be a sensitive diagnostic tool for pre-treatment disease classification. However, the ADC values increased in all irradiated sarcomas leading investigators to hypothesize that an increase in ADC values of soft tissue sarcomas after radiotherapy may be useful for evaluating therapy response.

A recent prospective study evaluating DW-MRI as a surrogate marker of tumour response to anti-cancer therapy in 23 soft-tissue sarcoma patients was reported (DUDECK et al. 2008). DW-MRI scans were acquired prior to and following initiation of regional or systemic chemotherapy. The mean scan interval between the pretreatment and follow-up imaging was about 2 months. It was found that an increase in sarcoma ADC values was always associated with a reduction of tumour volume and a decrease in ADC was always associated with a tumour volume increase. Thus changes in ADC values were found to be inversely correlated with morphologic changes. Overall, DW-MRI was reported to be useful for detecting treatment effects in patients with soft-tissue sarcomas. These findings provide the foundation and rationale to undertake additional clinical studies at shorter imaging intervals, so as to better understand the temporal changes in ADC values in response to treatment, in an effort to optimize and validate these initial studies to provide accurate and early prognostic information in this patient population.

10.4.7
Squamous Cell Carcinoma of the Head and Neck

The standard of care for patients with head and neck squamous cell carcinoma (HNSCC) is non-surgical organ preservation therapy (NSOPT) in order to preserve functionality (e.g. swallowing and speech) in the patient while maintaining the optimum survival rate. DW-MRI may be useful for providing information on tumour status following chemoradiotherapy in this patient population.

A prospective trial involving 15 patients with HNSCC was accomplished with DW-MRI measurements obtained at baseline and 3 weeks' posttreatment initiation of a NSOPT using concurrent radiation and chemotherapy (GALBÁN 2009). ADC maps were analysed by monitoring the percentage change in the whole-tumour mean ADC value and fDM. Serial ADC maps were spatially aligned using a deformable image registration algorithm.

The prognostic value of the percentage change in tumour volume, mean ADC value and fDM as a treatment response biomarker was assessed by correlating these with the tumour control assessed at 6 months. Examples of the application of these two different DW-MRI analysis approaches for two different patients treated for HNSCC are shown in Fig. 10.6. Both the primary tumour and metastatic lymph nodes could be easily identified on the T2-weighted, contrast-enhanced images and ADC maps. Voxel-by-voxel analysis using the fDM approach revealed regions where water mobility was increased after treatment. In addition, analysis of tumour ADC histograms revealed a significant increase in the mean ADC value 3 weeks after initiating treatment. However, statistical analysis of the patient cohort showed no correlation between the percentage change in mean ADC and tumour control at 6 months. In contrast, significant differences in fDM and the percentage change in tumour volume were observed between patients with pathologically different outcomes. These results revealed that DW-MRI when assessed by fDM has potential to provide both prognostic and spatial information related to chemoradiation treatment effects in head and neck cancer.

Recent work by others has also found that DW-MRI was useful as a surrogate biomarker for early treatment response (KIM et al. 2008). This study demonstrated, in a cohort of 33 patients with HNSCC that changes in the mean ADC of metastatic lymph nodes from pre-therapy to 1 week into chemoradiotherapy correlated with subsequent clinical or pathological disease response. Overall, changes in ADC values measured by DW-MRI may serve as a potential imaging biomarker for quantifying therapeutic efficacy in patients with HNSCC that can be incorporated into clinical head and neck cancer treatment protocols. DW-MRI also has the potential to aid the individualization of head and neck cancer treatment regimens. These results also reveal the ability to perform image registration in the head and neck region for fDM analysis.

10.4.8
Cervical Cancer

A recent study has evaluated DW-MRI as an early response indicator in women receiving chemoradiation for advanced cervical cancer (HARRY et al. 2008). In this study, 20 women with advanced cervical cancer

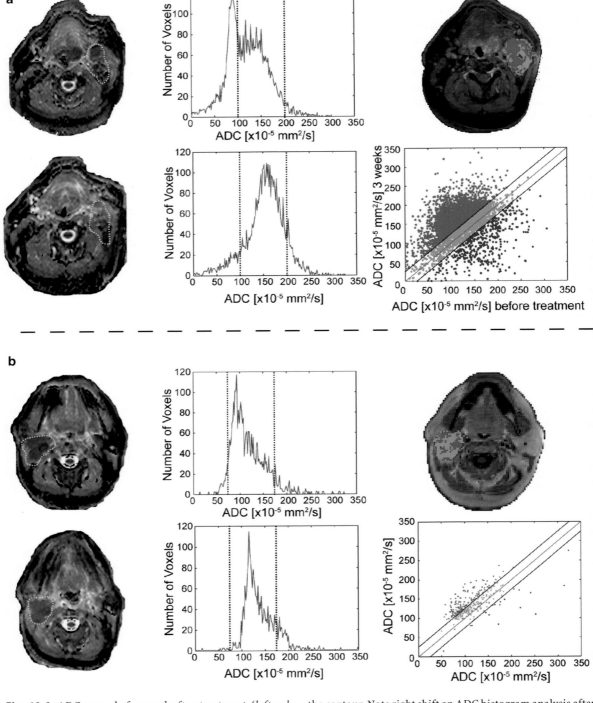

Fig. 10.6. ADC-maps before and after treatment (*left column*), ADC histograms over the entire tumour before and after treatment (*middle column*) and fDM analysis (*right column*) are provided for complete and partial responding patients. (**a**) Lymph node metastasis in level II shown in a patient diagnosed with HNSCC of the left base of the tongue. The lymph node metastasis is encompassed within the contour. Note right shift on ADC histogram analysis after treatment and significant changes on a voxel basis by fDM analysis. (**b**) A partial responder diagnosed with lymph node metastasis (encompassed) of HNSCC of the right tonsil. Note corresponding changes on ADC histograms and fDM map. All images and ADC histograms were acquired pretreatment and 3 weeks posttreatment initiation (GALBÁN et al. 2009)

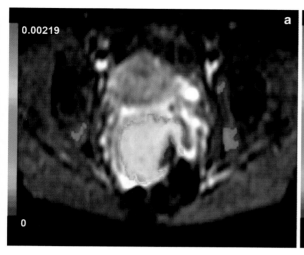
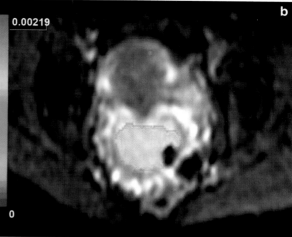

Fig. 10.7. Representative examples of ADC maps from a patient with an advanced cervical tumour (in colour) (**a**) prior to and (**b**) after 2 weeks of chemoradiation. A region of interest (ROI) is drawn around the tumour while avoiding an area of reduced signal intensity. (With kind permission HARRY et al. 2008)

were included in a prospective cohort. DW-MRI was carried out prior to chemoradiation, and repeated 2 weeks into therapy and again at the conclusion of therapy. The mean ADC values for each measurement were correlated with final tumour response as determined by volumetric assessment of tumour size using MR imaging and conventional clinical response. It was found that the ADC values after 2 weeks of therapy correlated with eventual MR response ($p = 0.048$) and clinical response ($p = 0.009$), as did the change in ADC values after 2 weeks of therapy ($p = 0.01$ for MR response; $p = 0.03$ for clinical response). Examples of ADC maps from a cervical cancer patient prior to and after 2 weeks of chemoradiation are shown in Fig. 10.7 revealing increased ADC values within the tumour. In the same study the investigators also reported on 12 women who underwent two separate pretreatment DW-MRI examinations to evaluate the reproducibility of the ADC measurement (HARRY et al. 2008). Reproducibility of ADC measurements were reported having a mean difference in ADC of −0.003 between consecutive pre-therapy MR imaging assessments and 95% confidence intervals of −0.12 and 0.11. Overall, this study provided evidence that DW-MRI has potential to serve as an early surrogate imaging biomarker of treatment response in advanced cervical cancers which may allow for the development of individualized regimens based upon the early response ADC metrics.

10.4.9
Rectal Cancers

Changes in DW-MRI in response to therapy have been evaluated in rectal cancers (DZIK-JURASZ et al. 2002; HEIN et al. 2003; KREMSER et al. 2003). Pretreatment ADC values in rectal cancer patients were found to be negatively correlated with tumour response and it was hypothesized that the presence of higher pretreatment ADC values reflected necrotic tumours that were resistant to therapy. The studies also found that following treatment, mean ADC values were consistently lower than prior to treatment initiation which was attributed to the possible increase in fibrosis and scar tissue in response to treatment. However, the ADC distribution for the therapeutically responding group showed a clear shift to higher ADC values following the first week of therapy (KREMSER et al. 2003). During subsequent weeks of therapy, the shift between the responder and non-responder group was gradually reduced indicating that for this tumour type, DW-MRI measurements in the first week of therapy may provide the most accurate information although further validation of this observation is required. This data highlights the fact that the timing of evaluation relative to treatment may be a key variable in the application of clinical diffusion MRI which should be carefully evaluated for a specific treatment and tumour type.

10.5

Summary

Results presented in this overview have been impressive as they have revealed that a significant body of work has been accomplished and published to date on the clinical evaluation of DW-MRI as a viable candidate for use as an early imaging biomarker of treatment response. Overall, each of the studies reviewed has uniformly presented data supporting the concept that DW-MRI can be used as an early surrogate biomarker for tumour response and that changes in diffusion values were detected in tumours responding to therapy (Table 10.1). This is in itself a remarkable finding especially when considering the myriad of tumour types, tumour sites, different MRI manufacturers, institutions and approaches to analysis reportedly used in these studies. The vast majority of studies showed that tumour ADC values tended to increase following successful intervention. In three of the studies presented in Table 10.1 a positive response was detected as a decrease in ADC rather than an increase; all of these studies were related to rectal cancer (Dzik-Jurasz et al. 2002; Hein et al. 2003; Kremser et al. 2003). Interpretation of these published results must be made with the understanding that changes within a tumour mass can occur dynamically over time during therapy and thus the timing of the acquired measurement may impact upon the finding or measured changes. For example, two of the studies involving rectal cancer (Hein et al. 2003; Kremser et al. 2003) in fact showed a brief, transient increase in ADC values in the first week posttreatment initiation followed by a decrease over the ensuing several weeks. It was confirmed by histology (Hein et al. 2003) that chemoradiation of rectal carcinoma resulted in increased interstitial fibrosis which could have a net effect of reducing ADC values in those tumour regions. In addition, it was pointed out by the authors that regions of obvious necrosis as observed by MR imaging within the tumour mass were also not included in the VOI definitions prescribed over the tumour mass which would bias the measurement to lower ADC values. The third study reporting a significant decrease in rectal cancer ADC values following treatment only measured pre-and posttreatment values (Dzik-Jurasz et al. 2002). Thus, as indicated in this and the previous study (Hein et al. 2003) the decrease was attributable to therapy-induced fibrosis in the responding tumours. Therefore, the three papers reporting decreased ADC values correlated with response to treatment were observed in rectal carcinomas which could be accounted for by scar tissue or fibrosis formation. The summation of the total data for clinical cancer studies reported to date shows that treatment-induced cell death can be detected in responding tumours as an increased ADC value in those regions. Heterogeneity of response within the tumour mass can complicate the analysis as well. Due to different acquisition and analytical post-processing protocols available to investigators, efforts have been made to reach a consensus to provide for standardization across institutions (Padhani et al. 2009). Standards are needed for data acquisition, post-image processing, timing of evaluation, and the method used to generate the quantifiable metrics used to report treatment response. Validation of DW-MRI is also needed: this will require a large, prospective, multi-institutional trial that applies DW-MRI in a standardized fashion between sites. Future opportunities may also be developed for expanding the clinical utility of DW-MRI which may include, for example, incorporation into adaptive chemo- and radiotherapy protocols to allow for alteration of agents or doses based on intra-therapy evaluation of early ADC changes or for quantifying multifocal disease response using whole-body DWI techniques (Kwee et al. 2008).

Acknowledgement   The authors of this chapter were supported in part by research grants from the NIH (U24CA83099, 1PO1CA85878 and 1P50CA93990).

References

Broet P, Scholl SM, de la Rochefordiere A et al (1999) Short and long-term effects on survival in breast cancer patients treated by primary chemotherapy: an updated analysis of a randomized trial. Breast Cancer Res Treat 58: 151–156

Buzdar AU, Ibrahim NK, Francis D et al (2005) Significantly higher pathologic complete remission rate after neoadjuvant therapy with trastuzumab, paclitaxel, and epirubicin chemotherapy: results of a randomized trial in human epidermal growth factor receptor 2-positive operable breast cancer. J Clin Oncol 23: 3676–3685

Byun WM, Shin SO, Chang Y et al (2002) Diffusion-weighted MR imaging of metastatic disease of the spine: assessment of response to therapy. AJNR Am J Neuroradiol 23: 906–912

Chang J, Powles TJ, Allred DC et al (1999) Biologic markers as predictors of clinical outcome from systemic therapy for primary operable breast cancer. J Clin Oncol 17: 3058–3063

Chenevert TL, Stegman LD, Taylor JM et al (2000) Diffusion magnetic resonance imaging: an early surrogate marker of therapeutic efficacy in brain tumours. J Natl Cancer Inst 92: 2029–2036

Choi H, Charnsangavej C, de Castro Faria S et al (2004) CT evaluation of the response of gastrointestinal stromal tumours after imatinib mesylate treatment: a quantitative analysis correlated with FDG PET findings. AJR Am J Roentgenol 183: 1619–1628

Cui Y, Zhang XP, Sun YS et al (2008) Apparent diffusion coefficient: potential imaging biomarker for prediction and early detection of response to chemotherapy in hepatic metastases. Radiology 248: 894–900

Dudeck O, Zeile M, Pink D et al (2008) Diffusion-weighted magnetic resonance imaging allows monitoring of anticancer treatment effects in patients with soft-tissue sarcomas. J Magn Reson Imaging 27: 1109–1113

Dzik-Jurasz A, Domenig C, George M et al (2002) Diffusion MRI for prediction of response of rectal cancer to chemoradiation. Lancet 360: 307–308

Einarsdottir H, Karlsson M, Wejde J et al (2004) Diffusion-weighted MRI of soft tissue tumours. Eur Radiol 14: 959–963

Galbán CJ, Mukherji SK, Chenevert TL, Meyer CR, Hamstra DA, Bland PH, Johnson TD, Moffat BA, Rehemtulla A, Eisbruch A and Ross BD. Parametric Response Map Analysis of DW-MRI Scans of Head and Neck Cancer Patients Provides for Early Detection of Therapeutic Efficacy. Translational Oncology (2009), 2(3): 184–190

Gianni L, Baselga J, Eiermann W et al (2005) Feasibility and tolerability of sequential doxorubicin/paclitaxel followed by cyclophosphamide, methotrexate, and fluorouracil and its effects on tumour response as preoperative therapy. Clin Cancer Res 11: 8715–8721

Hamstra DA, Chenevert TL, Moffat BA et al (2005) Evaluation of the functional diffusion map as an early biomarker of time-to-progression and overall survival in high-grade glioma. Proc Natl Acad Sci U S A 102: 16759–16764

Hamstra DA, Galbán CJ, Meyer CR et al (2008) Functional diffusion map as an early imaging biomarker for high-grade glioma: correlation with conventional radiologic response and overall survival. J Clin Oncol 26: 3387–3394

Harry VN, Semple SI, Gilbert FJ et al (2008) Diffusion-weighted magnetic resonance imaging in the early detection of response to chemoradiation in cervical cancer. Gynecol Oncol 111: 213–220

Hayashida Y, Yakushiji T, Awai K et al (2006) Monitoring therapeutic responses of primary bone tumours by diffusion-weighted image: initial results. Eur Radiol 16: 2637–2643

Hein PA, Kremser C, Judmaier W et al (2003) Diffusion-weighted magnetic resonance imaging for monitoring diffusion changes in rectal carcinoma during combined, preoperative chemoradiation: preliminary results of a prospective study. Eur J Radiol 45: 214–222

Huang CF, Chou HH, Tu HT et al (2008) Diffusion magnetic resonance imaging as an evaluation of the response of brain metastases treated by stereotactic radiosurgery. Surg Neurol 69: 62–68; discussion 68

Humphries PD, Sebire NJ, Siegel MJ et al (2007) Tumours in pediatric patients at diffusion-weighted MR imaging: apparent diffusion coefficient and tumour cellularity. Radiology 245: 848–854

Jaffe CC (2006) Measures of response: RECIST, WHO, and new alternatives. J Clin Oncol 24: 3245–3251

Jager HR, Waldman AD, Benton C et al (2005) Differential chemosensitivity of tumour components in a malignant oligodendroglioma: assessment with diffusion-weighted, perfusion-weighted, and serial volumetric MR imaging. AJNR Am J Neuroradiol 26: 274–278

Kamel R, Bluemke DA, Eng J et al (2006) The role of functional MR imaging in the assessment of tumour response after chemoembolization in patients with hepatocellular carcinoma. J Vasc Interv Radiol 17: 505–512

Kim S, Loevner LA, Quon H et al (2008) Monitoring response to chemoradiotherapy of squamous cell carcinoma of the head and neck using diffusion weighted MRI. In: International Society for Magnetic Reasonance in Medicine, Toronto

Kinoshita M, Hashimoto N, Goto T et al (2008) Fractional anisotropy and tumour cell density of the tumour core show positive correlation in diffusion tensor magnetic resonance imaging of malignant brain tumours. Neuroimage 43: 29–35

Koh DM, Scurr E, Collins DJ et al (2007) Predicting response of colorectal hepatic metastases: value of pre-treatment apparent diffusion coefficients. AJR Am J Roentgenol 188: 1001–1008

Kransdorf MJ, Murphey MD (2000) Radiologic evaluation of soft-tissue masses: a current perspective. AJR Am J Roentgenol 175: 575–587

Kremser C, Judmaier W, Hein P et al (2003) Preliminary results on the influence of chemoradiation on apparent diffusion coefficients of primary rectal carcinoma measured by magnetic resonance imaging. Strahlenther Onkol 179: 641–649

Kuerer HM, Newman LA, Smith TL et al (1999) Clinical course of breast cancer patients with complete pathologic primary tumour and axillary lymph node response to doxorubicin-based neoadjuvant chemotherapy. J Clin Oncol 17: 460–469

Kwee TC, Takahara T, Ochiai R et al (2008) Diffusion-weighted whole-body imaging with background body signal suppression (DWIBS): features and potential applications in oncology. Eur Radiol 18: 1937–1952

Le Bihan D (1991) Molecular diffusion nuclear magnetic resonance imaging. Magn Reson Q 7: 1–30

Le Bihan D, Breton E, Lallemand D et al (1988) Separation of diffusion and perfusion in intravoxel incoherent motion MR imaging. Radiology 168: 497–505

Le Bihan D. See the thinking brain: a story about water. Bull Mem Acad R Med Belg. 2008;163(1-2):105-21

Lee KC, Bradley DA, Hussain M et al (2007) A feasibility study evaluating the functional diffusion map as a predictive imaging biomarker for detection of treatment response in a patient with metastatic prostate cancer to the bone. Neoplasia 9: 1003–1011

Lidar Z, Mardor Y, Jonas T et al (2004) Convection-enhanced delivery of paclitaxel for the treatment of recurrent malignant glioma: a phase I/II clinical study. J Neurosurg 100: 472–479

Makris A, Powles TJ, Ashley SE et al (1998) A reduction in the requirements for mastectomy in a randomized trial of neoadjuvant chemoendocrine therapy in primary breast cancer. Ann Oncol 9: 1179–1184

Mardor Y, Pfeffer R, Spiegelmann R et al (2003) Early detection of response to radiation therapy in patients with brain malignancies using conventional and high b-value diffusion-weighted magnetic resonance imaging. J Clin Oncol 21: 1094–1100

Mardor Y, Roth Y, Lidar Z et al (2001) Monitoring response to convection-enhanced taxol delivery in brain tumour patients using diffusion-weighted magnetic resonance imaging. Cancer Res 61: 4971–4973

Mauriac L, MacGrogan G, Avril A et al (1999) Neoadjuvant chemotherapy for operable breast carcinoma larger than 3 cm: a unicentre randomized trial with a 124-month median follow-up. Institut Bergonie Bordeaux Groupe Sein (IBBGS). Ann Oncol 10: 47–52

Moffat BA, Chenevert TL, Lawrence TS et al (2005) Functional diffusion map: a noninvasive MRI biomarker for early stratification of clinical brain tumour response. Proc Natl Acad Sci U S A 102: 5524–5529

Nakayama T, Yoshida S, Fujii Y et al (2008) [Use of diffusion-weighted MRI in monitoring response of lymph node metastatic bladder cancer treated with chemotherary]. Nippon Hinyokika Gakkai Zasshi 99: 737–741

Padhani AR, Liu G, Mu-Koh D et al (2009) Diffusion-weighted magnetic resonance imaging as a cancer biomarker: consensus and recommendations. Neoplasia 11: 102–125

Pickles MD, Gibbs P, Lowry M et al (2006) Diffusion changes precede size reduction in neoadjuvant treatment of breast cancer. Magn Reson Imaging 24: 843–847

Robertson JF, Ellis IO, Pearson D et al (1994) Biological factors of prognostic significance in locally advanced breast cancer. Breast Cancer Res Treat 29: 259–264

Romond EH, Perez EA, Bryant J et al (2005) Trastuzumab plus adjuvant chemotherapy for operable HER2-positive breast cancer. N Engl J Med 353: 1673–1684

Sadeghi N, D'Haene N, Decaestecker C et al (2008) Apparent diffusion coefficient and cerebral blood volume in brain gliomas: relation to tumour cell density and tumour microvessel density based on stereotactic biopsies. AJNR Am J Neuroradiol 29: 476–482

Sasaki M, Yamada K, Watanabe Y et al (2008) Variability in absolute apparent diffusion coefficient values across different platforms may be substantial: a multivendor, multi-institutional comparison study. Radiology 249: 624–630

Sataloff DM, Mason BA, Prestipino AJ et al (1995) Pathologic response to induction chemotherapy in locally advanced carcinoma of the breast: a determinant of outcome. J Am Coll Surg 180: 297–306

Scholl SM, Fourquet A, Asselain B et al (1994) Neoadjuvant versus adjuvant chemotherapy in premenopausal patients with tumours considered too large for breast conserving surgery: preliminary results of a randomised trial: S6. Eur J Cancer 30A: 645–652

Schubert MI, Wilke M, Muller-Weihrich S et al (2006) Diffusion-weighted magnetic resonance imaging of treatment-associated changes in recurrent and residual medulloblastoma: preliminary observations in three children. Acta Radiol 47: 1100–1104

Sharma U, Danishad KK, Seenu V et al (2009) Longitudinal study of the assessment by MRI and diffusion-weighted imaging of tumour response in patients with locally advanced breast cancer undergoing neoadjuvant chemotherapy. NMR Biomed 22: 104–113

Slamon DJ, Romond EH, Perez EA (2006) Advances in adjuvant therapy for breast cancer. Clin Adv Hematol Oncol 4 (suppl 1): 4–9; discussion suppl 10; quiz 12 p following suppl 10

Strumberg D, Richly H, Hilger RA et al (2005) Phase I clinical and pharmacokinetic study of the novel Raf kinase and vascular endothelial growth factor receptor inhibitor BAY 43–9006 in patients with advanced refractory solid tumours. J Clin Oncol 23: 965–972

Theilmann RJ, Borders R, Trouard TP et al (2004) Changes in water mobility measured by diffusion MRI predict response of metastatic breast cancer to chemotherapy. Neoplasia 6: 831–837

Therasse P, Arbuck SG, Eisenhauer EA et al (2000) New guidelines to evaluate the response to treatment in solid tumours. European Organization for Research and Treatment of Cancer, National Cancer Institute of the United States, National Cancer Institute of Canada. J Natl Cancer Inst 92: 205–216

Thoeny HC, De Keyzer F, Chen F, Vandecaveye V, Verbeken EK, Ahmed B, Sun X, Ni Y, Bosmans H, Hermans R, van Oosterom A, Marchal G, Landuyt W. Diffusion-weighted magnetic resonance imaging allows noninvasive in vivo monitoring of the effects of combretastatin a-4 phosphate after repeated administration. Neoplasia. 2005,7:779-87.

Tomura N, Narita K, Izumi J et al (2006) Diffusion changes in a tumour and peritumoural tissue after stereotactic irradiation for brain tumours: possible prediction of treatment response. J Comput Assist Tomogr 30: 496–500

Uhl M, Saueressig U, van Buiren M et al (2006) Osteosarcoma: preliminary results of in vivo assessment of tumour necrosis after chemotherapy with diffusion- and perfusion-weighted magnetic resonance imaging. Invest Radiol 41: 618–623

Wolmark N, Wang J, Mamounas E et al (2001) Preoperative chemotherapy in patients with operable breast cancer: nine-year results from National Surgical Adjuvant Breast and Bowel Project B-18. J Natl Cancer Inst Monogr (30): 96–102

Yankeelov TE, Lepage M, Chakravarthy A et al (2007) Integration of quantitative DCE-MRI and ADC mapping to monitor treatment response in human breast cancer: initial results. Magn Reson Imaging 25: 1–13

Zelhof B, Pickles M, Liney G et al (2008) Correlation of diffusion-weighted magnetic resonance data with cellularity in prostate cancer. BJU Int 103: 883–888

DW-MRI Assessment of Treatment
Response to Minimally Invasive Therapy

11

ELENI LIAPI and IHAB R. KAMEL

SUMMARY

Minimally invasive interventional oncology therapies consist of various therapeutic catheter-based (such as transcatheter arterial chemoembolization) and percutaneous ablative approaches (such as radiofrequency ablation) using imaging for guidance to treat solid malignancies, and have recently emerged as a major therapeutic alternative against cancer. Monitoring tumour response to these therapies is currently performed by measuring changes in tumour size with contrast-enhanced computed tomography (CT) or magnetic resonance (MR) imaging. However, morphological tumour changes occur relatively late in the course of therapy, while functional changes can occur prior to tumour size changes. Since minimally invasive therapies cause tumour cell membrane destruction and/or obliteration of tumour microvessels, with subsequent alterations in the microscopic movement of water molecules, DW-MRI seems to be a potential non-invasive tool for measuring early functional tumour response to such therapies.

11.1

Introduction

Diffusion-weighted MR imaging (DW-MRI) is a functional imaging technique that explores the random motion of water molecules in the body (LE BIHAN 1988). DW-MRI was initially applied to the evaluation of ischaemic stroke for the detection of early changes within the brain before any visible conventional morphological abnormality could be seen (SCHAEFER et al. 2000). In the 1990s, the advent of the fast echo-planar MR imaging technique minimized the effect

ELENI LIAPI, MD
IHAB R. KAMEL, MD, PhD
The Russell H Morgan Department of Radiology and Radiological Sciences, The Johns Hopkins Hospital, Baltimore, MD 21287, USA

of gross physiologic respiratory and cardiac motion and DW-MRI of the abdomen became possible (TURNER 1990, 1991; NAMIMOTO et al. 1997). In this chapter, we focus on DW-MRI as a quantitative biomarker that is able to assess treatment response to minimally invasive interventional oncology therapies. Since DW-MRI is quick to perform (typically 1–5 min) and does not require the administration of contrast medium, DW-MRI sequences can be appended to existing imaging protocols without a significant increase in the examination time.

11.2
Minimally Invasive Treatments

The field of interventional oncology is built upon a growing number of minimally invasive treatments, which uses image guidance to treat solid malignancies. These novel treatment options have recently assumed greater importance in the battle against cancer. Minimally invasive treatments include catheter-based and percutaneous ablative treatments (LIAPI et al. 2007). Catheter-based therapies such as transcatheter arterial chemoembolization, a technique now widely applied to the treatment of hepatic malignancies, aims to deliver treatment to a target tumour volume by means of a percutaneously placed intra-arterial catheter within an artery that supplies the tumour (BROWN et al. 2006). As a result, the treatment, which is usually a mixture of vascular embolization particles (to reduce local blood flow) and therapeutic agent (e.g. chemotherapy or radio-pharmacy), can be directed locally to the site of disease. Transcatheter intra-arterial drug delivery has also been proposed for palliative treatment of bone, pulmonary, renal, oral cavity or anterior oropharynx tumours (CHIRAS et al. 2004; KONYA et al. 2004; KOVACS 2005; VOGL et al. 2005). By contrast, percutaneous tumour ablative therapies are represented by techniques such as radiofrequency ablation (RFA), high intensity focused ultrasound (HIFU) tumour ablation, thermal ablation, cryoablation and microware ablation. Of these, RFA is most widely used, especially for the treatment of liver tumours. However, these techniques have also rapidly expanded to include treatment of a variety of other solid tumours (renal, bone, prostate, lung, breast, and adrenal tumours) (MAYO-SMITH et al. 2004; BELAND et al. 2005; CALLSTROM et al. 2006; JINDAL et al. 2006; SUSINI et al. 2007).

Using such minimally invasive techniques, substantial tumour kill is usually achieved by directly applying chemicals or causing physical alterations to the solid malignancies (GOLDBERG et al. 2003). In comparison to traditional cancer treatments, these image-guided loco-regional therapies appear to have reduced morbidity and mortality, as well as lower procedural costs. In addition, they can be performed on an outpatient basis, repeated over time, and used in conjunction with other cancer treatments.

In part, the reasons for the successful and expanding use of minimally invasive therapies may be attributed to advances in radiological imaging, which has altered patients' management by offering not only early tumour detection but also effective monitoring of tumour response to therapy. Using novel imaging techniques, there is also the potential for individual early tailoring of therapy. The goal of any minimally invasive therapy is the complete ablation of any given tumour with minimal damage to the surrounding liver parenchyma. While cure is the ultimate clinical endpoint for any form of medical treatment, valid endpoints of measuring tumour response to therapy are also considered favourable endpoints for all minimally invasive therapies.

Standardized criteria for measuring tumour response to treatment have been established by the World Health Organization (WHO) and by the response evaluation criteria in solid tumours (RECIST). These guidelines use anatomic imaging with one- or two-dimensional diameter measurements to define tumour size for all aspects of cancer patient management from diagnosis and staging, to monitoring response to therapy and disease progression. However, these measurements are often inadequate for monitoring the acute effects of minimally invasive therapies, or interventional treatment that cause little or a slow reduction in tumour size (LIAPI et al. 2008). Hence, functional imaging modalities, such as DW-MRI, are currently being investigated as potential biomarkers for cancer therapies. Unlike anatomical imaging DW-MRI allows the detection of microstructural changes during treatment which can precede a change in tumour size.

11.3
The Advantages of DW-MRI in the Assessment of Tumour Response to Minimally Invasive Therapies

As any effective anti-cancer therapy, minimally invasive treatments such as chemoembolization or radioembolization result in tumour lysis, loss of cell membrane integrity, increased extracellular space, and therefore an increase in water diffusion, which can be detected by DW-MRI. DW-MRI has several potential advantages over other methods (e.g. CT, PET and tissue biopsy) for the evaluation of tumour response to therapy (THOENY et al. 2005):

- It is non-invasive, without ionizing radiation exposure, does not require contrast medium administration and has a relatively short examination time. The technique is easy to repeat, allowing close follow-up during and after cancer treatment.
- Image post-processing is less time-consuming for DW-MRI than for other methods (e.g. dynamic contrast-enhanced MR imaging (DCE-MRI)). In combination with conventional MR imaging, morphologic and functional changes can be assessed at the same examination.
- Diffusion-weighted MR imaging allows monitoring and evaluation of the entire tumour. This is important because of the heterogeneity that may occur within tumours. Tissue sampling is invasive and may not be representative of the entire tumour. Diffusion-weighted MR imaging provides quantitative information (ADC) that reflects microscopic structures and tissue organization; such as cell density, cell membrane integrity and tissue necrosis. Thus, viable tumour can potentially be differentiated from a necrotic tumour using DW-MRI. Tissue with high cellular density results in lower ADC, whereas necrotic tissue returns high ADC secondary to cell lysis and loss of membrane integrity (THOENY et al. 2005). Since DW-MRI is highly sensitive to molecular displacements, it may show biophysical intra-tumoural changes, even at the very early stages of treatment.
- As the quantitative parameter of DW-MRI, the ADC reflects not only diffusion but also perfusion of microvessels if a large range of b values ($b = 0, 50, 100, 150, 200, 250, 300, 500, 750$ and $1,000 \, s/mm^2$) is used. ADC measurements with low b values ($b < 100 \, s/mm^2$) may provide information related to perfusion effects, while ADC calculated using the higher b-values (e.g. $b = 500, 750, 1,000 \, s/mm^2$) shows mainly diffusion effects. Whenever desirable, the application of high b-values may reduce the influence of perfusion and may approximate true diffusion (THOENY et al. 2005).

11.4
Technical Considerations and Image Analysis

11.4.1
Image Acquisition

In the implementation of DW-MRI for assessment of tumour response, two main techniques can be used: breath-hold imaging and non-breath-hold imaging.

Breath-hold imaging allows a target volume (e.g. liver) to be rapidly assessed. The images retain good anatomic details and are usually not degraded by respiratory motion or volume averaging. Small lesions may be better perceived and the quantification of ADC is theoretically more accurate than with a non-breath-hold technique. The image acquisition time at each breath-hold is 20–30 s, and imaging is typically completed in a few breath-holds. The disadvantages of breath-hold imaging include a limited number of b-value images that can be acquired over the duration of a breath-hold, poorer signal-to-noise ratio compared with multiple averaging methods, and greater sensitivity to pulsatile and susceptibility artefacts (KOH et al. 2007).

Non-breath-hold spin-echo echo-planar imaging (EPI) combined with fat suppression is a versatile technique that can be used as a general purpose DW-MRI sequence in the body and for whole-body imaging. Multiple slice excitation and signal averaging over a longer duration improve the signal-to-noise and contrast-to-noise ratios. Thin sections can be achieved (4–5 mm), thus improving spatial resolution and enabling multiplanar image reformats. Furthermore, the longer acquisition time with non-breath-hold imaging provides flexibility in the use of multiple (>5) or of high b-values. Another advantage is the potential of this technique to be applied even in severely ill patients who are unable to hold their breath for more than 10 s. However, the image acquisition time using this technique is longer compared with breath-hold imaging, typically 3–6 min depending on the coverage required and the number of b-values used, and evaluation of tumour heterogeneity may be compromised by the degree of motion and volume averaging (KOH et al. 2007).

In our institution, breath-hold DW-MRI is the preferred method of image acquisition. Imaging is performed on a 1.5 T clinical MR scanner with a phased-array torso coil using breath-hold diffusion-weighted EPI. The typical scan parameters include: matrix = 128 × 128; slice thickness = 8 mm; interslice gap = 2 mm; b-values = 0 and 500 s/mm^2; TR = 5,000–6,500 ms; TE = 110 ms; receiver bandwidth = 64 kHz. This imaging protocol is always complemented by conventional unenhanced and contrast-enhanced MR imaging. DW-MRI measurements with ADC calculations are made using at least two b-values (e.g. b = 0 s/mm^2 and other b-values from 0 to 1,000 s/mm^2). The b-values of 500 and 750 s/mm^2 are most commonly applied in our practice to assess tumour response (Liapi et al. 2008; Kamel et al. 2009).

In the context of minimally invasive therapy, target lesions are lesions that have been treated. For response assessment, we currently perform ADC and anatomical size measurements according to the RECIST criteria (Therasse et al. 2000) on all target lesions. Non-target lesions may also be quantitatively evaluated and compared with target lesions.

The size of target lesions to be evaluated with DW-MRI however, may be limited by breathing and motion artefacts. We prefer to choose targeted lesions of >2 cm in diameter, so as to avoid degradation of the ADC evaluation by motion. Target liver lesions that are close to the diaphragm also pose a challenge to DW-MRI evaluation, as they are more sensitive to motion, susceptibility artefacts, as well as artefacts arising from the heart.

11.4.2
Measurement Time Points

DW-MRI measurements are performed at baseline (before treatment) and at regular intervals after treatment. The choice of measurement time points may be influenced by the nature of therapy or drug administered. In our institution, we usually perform DW-MRI at baseline and every 4–6 weeks after minimally invasive treatment. However, in selected instances, such as in patients receiving transarterial chemoembolization (TACE) for hepatocellular carcinoma (HCC), observed changes in ADC values can be seen as early as 24 h after treatment (Kamel et al. 2009). Statistically significant changes in ADC values have also been recorded at 1–2 weeks following TACE (Kamel et al. 2009) and at 1 month following treatment with ^{90}Y microspheres for irresectable HCC (Rhee et al. 2008). In patients with HCC, ethiodized oil, which is used in conjunction during TACE, does not create any artefacts or adversely affect the DW-MR imaging.

11.4.3
Image Analysis

Image analysis is performed by using dedicated software at the post-processing console and by positioning a region of interest (ROI) or volume of interest (VOI) over a section or volume of tumour. Volumetric measurements may be performed by summing up the results in individual ROIs in consecutive image sections and the results averaged. The individual voxel values in each ROI can also be used to generate ADC histograms. The histogram-based approach can also be helpful to visualize tumour response to treatment by a change in the shape or distribution of the histogram.

At our institution, we measure ADC values by placing a circular ROI on the ADC map corresponding to the level at which the tumour axial diameter is maximum, encompassing as much of the tumour as possible. We may also selectively place additional ROIs to interrogate region variations in the ADC values within large and heterogeneous tumours. The ROIs may be placed directly onto the ADC map or copied onto the map from those drawn on morphological or the b-value DW-MR images. In cases with significant geometric distortions, we may manually reposition the ROI based on anatomical references. When recording the results, we usually record the mean ADC value together with the standard deviation (SD). The SD provides an estimate of the variation in ADC values within the tumour ROI. We do not actively exclude regions of necrosis from our ROI. For comparison, we usually also place ROIs over other tissues (such as the liver, spleen or paraspinal muscles) to enable us to estimate the tumour-to-background signal ratios or used as controls.

11.4.4
Pre- and Post-Treatment ADC Evaluation

In order to maintain study design consistency and reproducibility, as well as being able to accurately measure tumour response after treatment, it is important to record measurements in a traceable and uniform manner. Study comparisons should be performed on a single workstation and always side-by-side. ROI positioning for ADC measurement should be recorded by saving the axial image showing all pertinent information (e.g. mean/median ADC value, SD). Selection of ROI positioning should be described in detail in the study design. As mentioned above, we prefer to place tumour ROI at the level of the tumour's maximum axial diameter. In this way, we are able to compare baseline to post-treatment studies in a uniform way.

For clinical trials, it is important to understand how the ADC value of a tumour varies over time with a particular treatment. As a tumour responds to treatment, the ADC is likely to rise, but this may undergo re-equilibrium after a period of time, leading to a decrease in the ADC (KOH et al. 2007). Hence, optimal timing of the measurement is important to maximize the chance of detecting a significant treatment effect.

11.5
Application of ADC for the Assessment of Minimally Invasive Therapies in Oncology

Following treatment with transcatheter arterial chemoembolization, the integrity of cancerous cell membranes is compromised by the lack of nutrients with vascular shutdown and the direct cytotoxic chemotherapeutic effect. Subsequently, the fractional volume of the interstitial space increases, due to apoptosis and cell loss (GESCHWIND et al. 2000). These changes increase the mobility of free water in the damaged tissue, which is reflected by an increase in the ADC value. Thus, successful therapy is expected to lead to a concomitant increase in ADC, a feature that has been observed in animal and human studies.

Following treatment, changes in ADC may be heterogeneous within a tumour (i.e. may be more pronounced in the tumour periphery than in the centre) (GESCHWIND et al. 2000). However, it is the ADC of the entire tumour that is usually used to provide information on the changes in the tumour microenvironment in response to treatment. Measuring ADC over the entire tumour may also minimize selection bias of the investigator when evaluating the tumour. Separate analysis of the centre and periphery of tumour could provide more detailed and precise information of response to treatment (THOENY et al. 2005).

11.5.1
Preclinical Studies

The results of animal studies have shown that following minimally invasive therapies, an increase in the ADC value may be observed in those responding to treatment (GESCHWIND et al. 2000; DENG et al. 2006a,b;

YOUN et al. 2008). Furthermore, treatment effects can be observed within the first 24 h after initiating treatment due to initial apoptosis and cellular swelling, which results in a transient decrease in the ADC. Cellular swelling is followed by a reduction of cell volume through the process of membrane blebbing and cell lysis. As a result, increased displacement of water molecules occurs in the extracellular space and water may also move more freely between intracellular and extracellular compartments. Further increases in water diffusion are attributable to treatment-induced necrosis (GESCHWIND et al. 2000) (Fig. 11.1). Changes in water diffusion might be seen before changes in tumour volume and, thus, DW-MRI has the potential to be an early biomarker of therapy response. A list of studies evaluating the use of ADC for the assessment of treatment response in animal models is summarized in Table 11.1.

11.5.2
Clinical Studies

There is a growing appreciation that measurement of response is often inadequately addressed by RECIST when tumours are treated with novel molecularly targeted agents or by interventional oncology therapies. These types of treatment can result in a meaningful clinical impact without significantly changing the tumour dimensions (KAMEL et al. 2003; LIAPI et al. 2008).

Functional MR imaging using DW-MRI has been used to evaluate tumour response after transarterial chemoembolization (TACE) in HCC (KAMEL et al. 2003, 2006; CHEN 2006), neuroendocrine metastases (LIAPI et al. 2008), breast metastases(BUIJS et al. 2007), ocular melanoma metastases(BUIJS et al. 2008) and metastatic leiomyosarcoma (VOSSEN et al. 2008). In an initial clinical study, patients with HCC underwent chemoembolization followed by resection, and a direct correlation was found between increasing ADC and increasing necrosis within the surgical specimens ($r = 0.95$; $p < 0.05$) (KAMEL et al. 2003). Following this study, other studies confirmed that individuals with HCC who responded to chemoembolization treatment showed a significant increase in the ADC values after therapy (KAMEL et al. 2003, 2006; BUIJS et al. 2007, 2008; LIAPI et al. 2008; VOSSEN et al. 2008). Interestingly, a significant increase in the ADC values following TACE in patients with HCC could be seen as early as 12–24 h after treatment in patients who were subsequently defined as responders by RECIST criteria (KAMEL et al. 2009).

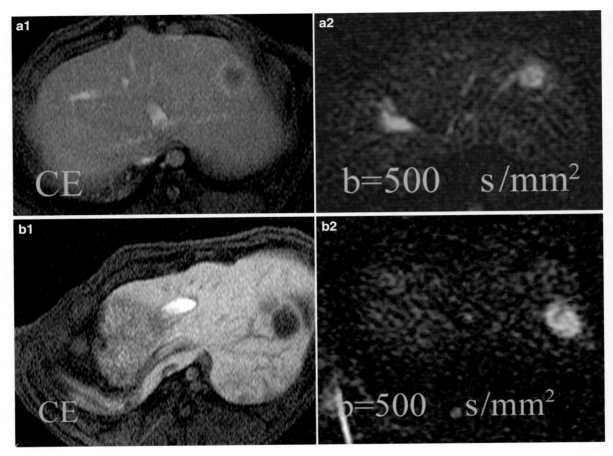

Fig. 11.1. Axial contrast-enhanced T1-weighted images of rabbit liver implanted with VX-2 and corresponding axial DW-MR images ($b = 500\,\text{s/mm}^2$) (**a**) before and (**b**) 24 h after chemoembolization. The mean ADC value increased from 1.65×10^{-3} to $1.91 \times 10^{-3}\,\text{mm}^2/\text{s}$ (*not shown*)

Table 11.1. Preclinical studies evaluating DW-MRI as a surrogate for treatment response

Study	Tumour type	Type of minimally invasive therapy	Timing	Conclusion
Preclinical				
Geschwind et al. (2000)	VX-2	TACE	2–3 days	ADC values were significantly higher in the area of tumour necrosis than in the area of viable tumour
Yuan et al. (2007)	VX-2	TACE	6–48 h	With low *b*-values (100 s/mm²) ADC values were lowest at 16 h after TACE
Youn et al. (2008)	VX-2	TACE	1 week	The ADC values of necrotic tumours were significantly higher than those in viable tumours ($p < 0.01$)
Ohira et al. (2009)	VX-2	Radiofrequency ablation	3 days	The ADC value of ablated VX2 tumours ($1.52 \pm 0.24 \times 10^{-3}\,\text{mm}^2/\text{s}$) was significantly higher than that of untreated tumours ($1.09 \pm 0.12 \times 10^{-3}$; $p < 0.05$)
Ohira et al. (2009)	VX-2	Radiofrequency ablation	3 days	Both ADC value and FDG-PET are potentially useful markers for monitoring the early effects of RFA

However, in a more recent study evaluating DW-MRI as a predictor of HCC recurrence after TACE, DW-MRI was found not to be a reliable predictor of local HCC recurrence after TACE as compared with gadolinium-enhanced MR imaging (Goshima et al. 2008).

Diffusion-weighted imaging has been also utilized in the assessment of patients with HCC and colorectal hepatic metastases following radioembolization (Kamel et al. 2007, 2009; Rhee et al. 2008). In these studies, responders showed a significant increase in the ADC values after TACE. Table 11.2 summarizes the various clinical studies applying DW-MRI after interventional oncological therapies that have been reported in the published literature. Clinical examples of DW-MR imaging for evaluating the effects of chemoembolization are shown in Figs. 11.2–11.4.

Table 11.2. Clinical studies evaluating DW-MRI as a surrogate for treatment response

Study	Tumour type	Type of minimally invasive therapy	Timing	Conclusion
Clinical				
Kamel et al. (2003)	HCC	TACE	27–42 days	ADC values were greater in non-enhancing (presumed necrotic) tumours than in enhancing (presumed viable) tumours. These values had a high correlation with the degree of tumour necrosis at pathology ($r = 0.95$)
Liapi et al. (2005)	Uterine fibroids	Embolization	99–239 days	Decrease in ADC late after treatment in treated fibroids ($p < 0.01$) but not in surrounding normal tissue
Jacobs et al. (2005)	Uterine fibroids	High-frequency ultrasound	Early and 6 months	Initial decrease in ADC ($p = 0.001$) followed by late increase ($p < 0.001$) in treated lesions
Deng et al. (2006 b)	HCC	^{90}Y microspheres	29–70 days	Tumour ADC increased significantly approximately 40 days after ^{90}Y microspheres administration
Kamel et al. (2006)	HCC	TACE	4–6 weeks	Increased ADC ($p < 0.03$) and decrease in AFP but no response by RECIST
Kamel et al. (2007)	HCC	^{90}Y microspheres	4 weeks	Increased ADC in treated ($p < 0.001$) but not untreated lesions
Rhee et al. (2008)	HCC	^{90}Y microspheres	1 and 3 months	The mean baseline ADC significantly increased at 1 month ($p = 0.02$) and at 3 months ($p = 0.02$)
Buijs et al. (2007)	Metastatic breast cancer	TACE	54 ± 33 days	Mean tumour ADC increased by 27% ($p < 0.0001$) after TACE
Kim et al. (2008)	Prostate cancer	High-frequency ultrasound	3–26 months	For prediction of local tumour progression of prostate cancer. DCE-MRI was more sensitive than T2-weighted MRI with DW-MRI, but T2-weighted MRI with DWI-MRI was more specific than DCE-MRI
Liapi et al. (2008)	Neuroendocrine hepatic metastases	TACE	206 ± 201 days	Tumour ADC values increased after treatment ($p < 0.0001$)
Vossen et al. (2008)	Metastatic leiomyosarcoma	TACE	141 ± 67 days	After TACE, mean tumour ADC increased by 20% ($p = 0.0015$)
Buijs et al. (2008)	Metastatic ocular melanoma	TACE	21–45 days	The mean tumour ADC increased 48% after TACE ($p = 0.0003$)
Kamel et al. (2009)	HCC	TACE	24 h and every week for 4 weeks	The increase in tumour ADC value was significant 1–2 weeks after therapy ($p = 0.004$), borderline significant 3 weeks after therapy

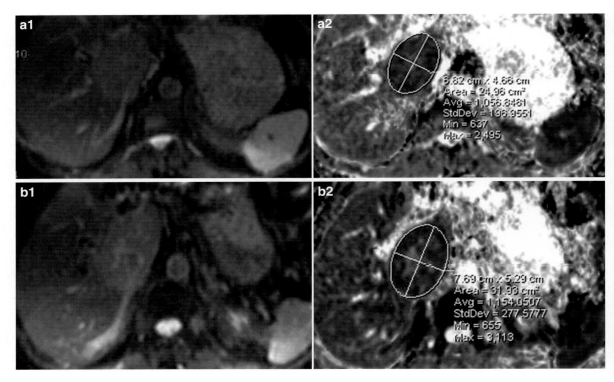

Fig. 11.2. (a1, b1) Axial DW-MRI at $b = 750$ s/mm² and corresponding **(a2, b2)** ADC maps of a hepatocellular carcinoma **(a1, a2)** before and **(b1, b2)** after chemoembolization, as well as initial increase in size of the tumour. The tumour eventually decreased in size 3 months following treatment

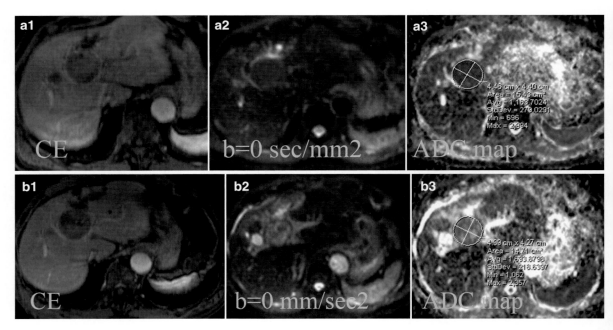

Fig. 11.3. '(a1, b1) Contrast enhanced T1-weighted images, **(a2, b2)** axial DW-MRI acquired at $b = 0$s/mm² and **(a3, b3)** corresponding ADC maps of a hepatocellular carcinoma **(a1-a3)** before and **(b1-b3)** 6 weeks after chemoembolization. There is also diminished enhancement in the tumour on the T1-weighted contrast enhanced imaging

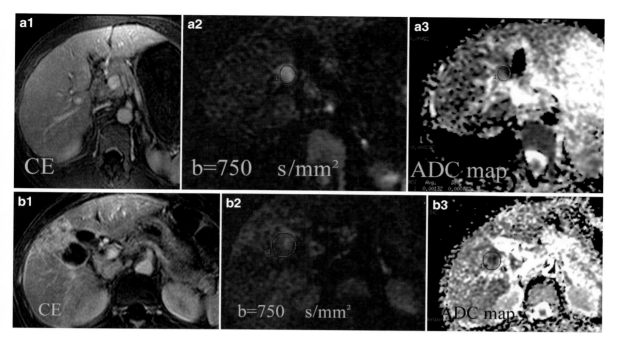

Fig. 11.4. Contrast-enhanced axial T1-weighted images, axial DW-MRI index image ($b = 750\,s/mm^2$) and corresponding ADC map of a hepatocellular carcinoma (**a1, a3**) before and (**b1, b3**) 4 weeks after chemoembolization. Note the increase in the ADC value after chemoembolization (from 1.91×10^{-3} to $2.43 \times 10^{-3}\,mm^2/s$)

A recent study evaluated the diagnostic performance of DCE-MRI and T2-weighted MR imaging with DW-MRI for predicting local tumour progression after high-intensity focused ultrasonic ablation of localized prostate cancer (KIM et al. 2008). Interestingly, for the prediction of local tumour progression of prostate cancer after high-intensity focused ultrasonic ablation, DCE-MRI was more sensitive than T2-weighted MR imaging combined with DW-MRI, but T2-weighted MR imaging combined with DW-MRI was more specific than DCE-MRI.

DW-MRI has also been used for the assessment of response to minimally invasive treatment of uterine fibroids (JACOBS 2005; LIAPI et al. 2005). Two studies addressed the use of DW-MRI after embolization or focused ultrasound ablation, and in both studies, an increase in the mean ADC value was detected in treated lesions, but differences in the timing of follow-up imaging limited the ability to interpret these data in terms of temporal evolution of the treatment response.

Studies exploring the potential for using DW-MRI for the early detection of therapeutic-induced changes in tumours are ongoing. One of the most interesting findings associated with the use of DW-MRI in cancer patients has been that ADC measurements appear to be able to predict the response of tumour to chemotherapy and radiation treatment, presumably depending on the type of treatment and the histology of tumours. This ability of DW-MRI to predict response of tumour to interventional oncological treatments has yet to be defined. Currently, there is little published data regarding the role of DW-MRI in the evaluation of disease recurrence after interventional oncological treatment; a single study showed that DW-MRI was not found to be a reliable predictor of local HCC recurrence after TACE as compared with gadolinium-enhanced MR imaging (GOSHIMA et al. 2008).

11.6
Future Developments

As the development and testing of new acquisition protocols continues to evolve, there is little doubt that DW-MRI will continue to play an important role in evaluating tumour response to minimally invasive therapies. Moreover, as the application of minimally invasive therapies expands, DW-MRI will grow to meet the needs of assessment of tumour response to such therapies.

Recently, RFA has been successfully employed for the treatment of small primary lung tumours and lung metastases in patients who are medically inoperable. Currently, fluorodeoxyglucose PET/CT, contrast-enhanced CT and conventional MR imaging are being used to assess tumour response to RFA. The recent interest in developing suitable MR techniques for the imaging of pulmonary nodules has led to the successful employment of the respiratory-triggering technique for diffusion-weighted imaging (TANAKA et al. 2009). In the near future, assessment of lung tumour response to RFA may be feasible with DW-MRI.

For monitoring thermal therapy, DW-MRI is also known to be temperature-dependent. However, in vivo studies of DW-MRI thermometry have been limited due to its high motion sensitivity. An initial study in canine prostates treated with cryoablation and high-intensity frequency ultrasound, the ADC decreased by 36% in thermally ablated prostate tissue, with no difference between tissues ablated with freezing and heating (CHEN et al. 2008). In the future, the possibility of performing temperature measurement (thermometry) using DW-MRI in the body will be further exploited and may help to monitor types of interventional therapies such as liver RFA or cryoablation in vivo during the procedure.

DW-MRI may effectively monitor early changes in tumour cellularity that are reflective of treatment response (KAMEL et al. 2009). Because the display of diffusion maps retains the anatomical spatial orientation of the diffusion values, DW-MRI also provides the possibility of assessing the regional/spatial heterogeneity of therapeutic response within a tumour. The heterogeneity of response may be accentuated in minimally invasive therapies such as TACE or radioembolization. Mapping of tumour heterogeneity and tumour response may be possible using ADC histograms and separately analysing viable and necrotic parts of tumours by appropriate ADC thresholds or by applying tissue segmentation based on information derived from other functional imaging techniques.

11.7

Conclusion

There is tremendous potential for ADC derived from DW-MRI to become an important surrogate biomarker for cancer therapeutic efficacy of minimally invasive therapies. The ability of ADC to become an accepted surrogate of therapeutic efficacy depends not only on its correlation with therapeutic efficacy

but also on its ability to predict response. Research is currently underway to determine whether the observed changes in tumour diffusion are a universal response to tumour cell death via a variety of interventions and to more fully delineate the prognostic value of DW-MRI in both an experimental and clinical setting. Evaluating ADC changes in preclinical models and correlation with histopathology will also be vital to improve our understanding of how universal ADC changes can be in assessing and predicting the effects of minimally invasive therapies.

References

Beland MD, Dupuy DE, Mayo-Smith WW (2005) Percutaneous cryoablation of symptomatic extraabdominal metastatic disease: preliminary results. Am J Roentgenol 184: 926–930

Brown DB, Geschwind J-FH, Soulen MC, et al (2006) Society of interventional radiology position statement on chemoembolization of hepatic malignancies. J Vasc Interv Radiol 17: 217–223

Buijs M, Kamel IR, Vossen JA et al (2007) Assessment of metastatic breast cancer response to chemoembolization with contrast agent enhanced and diffusion-weighted MR imaging. J Vasc Interv Radiol 18: 957–963

Buijs M, Vossen JA, Hong K et al (2008) Chemoembolization of hepatic metastases from ocular melanoma: assessment of response with contrast-enhanced and diffusion-weighted MRI. AJR Am J Roentgenol 191: 285–289

Callstrom MR, Atwell TD, Charboneau JW et al (2006) Painful metastases involving bone: percutaneous image-guided cryoablation–prospective trial interim analysis. Radiology 241: 572580

Chen CY (2006) Early response of hepatocellular carcinoma to transcatheter arterial chemoembolization: choline levels and MR diffusion constants–initial experience. Radiology 239: 448–456

Chen J, Daniel BL, Diederich CJ et al (2008) Monitoring prostate thermal therapy with diffusion-weighted MRI. Magn Reson Med 59: 1365–1372

Chiras J, Adem C, Vallee J-Nl et al (2004) Selective intra-arterial chemoembolization of pelvic and spine bone metastases. Eur Radiol 14: 1774

Deng J, Miller FH, Rhee TK et al (2006a) Diffusion-weighted MR imaging for determination of hepatocellular carcinoma response to yttrium-90 radioembolization. J Vasc Interv Radiol 17: 1195–1200

Deng J, Rhee TK, Sato KT et al (2006b) In vivo diffusion-weighted imaging of liver tumor necrosis in the VX2 rabbit model at 1.5 Tesla. Invest Radiol 41: 410–414

Geschwind JF, Artemov D, Abraham S et al (2000) Chemoembolization of liver tumor in a rabbit model: assessment of tumor cell death with diffusion-weighted MR imaging and histologic analysis. J Vasc Interv Radiol 11: 1245–1255

Goldberg SN, Charboneau JW, Dodd GD III et al (2003) Image-guided tumor ablation: proposal for standardization of terms and reporting criteria. Radiology 228: 335–345

Goshima S, Kanematsu M, Kondo H et al (2008) Evaluating local hepatocellular carcinoma recurrence post-transcatheter arterial chemoembolization: is diffusion-weighted MRI reliable as an indicator? J Magn Reson Imaging 27: 834–839

Jacobs MA (2005) Uterine fibroids: diffusion-weighted MR imaging for monitoring therapy with focused ultrasound surgery–preliminary study. Radiology 236: 196–203

Jindal G, Friedman M, Locklin J et al (2006) Palliative radiofrequency ablation for recurrent prostate cancer. Cardiovasc Intervent Radiol 29: 482–485

Kamel I, Liapi E, Reyes D et al (2009) Unresectable hepatocellular carcinoma: serial early vascular and cellular changes after transarterial chemoembolization as detected with MR imaging. Radiology; 250:466-73.

Kamel IR, Bluemke DA, Eng J et al (2006) The role of functional MR imaging in the assessment of tumor response after chemoembolization in patients with hepatocellular carcinoma. J Vasc Interv Radiol 17: 505–512

Kamel IR, Bluemke DA, Ramsey D et al (2003) Role of diffusion-weighted imaging in estimating tumor necrosis after chemoembolization of hepatocellular carcinoma. Am J Roentgenol 181: 708–710

Kamel IR, Liapi E, Reyes DK et al (2009) Unresectable hepatocellular carcinoma: serial early vascular and cellular changes after transarterial chemoembolization as detected with MR imaging. Radiology 250: 466–473

Kamel IR, Reyes DK, Liapi E et al (2007) Functional MR imaging assessment of tumor response after 90Y microsphere treatment in patients with unresectable hepatocellular carcinoma. J Vasc Interv Radiol 18: 49–56

Kim CK, Park BK, Lee HM et al (2008) MRI techniques for prediction of local tumor progression after high-intensity focused ultrasonic ablation of prostate cancer. Am J Roentgenol 190: 1180–1186

Koh DM, Collins DJ (2007) Diffusion-weighted MRI in the body: applications and challenges in oncology. AJR Am J Roentgenol 188: 1622–1635

Konya A, Van Pelt CS, Wright KC (2004) Ethiodized oil-ethanol capillary embolization in rabbit kidneys: temporal histopathologic findings. Radiology 232: 147–153

Kovacs AF (2005) Chemoembolization using Cisplatin crystals as neoadjuvant treatment of oral cancer. Cancer Biother Radiopharm 20: 267–279

Le Bihan D (1988) Separation of diffusion and perfusion in intravoxel incoherent motion MR imaging. Radiology 168: 497–505

Liapi E, Georgiades CC, Hong K et al (2007) Transcatheter arterial chemoembolization: current technique and future promise. Tech Vasc Interv Radiol 10: 2–11

Liapi E, Geschwind JF, Vossen JA et al (2008) Functional MRI evaluation of tumor response in patients with neuroendocrine hepatic metastasis treated with transcatheter arterial chemoembolization. AJR Am J Roentgenol 190: 67–73

Liapi E, Kamel IR, Bluemke DA et al (2005) Assessment of response of uterine fibroids and myometrium to embolization using diffusion-weighted echoplanar MR imaging. J Comput Assist Tomogr 29: 83–86

Mayo-Smith WW, Dupuy DE (2004) Adrenal neoplasms: CT-guided radiofrequency ablation–preliminary results. Radiology 231: 225–230

Namimoto T, Yamashita Y, Sumi S et al (1997) Focal liver masses: characterization with diffusion-weighted echo-planar MR imaging. Radiology 204: 739–744

Ohira T, Okuma T, Matsuoka T et al (2009) FDG-MicroPET and diffusion-weighted MR image evaluation of early changes after radiofrequency ablation in implanted VX2 tumors in rabbits. Cardiovasc Intervent Radiol 32: 114–120

Rhee TK, Naik NK, Deng J et al (2008) Tumor response after yttrium-90 radioembolization for hepatocellular carcinoma: comparison of diffusion-weighted functional MR imaging with anatomic MR imaging. J Vasc Interv Radiol 19: 1180–1186

Schaefer PW, Grant PE, Gonzalez RG (2000) Diffusion-weighted MR imaging of the brain. Radiology 217: 331–345

Susini T, Nori J, Olivieri S et al (2007) Radiofrequency ablation for minimally invasive treatment of breast carcinoma. A pilot study in elderly inoperable patients. Gynecol Oncol 104: 304–310

Tanaka R, Horikoshi H, Nakazato Y et al (2009) Magnetic resonance imaging in peripheral lung adenocarcinoma: correlation with histopathologic features. J Thorac Imaging 24: 4–9

Therasse P, Arbuck SG, Eisenhauer EA et al (2000) New guidelines to evaluate the response to treatment in solid tumors. J Natl Cancer Inst 92: 205–216

Thoeny HC, De Keyzer F, Chen F et al (2005) Diffusion-weighted MR imaging in monitoring the effect of a vascular targeting agent on rhabdomyosarcoma in rats. Radiology 234: 756–764

Turner R (1990) Echo-planar imaging of intravoxel incoherent motion. Radiology 177: 407–414

Turner R (1991) Echo-planar imaging of diffusion and perfusion. Magn Reson Med 19: 247–253

Vogl TJ, Wetter A, Lindemayr S et al (2005) Treatment of unresectable lung metastases with transpulmonary chemoembolization: preliminary experience. Radiology 234: 917–922

Vossen JA, Kamel IR, Buijs M et al (2008) Role of functional magnetic resonance imaging in assessing metastatic leiomyosarcoma response to chemoembolization. J Comput Assist Tomogr 32: 347–352

Youn BJ, Chung JW, Son KR et al (2008) Diffusion-weighted MR: therapeutic evaluation after chemoembolization of VX-2 carcinoma implanted in rabbit liver. Acad Radiol 15: 593–600

Yuan YH, Xiao EH, Liu JB et al (2007) Characteristics and pathological mechanism on magnetic resonance diffusion-weighted imaging after chemoembolization in rabbit liver VX-2 tumor model. World J Gastroenterol 13: 5699–5706

Evaluation of Lymph Nodes Using DW-MRI

J. M. Froehlich and Harriet C. Thoeny

J. M. Froehlich, PhD
Harriet C. Thoeny, MD
Department of Diagnostic, Pediatric and Interventional
Radiology, University Hospital of Bern, Freiburgstrasse 10,
3013 Bern, Switzerland

SUMMARY

Presence of lymph node metastases and thus pre-diction of nodal malignancy remains one of the most important challenges in treatment and prognosis of patients with cancer. Diffusion-weighted MR imaging (DW-MRI) can identify differences in molecular water mobility in the extracellular spaces, reflecting cellular organization and density, microstructure and microcirculation. Improvements in DW-MRI techniques have overcome most of the drawbacks and limitations of whole-body imaging and enables nodal characterization. The generally higher cellularity of malignant lymph nodes facilitates their detection on high *b*-value DW-MR images, even in lymph nodes which are normal in size. Using quantitative ADC evaluation, pre-surgical assessment based on ADC threshold values may be valuable but must be interpreted with caution given the varying cut-off values for malignancy published in the literature. Moreover, necrotic areas, often encountered with squamous cell carcinomas, and inflammatory nodal hyperplasia accompanied by increased cellularity and nodal heterogeneity remain limitations when ADC values are applied to characterize nodal disease. ADC mapping relative to the primary tumour or standardized to reference structures such as the renal cortex, together with increased spatial resolution may further improve the diagnostic performance of DW-MRI. In the future, combining DW-MRI with lymphotrophic agents such as ultrasmall superparamagnetic iron oxide particles (USPIO) may enhance detection and characterization of lymph nodes. The pre-surgical planning for lymphadenectomy, radiotherapy

▷

and follow-up of oncological patients will profit from well-conducted DW-MRI studies even though histopathology remains the gold standard for nodal staging. The impact of DW-MRI on clinical practice for confident identification and risk stratification of patients for nodal metastases remains to be clarified.

12.1
Introduction

Early identification and accurate staging of lymph node metastases is a challenging problem for the radiologist as it has major impact on prognosis, treatment and follow-up of oncological patients. Accurate nodal staging informs on disease survival and the selection of the most appropriate treatment strategy.

Clinical examination is frequently limited for nodal assessment and precise definition of nodal involvement is reliant on imaging modalities, such as computed tomography (CT), conventional MR imaging, ultrasonography (US), positron emission tomography (PET) and the fusion of PET and CT. Despite many attempts and/or techniques to improve the diagnostic accuracy, the main criteria for determining malignant nodal involvement are still largely based on their morphological appearances on imaging, such as nodal size, shape, borders (lobulated or spiculated), extracapsular spread and abnormal internal architecture (such as central necrosis). The sensitivities and specificities of employing such criteria to determine nodal metastases vary between studies and tumour types, and are influenced by the mean size of the normal nodal population associated with the type and location of cancer as well as the adopted cut-off value. In clinical practice, despite the varying accuracy of applying size measurement criteria for nodal assessment, CT evaluation of nodal size is widely adopted and is considered to be one of the most consistent and convenient methods for nodal evaluation. Part of the reason is likely due to the wide availability of CT, which is usually employed to stage the primary tumour. The associated lymph nodes are also "in view" for radiological assessment even though nodal assessment may sometimes be limited or poor on CT.

High-resolution MR imaging at higher field strength (3 T), improved surface coils and development of lymphotrophic contrast media based on iron oxide or gadolinium, hold the potential to improve the detection and characterization of metastatic nodes using MR imaging (KING et al. 2004). But neither CT nor MR imaging can accurately differentiate between benign and malignant lymph nodes, especially in smaller size nodes (5–10 mm) so that lymph node dissection remains the most accurate and reliable method of assessing nodal involvement. However, lymphadenectomy or even lymph node biopsy are invasive and it is well established that not all patients are at the same risk of harbouring lymph node metastases (BRIGANTI 2009). Therefore, a technique which allows preoperative identification of patients with increased risk of nodal disease or patients with node positive disease, who may benefit from lymph node dissection, is warranted. Radiotherapy planning would also profit from an increased diagnostic accuracy. New criteria other than size may further extend lymph node staging accuracy by applying morphological interpretation based on an understanding of the microstructural changes in normal-sized nodes associated with micrometastases.

DW-MRI has become widely available over recent years and seems to hold promise as a powerful functional imaging tool in oncology, for identifying metastatic disease including nodal staging (PADHANI et al. 2009). Recent technical advances allow DW-MRI to be used for body applications and visualization of smaller structures such as lymph nodes. The technique has been shown to improve discrimination between benign and malignant lesions and better definition of malignant spread in cervical, abdominal and pelvic tumours. Thus, DW-MRI has the potential to provide unique information that reflects microstructural alterations in lymph nodes, which may improve patient care, although the technique is still in need of further validation, technical quality assurance and more clinical comparative data (PADHANI et al. 2009). The aim of this chapter is to review critically the role of DW-MRI in lymph node imaging and provide an outlook regarding its future potential.

12.2
Imaging Techniques for Lymph Node Staging

The gold standard for diagnosing lymph node invasion by malignancy is histopathological analysis following lymphadenectomy. Higher diagnostic accuracy is achieved when extended nodal dissection is performed but at an increased risk of complications by exposing the patient to dissection-related sequelae and morbidity (Briganti 2009; Heidenreich et al. 2002). For this reason, non-invasive imaging by CT, MR imaging, US, PET or PET/CT to identify probable nodal involvement is important to streamline surgical resection protocol, including the use of sentinel lymph node diagnostic algorithms in certain tumour types. It is widely accepted that none of these imaging modalities are entirely satisfactory. As stated above, this is due to the limited diagnostic accuracy of morphological criteria, such as nodal size, shape and presence of necrosis. Even the pattern of nodal contrast enhancement at CT or MR imaging has met with similar limitations (Bellin et al. 2003).

To date, there is no consensus with regards to the optimal diagnostic work-up for lymph node staging. Practice varies between countries and hospitals, adopting different size and morphological criteria, which is influenced by local medical experience and imaging equipment. Although metabolic imaging using FDG-PET or single photon emission CT (SPECT) have been shown to have a high diagnostic accuracy in certain tumour types, these are not widely available and can be expensive. These techniques are also inherently low in spatial resolution and may lack specificity. Furthermore, clinical studies evaluating the diagnostic accuracy of FDG-PET/CT for lymph node imaging have sometimes derived conflicting results (Helwig et al. 2009; Escalona et al. 2009; Crippa et al. 2004; Fehr et al. 2004; Lovrics et al. 2004; Wahl et al. 2004; Stadhaus et al. 2005; Schiavina et al. 2008; Goerres et al. 2003; Vermeersch et al. 2003; Facey et al. 2007).

A meta-analysis comparing the diagnostic performances of MR imaging and CT for lymph node staging in gynaecological, lung, rectal, head and neck, breast, urinary bladder and prostatic cancer was performed during the European Phase III trial of nodal staging using ultrasmall superparamagnetic nanoparticles of iron oxide (USPIO) contrast medium (Hamm et al. 2007). A few studies compared results using MR imaging and CT. No significant difference was found between the odds ratios (OR) of the MR imaging and CT in lymph node staging, i.e. OR MR imaging = 11.8 [5.9–23.8] and OR CT = 11.1 [6.1–20.1] ($p = 0.85$). The results stratified by tumour types were also not significantly different (gynaecological cancer $p = 0.28$, lung cancer $p = 0.81$, rectum cancer $p = 0.64$, head and neck cancer $p = 0.68$).

Lymphotrophic contrast medium (e.g. USPIO) taken up by the mononuclear cells provide functional data which have been shown to improve the sensitivity and specificity of MR imaging. Metastatic lymph nodes do not show any significant signal change 24–36 h after intravenous administration of USPIO, whereas normal or inflammatory lymph nodes demonstrate signal decrease on T2/T2*-weighted sequences. Based on such interpretation and when compared with histopathology, USPIO-enhanced MR imaging could improve the diagnostic sensitivity, specificity, diagnostic accuracy, PPV and NPV of nodal staging compared with unenhanced MR imaging in a Phase III study, although not when the data was systematically pooled and analysed together (Table 12.1). Major drawbacks of this pilot study were the high degree of reader variability, technical constraints and difficulties in histopathological correlation with MR imaging. More significant findings were corroborated in subsequent studies in different anatomical regions (Harisinghani et al. 2003, 2006; Heesakkers et al. 2008, 2009; Rockall et al. 2005). In a recent multi-centre prostate cancer trial, patients were found to benefit from the USPIO-enhanced MR imaging for nodal assessment (Heesakkers et al. 2009). The diagnostic performance of unenhanced MR imaging compared with USPIO-enhanced MR imaging in pelvic cancers (prostate, uterus or bladder) showed improved sensitivity using USPIO contrast medium (Hamm et al. 2007) compared with histology as gold standard (Table 12.1). Perhaps not surprisingly, the diagnostic performance using USPIO-enhanced MR imaging was still found to be reader dependant, emphasizing the need to be familiar with the technique prior to clinical adoption.

Overall, even though newer imaging methods such as PET–CT and USPIO-enhanced MR imaging seem to improve the preoperative detection of metastatic lymph nodes in various cancer types compared to conventional cross-section imaging, their limited availability, high costs and sometimes cumbersome analysis means that the detection and characterization of

Table 12.1. Results of diagnostic performance for staging lymph nodes in pelvic cancers on a patient level in comparison to histopathology for plain MRI and USPIO-enhanced MRI

	Sensitivity	Specificity	PPV	NPV
Plain MRI (%)	27.8–54.4	85.2–94.7	58.7–66.7	78–82.9
USPIO-enhanced MRI (%)	53.0–61.8	78.3–90.8	49.2–68.6	83.5–85.1

malignant nodal disease remains an important clinical challenge.

Detection and Characterization of Lymph Nodes Using DW-MRI

DW-MRI is a non-invasive technique capable of characterizing the mobility of water protons on a cellular scale. The degree of signal loss at a particular diffusion weighting (b-value) reflects the degree of water motion. Using low b-values (e.g. <100 s/mm^2) yields T2-weighted and perfusion dependent images, while higher b-value informs on tissue diffusivity with relative signal preservation in hypercellular tissues demonstrating impeded water diffusion. Typically, tissues with high cellularity such as lymph nodes (Figs. 12.1a and 12.2a) and tumours will appear with a high signal intensity on the high b-value images and return low ADC values. By contrast, non-tumorous tissues such as oedema, inflammation and necrosis are characterized by low cellularity and increased ADC values. Reduced ADC values may also be observed in fibrosis.

Metastatic lymph nodes often have increased cellular density and consequently lower ADC; although, some metastatic disease can result in central nodal necrosis and ADC increase (KWEE et al. 2008). ADC measurements may be helpful in discriminating between malignant and non-malignant lymph nodes, independently of nodal size. Nevertheless, inter- and intra-observer reproducibility of nodal ADC measurements still needs to be determined to ensure that serial comparison of measurements is clinically meaningful (KWEE et al. 2009).

12.3.1
Technical Requirements

Improvements in image acquisition (parallel imaging, segmented k-space acquisition with propeller techniques, ECG or respiratory triggering) allow fast data acquisition with fewer artefacts, resulting in significant improvement in image quality of DW-MRI of the body including lymph nodes. The administration of antiperistaltic drugs can help to reduce bowel-related motion artefacts. The application of fat suppression (TAKAHARA et al. 2004) also helps in nodal visualization (Figs. 12.1–12.3) by suppression of the

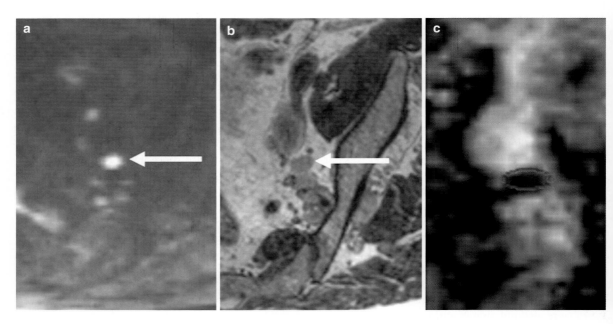

Fig. 12.1. 3T images (Trio, Siemens Medical Imaging, Erlangen, Germany) of the pelvic region in a patient with prostate cancer. (**a**) A high signal intensity node (*arrow*) is visible on the axial DW-MR high b-value images (b = 1,000 s/mm^2). (**b**) Axial reconstruction of the T2-weighted cross-section image. The lymph node seen in (**a**) is round but not enlarged (5 × 7 mm) (*arrow*). (**c**) Mean ADC value of lymph node (*red circle*) was 0.65 × 10^{-3} mm^2/s highly suspicious for malignancy. In this patient, lymph node characterization based on the ADC value was correct and was confirmed by histopathology

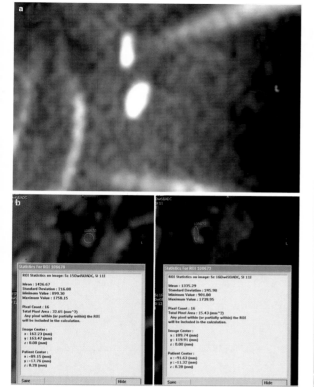

Fig. 12.2. A 51-year-old male volunteer who underwent DW-MRI of the axilla. (**a**) Two hyperintense axillary nodes are visible on the high b-value image ($b = 900\,s/mm^2$) acquired on a 3T Philips scanner (Achieva, Philips Medical Imaging, Best, The Netherlands). (**b**) Calculation of the mean ADC value for two regions of interest (16 pixels each, *red circles*) on two different image sections of the same lymph node. The mono-exponential fit yielded ADC-values of 1.43×10^{-3} and 1.33×10^{-3} mm^2/s respectively

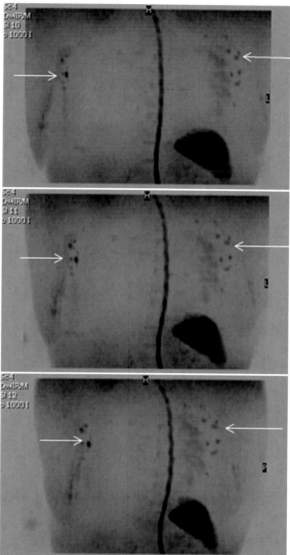

Fig. 12.3. Inversed grey-scale DW-MR image (1.5 T; Achieva Philips Medical) with background body signal suppression (DWIBS) of a 48-year-old male volunteer. 3D maximum intensity projection images of the thorax and upper abdomen. The spleen (hypointense *triangular structure* on the *right*) and normal axillary lymph nodes (*arrows*) are visible, as is the spinal cord

background signal. The averaging of several repetitive acquisitions of the same image section contributes to a better image quality. Higher field strengths (3 vs. 1.5 T) and/or dedicated receiver coils may be invested towards an increase in spatial resolution, shortening of acquisition time or improved signal-to-noise ratio. In most regions of the body, axial DW-MRI acquisition yields better image quality with fewer artefacts. To enable nodal ADC quantification, a minimum number of pixels per node must be evaluated to ensure a reliable result (Fig. 12.2). Slice orientation also defines the in-plane spatial resolution which is usually higher than the through-plane resolution (Table 12.2).

In clinical practice, DW-MRI of the lymph nodes is performed using at least two or more b-values. For practical reasons a low b-value image of 0 or 50 s/mm^2 is acquired, which results in T2-weighted images with b = 0 s/mm^2 or blood-flow suppressed images at a b-value of 50 s/mm^2. A Higher b-values of 800–1,000 s/mm^2 are applied to eliminate background signal to make the cellular lymph nodes more conspicuous. In addition to nodal tissue, small foci of hyperintensity may result from neural tissues and other glandular tissues (Fig. 12.3). Therefore, correlation of hyperin-

Table 12.2. Typical parameters of DW-MRI sequences used for nodal imaging

	Head–neck (axial) (24)	Pelvic region (axial) (24)	Pelvic region (axial)/3T	Head–neck (axial) (26)
Repetition time (ms)	8,612	6,962	4,700	7,100
Echo time (ms)	78	78	59	84
Inversion time (ms)	180	180 (CHESS)		
Slices	60	60		44
Slice thickness (mm)	4.0	4.0	4.0	4.0/gap 10%
FOV (mm)	450 × 366	450 × 366	330 × 330	200 × 250
rFOV (%)	81.3	81.3		
Matrix	256	256	128	104 × 128
Scan percentage	78.2	78.2		
Phase-encoding				
Half-scan factor	0.651	0.651		
EPI factor	43	43		
Bandwidth (Hz)	1,874.3	1,874.3		1,502
b-values (s/mm^2)	0, 1,000	0, 1,000	0, 500, 1,000	0, 50, 100, 500, 750, 1,000
Averages	3	3	6	3
SENSE factor	2	2		
Voxel size (mm)	3.52 × 4.5 × 4.0	3.52 × 4.5 × 4.0	2.58 × 2.58 × 4.0	2.0 × 2.0 × 4.0
Acquisition time	4 min 44 s	3 min 50 s	4 min 23 s	5 min 19 s

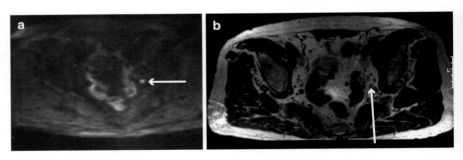

Fig. 12.4. A 63-year-old male patient with prostate cancer imaged on a 3T MR machine (Trio, Siemens Medical). (**a**) Hyperintense structure (*arrow*) on the high b-value image (1,000 s/mm^2) corresponding to a lymph node. (**b**) Correlation of hyperintense structure to a lymph node on the T2-weighted turbo spin-echo morphological image (*arrow*)

tense structures to morphological images is required for anatomical localization (Figs. 12.4 and 12.5). For calculation of an accurate ADC value, acquisition of several b-values is warranted. As discussed in previous chapters, bi-exponential fitting of the signal intensity at the respective b-value allows differentiating water movement in vessels at lower b-values (perfusion) in contrast to water movement corresponding to true diffusion. Therefore, several b-values from 0 to 100 s/mm^2 (perfusion-dependant) and from 100 to 1,000 s/mm^2 (true diffusion-dependant) can be recommended. Areas of impeded diffusion have lower ADC values compared with cystic structures. Clearly, one of the challenges in nodal ADC

Fig. 12.5. 3T DW-MRI of a 60-year-old male patient with bladder cancer with several hyperintense structures on (**a**) the high *b*-value (1,000 s/mm²) image. The *red encircled structure* corresponds to a malignant lymph node (ADC value = 0.84×10^{-3} mm²/s) while the posteriorly placed structures (*green circle*) were found to be sacral nerves, confirmed using the T2-weighted (**b**) axial, (**c**) coronal (nerves highlighted with *arrow*) and (**d**) parasagittal reconstruction. In this case, the lymph node (*red circle*) was found to be malignant and was correctly staged by DW-MRI (true-positive)

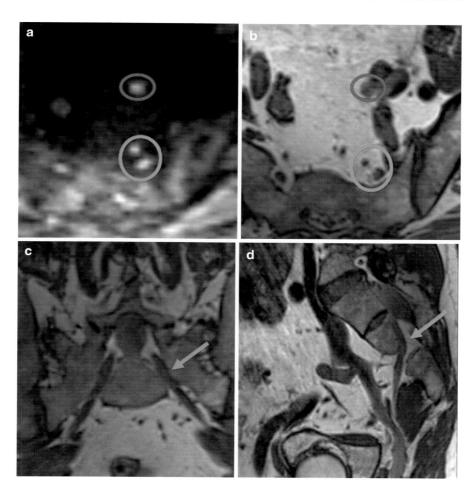

Fig. 12.6. A 53-year-old female patient with a cervical carcinoma. (**a**) Axial T2-weighted Turbo Spin-Echo image (1.5 T) of enlarged left external iliac node (*arrow*) and (**b**) corresponding ADC map showing lymph node (*arrow*) derived from DW-MRI. On the ADC map the lymph node has a hyperintense rim and hypointense central zone with a rather low ADC of 0.73×10^{-3} mm²/s. The node was confirmed to be malignant. (Courtesy Kubik and Chilla, Department of Radiology, Kantonsspital Baden, Switzerland.)

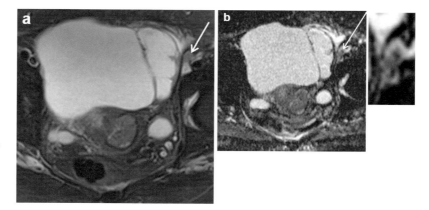

quantification is the relatively small size of lymph nodes, making ADC by region of interest analysis susceptible to partial volume effects and heterogeneity of the ADC values within the single node (Fig. 12.6). These are limitations which should be actively addressed in the future.

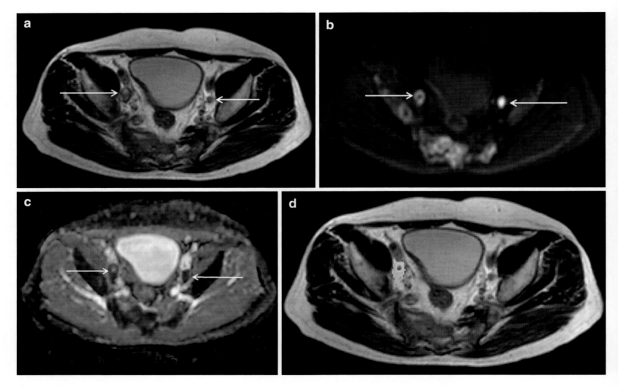

Fig. 12.7. A 73-year-old male with prostate cancer and pelvic lymph node metastases undergoing chemotherapy which was monitored using DW-MRI on a 3 T MR system. (**a**) T2-weighted image shows bilateral obturator lymph node (*arrows*). (**b**) On the high *b*-value image (800 s/mm²), the two lymph nodes are hyperintense (*arrows*), but a more variegated appearance is observed on the *right*. (**c**) The nodes return relatively low ADC values (*arrows*). (**d**) The coloured voxel-per-voxel analysis of the ADC calculated from the DW-MRI images (five *b*-values ranging homogeneously from 0 to 800 s/mm²) for the lymph node on the right revealed high intra-nodular variability of the ADC values ranging from 0.685 to 1.85×10^{-3} mm²/s. This case illustrates the potential of using high-resolution imaging and more detailed sub-nodal analysis for assessing partial invasion. (Courtesy: A Gutzeit, Department of Radiology, Kantonsspital Winterthur, Switzerland; ADC colour coding: courtesy Reischauer, Institute for Biomedical Engineering, Polytechnical High School, Zurich, Switzerland)

12.3.2
Qualitative Analysis

Evaluation of DW-MR images of lymph nodes consists of initially a qualitative step, whereby the high *b*-values images are screened for bright signal spots. These round or slightly elongated spots should not be part of a continuous structure visible on several image sections but only displayed on one or two image sections. Cross-checking with the anatomical images is essential and high *b*-value images should never be interpreted alone. Once a bright spot is determined on the high *b*-value images (Figs. 12.1, 12.4 and 12.5), it should be correlated and confirmed to be a node on the anatomical images. Grey-scale inversion may be used to display areas of impeded diffusion as dark foci against a bright background (Fig. 12.3) thus resembling PET imaging. The display preference is subjec- tive as the signal is essentially non-quantitative and does not modify the diagnosis. Datasets might also be visualized by ascribing a colour scale to the *b*-value images and fusing these with the grey-scale anatomical images. It must be emphasized that high *b*-value images are helpful as a quick survey for the presence and location of lymph node (node mapping) and increase the visibility of potentially suspicious nodes.

The brightness of lymph nodes on high *b*-value images must not be over-interpreted even though it may be a sign of malignancy, especially when closely associated with the primary neoplasms (Figs. 12.5 and 12.7). This is because normal nodes can exhibit a range of high signal intensities. In addition, reactive nodal hyperplasia can result in increased cellularity and nodal signal intensity on DW-MRI. By contrast, fibrotic proliferation and nodal lipomatosis may also confound interpretation (Fig. 12.8). If nodal signal

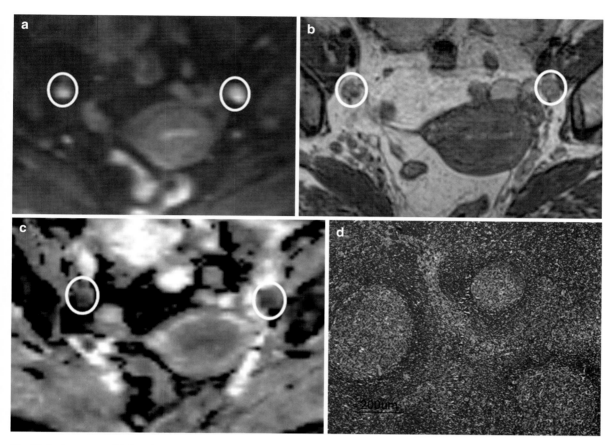

Fig.12.8. A 50-year-old female patient with bladder cancer who underwent tumour resection and extended lymph-adenectomy following staging MR imaging at 3 T. (**a**) Two enlarged external iliac nodes (*circled*) are visible on the axial DW-MR image (*b*-value = 1,000 s/mm²). (**b**) Corresponding T2-weighted image in the same image plane as (a) showing the anatomical location of nodes (*circled*). (**c**) Axial ADC map with a mean ADC value of 0.82 × 10⁻³ mm²/s for the nodes. This value was defined as malignant in our series (<0.90 × 10⁻³ mm²/s). (**d**) Histopathology showed residual lymphoreticular tissue with follicular hyperplasia in both enlarged lymph nodes (H& E stain of one lymph node shown here). In this case quantitative DW-MRI led to false-positive results

intensity is to be used as a guide, comparison with the signal intensity of lymph nodes that are known to be benign can be helpful. For example, in the pelvis, inguinal nodes are often benign in a substantial proportion of patients with pelvic malignancies. Hence, pelvic lymph nodes showing relatively higher signal intensity on DW-MRI than normal inguinal nodes may be further scrutinized.

12.3.3
Quantitative Analysis: ADC Measurement

The second step of evaluation following qualitative analysis is ADC measurement of suspicious lymph nodes. ADC measurements can be targeted towards lymph nodes that are suspicious by morphological criteria (size, shape and borders) or increased brightness on the high *b*-value images. As lymph nodes are often small in size, direct survey of the ADC maps are often unhelpful. In order to quantify nodal ADC, meticulous alignment of the morphological (e.g. 3D volumetric dataset) with the ADC map should be performed. In our experience, susceptibility, motion artefacts and geometric distortion between the acquisitions of two sequences may require image registration or manual adjustment. Another useful technique is to co-register the low *b*-value images of suspicious lymph nodes with the ADC maps. Enlarged lymph nodes (>10 mm) are easier to assess and may even be distinguishable on the ADC maps alone by their lower ADC values (Figs. 12.7 and 12.9b). Some authors recommend the exclusion of nodes smaller than 4 mm in the maximum diameter from analysis because of the difficulty in obtaining reliable ADC quantification. In certain instances, it may be possible to distinguish partially replaced lymph nodes, with the nodal cortex returning different ADC values compared with the tumour-replaced central zone (Fig. 12.6).

Quantitative analysis of DW-MRI using ADC values can be performed either by:

(a) Region of interest analysis. This is performed to record the mean or median ADC value. Histogram analysis of the distribution of ADC values within the region of interest can also be performed (Figs. 12.1 and 12.2).
(b) Voxel-wise analysis. When imaging has been performed at high spatial resolution, with a sufficient large number of image voxels, it may be possible to derive functional diffusion maps (Fig. 12.7).

Calculation of ADC values ideally should be performed on a voxel-per-voxel basis. The choice of data-fitting algorithm (e.g. monoexponential vs. bi-exponential) would depend on the available software and local expertise. Mean ADC value calculated across an entire lymph node derived from just two b-values may not be as accurate as one derived using a range of b-values. Furthermore, there is also relatively low inter- and intra-observer reproducibility of the nodal ADC measurements, which may limit the use of ADC values for discriminating between malignant and non-malignant lymph nodes (KWEE et al. 2009). Figure 12.7 demonstrates the high variability of ADC values within a single lymph node ranging from clearly malignant to benign partitions. Mean values calculated across the entire lymph node alone may therefore miss partial malignant invasion.

There is still controversy regarding the usefulness of nodal ADC value alone as a discriminator for metastatic nodal involvement. Nodal hyperplasia and central necrosis in lymph nodes are well-recognized pitfalls for nodal evaluation in the head and neck region. In the neck, lymphomatous nodal infiltration results in significantly lower ADC values compared with metastatic ones (VANDECAVEYE et al. 2009; SUMI et al. 2003, 2006; DE BONDT et al. 2009). Squamous cell carcinomas, which are the most frequently encountered tumours in the head and neck area, tend to undergo necrosis which leads to an increase in ADC values with tumour involvement. Hence, in order to enhance diagnostic specificity, ADC and DW-MRI evaluation should be made alongside morphological imaging, including the use of contrast-enhanced

Table 12.3. Assessment of malignancy based on ADC values determined by using higher b-values ranging from 100 to 1,000 s/mm² for pelvic tumours (see Figs. 12.3–12.5 and 12.7)

	Malignant	Indeterminate or needing additional criteria	Benign
ADC-values (mm²/s)	$<0.900 \times 10^{-3}$	$0.900–1.000 \times 10^{-3}$	$>1.000 \times 10^{-3}$

imaging sequences. It has been suggested that excluding necrotic areas of lymph nodes from analysis may help to improve ADC determination (DE BONDT et al. 2009). A necrotic area in a lymph node may be defined on conventional imaging as a hyperintense region on T2-weighted images and hypointense area on contrast-enhanced T1-weighted images. A practical predictive classification or cut-off scheme based on ADC values for non-necrotic pelvic lymph nodes is suggested in Table 12.3.

Interpretation of ADC values and their significance must take into account the quality of the ADC data. Enlarged lymph nodes with sufficiently large number of image voxels may even allow ADC mapping on a sub-nodal basis (Fig. 12.7). ADC values of normal-sized lymph nodes, due to the challenges of reliable ADC measurement as a result of small nodal size and potential artefacts must always be critically appraised. The smaller the region of interest, the more likely that partial volume effects will influence the measurements leading to inaccurate results. For these reasons, it has been suggested that (for the evaluation of pelvic lymph nodes), besides the clear cut-off values of 0.90 $\times 10^{-3}$ mm²/s for malignancy and 1.00 $\times 10^{-3}$ mm²/s for benign lymph nodes, there could be an in-between range of indeterminate ADC values (Table 12.3) where other imaging criteria should be carefully considered. Another promising approach compared the nodal ADC values with those of the primary tumour, which should share similar pathological characteristics (e.g. similar cellular architecture). Malignant nodes are more likely to approximate the ADC values of the primary tumour and thus help to improve nodal characterization (WHITTAKER et al. 2009) (Fig. 12.9). Some investigators have also suggested the potential value of the minimum ADC values within a region of interest instead of the mean values for nodal characterization. All these approaches demonstrate a lack of firm evaluation and characterization criteria for nodal assessment using DW-MRI although there is currently substantial research being conducted in this area (PADHANI et al. 2009).

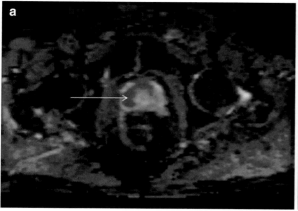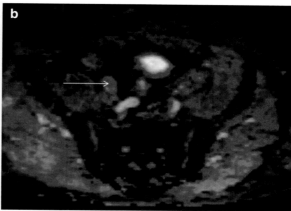

Fig. 12.9. A 53-year-old patient with prostate cancer imaged on a 3 T MR system. (**a**) ADC map of the primary tumour (*arrow*) and (**b**) suspicious right external iliac lymph node (*arrow*). The ADC values of the primary tumour and lymph node were mea-sured to be $0.82 \pm 0.12 \times 10^{-3}$ and $0.84 \pm 0.09 \times 10^{-3}$ mm^2/s, respectively. The near identical ADC values of the node relative to the primary tumour was suggestive of nodal malignancy. In this case, malignant nodal disease was confirmed at surgery

Clinical Applications of Diffusion-Weighted MR Imaging of Lymph Nodes

A recent review analysed the value of ADC for nodal characterization (KWEE et al. 2009). In the vast majority of the studies (11/13) ADC measurements proved to be helpful for nodal assessment. The reported ADC values of benign and malignant nodes varied widely: metastatic lymph nodes ranging between 0.41 and 1.84×10^{-3} mm^2/s; malignant lymphoma from 0.223 to 0.97×10^{-3} mm^2/s, benign lymphadenopathy between 0.302 and 1.64×10^{-3} mm^2/s and non-malignant lymph nodes from 0.75 to 2.38×10^{-3} mm^2/s. Kwee et al. explained these variations by different histological subtypes included in the studies (with differing ADCs due to differences in cellular architecture), differences in the imaging sequences and parameters (mainly different choice of *b*-values) and the different methods by which ADCs are measured. It is possible that software and hardware for image analysis may also have contributed some degree to the measurement variability.

In their own series analysing the short-term ADC reproducibility within normal lymph nodes of young volunteers, these authors revealed relatively large intra- and inter-observer variability frequently exceeding the absolute differences between nodal pathologies and normal values (KWEE et al. 2009). The use of only two *b*-values may have contributed to the degree of error. Based on the published literature, although it seems that ADC measurements can be helpful towards nodal characterization, it is still too early to be certain of its use in clinical practice. More studies are required, including longitudinal studies and its use for monitoring therapy outcome. Nevertheless, a number of published studies have testified the potential of the technique (Table 12.4).

12.4.1
Head and Neck

In cases of tumours growing close to the midline or patients with extensive ipsilateral nodal meta-static involvement, the exclusion of contralateral nodal spread is pivotal for treatment planning (VANDEKAVEYE et al. 2009; SUOGLU et al. 2002). Several investigators have studied the use of DW-MRI in the head and neck to evaluate visible lymph nodes and have found that the ADC values were significantly lower in malignant nodes than in benign nodes (VANDEKAVEYE et al. 2009; DE BONDT et al. 2009). King et al. were even able to distinguish squamous cell carcinoma (1.057×10^{-3} mm^2/s) from nasopharyngeal carcinoma (0.802×10^{-3} mm^2/s) and lymphoma (0.664×10^{-3} mm^2/s) based on mean ADC-values ($p < 0.001$) (KING et al. 2007). The ADC criterion was found to have the highest discriminatory value for distinguishing between lymph nodes with and without metasta-ses in this study, which included small lymph nodes.

Table 12.4. Overview of published studies using DW-MRI for nodal characterization

Region b-values in s/mm²	Nodal pathology (number)	Mean ADC in 10^{-3} mm²/s
Cervical LN Neck 500–1,000	Metastatic (25) Benign lymphadenopathy (25) Lymphoma (5)	0.41 ± 0.105 0.302 ± 0.062 0.223 ± 0.056
Neck 500–1,000	Metastatic (24) Benign lymphadenopathy (35) Lymphoma(14)	1.167 ± 0.447 0.652 ± 0.101 0.601 ± 0.427
Cervical LN neck 0–1,000	Metastatic (51) Benign lymphadenopathy (15) Lymphoma (21)	1.09 ± 0.11 1.64 ± 0.128 0.97 ± 0.27
Cervical LN neck 0, 100, 200, 300, 400, 500	Metastatic (SCC) (18) Metastatic (NPC) (17) Lymphoma (8)	1.057 ± 0.169 0.802 ± 0.128 0.664 ± 0.071
Cervical LN enlarged >10 mm 0–500–1,000	Metastatic (25) Benign lymphadenopathy (24) Lymphoma (6)	0.78 ± 0.09 1.24 ± 0.16 0.64 ± 0.09
Head and neck squamous cell carcinoma 0–1,000	Metastatic (26) Non-malignant (191)	0.85 ± 0.19 1.2 ± 0.24
Head and neck squamous cell carcinoma 0–1,000	Metastatic (74) Non-malignant (227)	0.85 ± 0.27 1.19 ± 0.22
Head and Neck Pelvic region 0–1,000	Non-malignant (20) Four measurements	1.15–1.18 ± 0.275
Non-small cell lung cancer 0–500–1,000	Non-malignant (698 LN) Malignant (36)	
Thorax 0–1,000	Metastatic (4/5) Without metastases: 36/37	High NPV: 97%
Esophageal cancer 0–1,000	Metastatic (NR) Non-malignant (NR)	1.46 ± 0.35 1.15 ± 0.25
Abdomen 0–600	Metastatic (16) Non-malignant (40)	1.84 ± 0.37 2.38 ± 0.29
Uterine cervical 0–1,000	Metastatic (30) Non-malignant (220)	0.7651 ± 0.1137 1.0021 ± 0.1859
Pelvis, gynaecological 0–800	Metastatic (7) Non-malignant (134)	1.4 ± 0.4 1.3 ± 0.24
Pelvis, bladder prostate 0–500–1,000	Metastatic (10) Non-malignant (29)	Malignant <0.9 Ambiguous 0.9–1.0 Benign >1.0
Cervical and uterine LN 0–1,000	Metastatic (12) Non-malignant	0.83 ± 0.15 0.75 ± 0.19
Cervical cancer LN	Metastatic (16 LN) Non-malignant (51 LN)	0.77 ± 0.13 1.07 ± 0.16
Uterine cervical LN 0–1,000	Metastatic (29) Non-malignant (226)	0.748 ± 0.16 0.996 ± 0.196

Statistics	References, comments
1 vs. 2: $p < 0.01$ 1 vs. 3: $p < 0.01$ 2 vs. 3: $p < 0.05$	SUMI et al. (2003)
1 vs. 2: $p < 0.001$ 1 vs. 3: $p < 0.001$ 2 vs. 3: $p < 0.01$	SUMI et al. (2006)
1 vs. 2: $p < 0.04$ 1 vs. 3: NS 2 vs. 3: $p < 0.04$	ABDEL RAZEK et al. (2006)
1 vs. 2; $p < 0.001$ 1 vs. 3: $p < 0.001$ 2 vs. 3: $p < 0.04$	KING et al. (2007)
1 vs. 2: $p < 0.05$ 1 vs. 3: $p < 0.05$ 2 vs. 3: $p < 0.05$	HOLZAPFEL et al. (2008)
1 vs. 2: $p < 0.05$	DE BONDT et al. (2009) Optimal ADC threshold 1.0×10^{-3} mm^2/s
1 vs. 2: $p < 0.0001$	VANDECAVEYE et al. (2009)
	KWEE et al. (2009)
$p < 0.002$ PET vs. DW-MRI	NOMORI et al. (2008) Cut-off: 1.6×10^{-3} mm^2/s
	HASEGAWA et al. (2008)
1 vs. 2: $p < 0.0001$	SAKURADA et al. (2009)
1 vs. 2: $p < 0.0005$	AKDUMAN et al. (2008)
1 vs. 2: $p < 0.001$	KIM et al. 2008
1 vs. 2: $p = 0.28$	NAKAI et al. (2008)
Sens: 80% Spec: 79% PPV: 57% NPV: 92% Diagnostic Accuracy: 79%	TRIANTAFYLLOU et al. (2009) Threshold $0.9–1.0 \times 10^{-3}$ mm^2/s
1 vs. 2: $p = 0.639$ 1 vs. 2: $p < 0.0001$ with relative ADC	LIN et al. (2008) Sensitivity 83%, specificity 99% when using relative ADC values
$p < 0.01$	XUE et al. (2008)
1 vs. 2: $p < 0.01$	PARK et al. (2009)

Interestingly, Vandecaveye et al. reported low ADC values also in partially invaded malignant lymph nodes from head and neck cancers, ascribed to the presence of keratinization and/or peritumoral nodal reactivity (VANDEKAVEYE et al. 2009). The presence of keratin which is specific to metastases of squamous cell carcinoma may intensify ADC decrease in metastatic lymph nodes (VANDEKAVEYE et al. 2009; SUOGLU et al. 2002; WHITE et al. 2006). In other studies including patients with enlarged lymph nodes due to lymphoma, squamous cell carcinoma or nasopharyngeal carcinomas, the lowest ADC values were reported for lymphomas compared to the other histological subtypes (KING et al. 2007). This observation is likely related to the hypercellular nature of the lymphomatous disease and the presence of necrosis which occurs commonly in squamous cell head and neck carcinomas (SUMI et al. 2003, 2006; KING et al. 2007). Similar observation was reported within lymph nodes of oesophageal squamous cell carcinoma (HASEGAWA et al. 2008). In another study by de Bondt et al. in patients with head and neck cancers, the optimal ADC threshold for distinguishing malignant from benign nodes appeared to be 1.0×10^{-3} mm^2/s when the MR size criteria and MR morphology were assessed in combination (DE BONDT et al. 2009). Lymph nodes with ADC values below this cut-off value were highly likely to be malignant, while those with ADC values above this threshold were likely to be benign.

12.4.2
Lung

Hasegawa et al. report a NPV of 97% for excluding mediastinal lymph node metastases in their series of 42 patients with non-small-cell lung cancer when using diffusion-weighted images at a b-value of 1,000 together with T2-weighted images (HASEGAWA et al. 2008). Mediastinal lymph node metastasis was defined as a focus of low signal intensity on the ADC map, corresponding to a visible lymph node on DW-MRI and T2-weighted image (HASEGAWA et al. 2008). Apparently, the qualitative high b-value images were useful to quickly distinguish which lymph nodes were suspicious. Nomori et al. report an accuracy of N staging in their cohort of 88 patients with non-small-cell lung cancer of 89% with DW-MRI, which was significantly higher than the 78% obtained using PET–CT (NOMORI et al. 2008). The main reason for the superiority in N staging by DW-MRI was ascribed to a lower false-

positive rate resulting from lymphadenitis, which increased tracer uptake on PET–CT.

12.4.3
Upper Abdomen

In the single retrospective series of Akduman et al. including a large variety of primary tumours (oesophageal cancer, hepatocellular carcinoma, small-cell lung cancer, cholangiocarcinoma, pancreatic carcinoma, gastric carcinoma, renal cell carcinoma) higher mean ADC values ($2.38 \pm 0.29 \times 10^{-3}$ mm^2/s) were measured for benign lymph nodes compared to malignant ones ($1.87 \pm 0.34 \times 10^{-3}$ mm^2/s) (AKDUMAN et al. 2008). The authors also discussed inflammatory processes that could potentially result in higher ADC values in the benign lymph nodes. However, the authors found no useful ADC cut-off values which could be applied to differentiate between benign and malignant lymph nodes. Contrary results were reported in another cohort of 24 patients with oesophageal cancer, with significantly higher ADC values observed in metastatic lymph nodes (1.46×10^{-3} mm^2/s) compared with 1.15×10^{-3} mm^2/s in non-metastatic nodes, but there was overlap in the ADC values (HASEGAWA et al. 2008). This discrepancy may be explained by the fact that lymph nodes from squamous cell carcinomas tend to undergo necrosis which can lead to an increase in ADC value.

12.4.4
Pelvis

12.4.4.1
Female Tumours

The presence of lymph node metastasis is an important prognostic factor for patients with cervical and uterine cancers since it influences the 5-year survival and affects treatment planning (LUTMAN et al. 2006; KODAMA et al. 2009). The application of DW-MRI for discriminating between benign and malignant lymph nodes in female patients with pelvic tumours is emerging in the published literature. Several approaches combining different ways of ADC assessment with morphological MR criteria have been proposed. LIN et al. reported a significantly lower relative ADC value in metastatic nodes compared to benign ones in their 50 patients evaluated at 3 T (LIN et al. 2008). The relative ADC values were calculated with reference to the primary tumour. Interestingly, no significant difference was found between benign and malignant nodes where absolute ADC values were employed (NAKAI et al. 2008). The relative ADC value assumes that regional lymph nodes invaded by tumour cells would display similar cellularity and/or microarchitecture and hence ADC values to the primary tumour. Whittaker et al. propose an alternative method of identifying suspicious lymph nodes using very high b-value ($>1,500$ s/mm^2) images by comparing the relative signal intensity of nodes to those that they presume to be benign (e.g. groin nodes in patients with endometrial or cervical cancer) (WHITTAKER et al. 2009). However, central necrosis in lymph node, which can lead to signal suppression on high b-value imaging, is a potential pitfall which must be recognized. Park et al. achieved a high area under the ROC curve for distinguishing malignant from benign lymph nodes using the renal cortex ADC as an appropriate reference tissue to calculate a so-called relative ADC (PARK et al. 2009). Thoeny et al. had previously shown that the ADC of the renal cortex is highly reproducible with little difference between measurements over a 6-month interval (1.67×10^{-3} vs. 1.63×10^{-3} mm^2/s) (THOENY et al. 2005). Visibility of lymph nodes may be increased in the presence of ascites or paucity of pelvic fat. As previously discussed, high spatial resolution of DW-MRI may help to distinguish distinct zones within a lymph node, and hence help to identify partial malignant invasion (Figs 12.6 and 12.7).

12.4.4.2
Prostate and Bladder Cancers

Recently, one group presented a series of 40 patients with prostate and bladder cancers, who underwent extended pelvic lymphadenectomy and surgery of the primary tumour (TRIANTAFYLLOU et al. 2009). Discrimination of brighter, ambiguous lymph nodes on high b-value was done by classifying them according to their ADC values. Those with an ADC beyond 0.9×10^{-3} mm^2/s were judged as definitely malignant, those between 0.9 and 1.0×10^{-3} mm^2/s as ambiguous and to follow more closely, while those above 1.0×10^{-3} mm^2/s were scored as benign (Table 12.3). Histopathology revealed 29 patients as negative, while ten were positive. A rather high number of six false-positives resulted from lipomatosis follicular hyperplasia (Fig. 12.8), or sinus histiocytosis on histology. Overall, a sensitivity of 80%, a specificity of 79%, a PPV of 57%, a NPV of 92% and a diagnostic accuracy

of 79% resulted using these threshold values. The high NPV with only two false-negative patients, one patient with a mean nodal ADC of 1.02×10^{-3} mm^2/s and another with a missed small metastasis, which could be detected retrospectively confirm the high predictive value of DW-MRI (Fig. 12.10). Clearly, micrometastases are still currently beyond the limits of the spatial resolution of DW-MRI to confidently detect.

12.4.4.3
Colorectal Cancer

Detection of nodal dissemination is extremely important for staging and further treatment in patients with colorectal cancer. Staging of lymph node metastases thus differentiates between pN0 with no regional lymph node metastases, pN1 with metastases in one to three regional lymph nodes and pN2 with metastases in four or more regional lymph nodes. Despite the difficulties of detecting nodal involvement in the retroperitoneum due to small size of normal lymph nodes, DW-MRI when used with an inversion-pulse fat saturation was found to result in a superior detection rate of lymph node metastases compared to FDG-PET (ONO et al. 2009). In a small series with 27 patients and 23 tumours with lymph node involvement, DW-MRI and FDG-PET exhibited a sensitivity of 80/30%, their specificity was 76.9/100% and their accuracy 78.3 vs. 69.9%, respectively (ONO et al. 2009).

12.5

Potential Pitfalls and Limitations

Potential pitfalls and limitations of DW-MRI for nodal assessment should be borne in mind when applying the technique for evaluation. The salient points are listed below.

- Small nodes (<2 mm in short axis diameter) may be visualized using DW-MRI and anatomically localized, but the presence of malignant disease cannot be always established using the technique (TRIANTAFYLLOU et al. 2009).
- The ADC measurements of normal-sized lymph nodes may be degraded by partial volume effects.
- Lymph nodes involved by lymphoma and metastatic nodes both show low ADC values, thus limiting the application of the technique in characterizing the aetiology of the low ADC value.

Fig. 12.10. A 63-year-old male patient with prostate cancer evaluated on a 3 T MRI system for lymph node characterization. (**a**) Axial DW-MRI of a single bright lymph node (*encircled*) in the internal iliac region with a cross-section diameter of 4 × 5 mm. This lymph node was missed during initial staging. Retrospective quantitative analysis revealed an ADC-value of 0.82×10^{-3} mm²/s. (**b**) axial T2-weighted, (**c**) coronal T2-weighted and (**d**) parasagittal T2-weighted reconstruction of the same lymph node. Prospective staging was false-negative but retrospective analysis allowed the malignant node to be identified. However, the ADC measurement was approaching the limits of feasibility because of the small nodal size

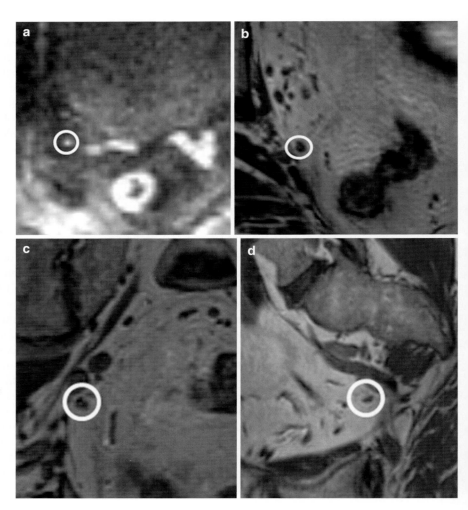

- Necrotic areas in neoplastic nodes may lead to false-negative results due to the resultant ADC increase (e.g. squamous cell carcinomas) (VANDECAVEYE et al. 2009). Necrotic deposits therefore must be excluded by comparing the ADC maps with the morphological images.
- Decrease in nodal ADC value may result from nodal reactive changes, leading to spurious diagnosis of metastatic burden (VANDECAVEYE et al. 2008, 2009).
- False-positives may result from apparent impeded diffusion due to haemorrhage or haematoma, which limits the use of DW-MRI after biopsy (VANDECAVEYE et al. 2008; CHOI et al. 2007; SILVERA et al. 2005).
- Instrumental factors such as image noise, motion artefacts, errors related to diffusion gradient applications, susceptibility artefacts or eddy current effects can lead to systematic or random ADC quantification errors.

- Micrometastases in smaller lymph nodes with insufficient intra-nodal tumour burden may not impede water diffusion (VANDECAVEYE et al. 2009) and can therefore lead to false-negative results.
- The robustness of the fat saturation techniques can influence the outcome of studies and must be checked.

12.6
Hybrid MR Imaging Techniques

As with other applications, future standardization of nodal interpretation with DW-MRI using an optimal choice of *b*-values may improve nodal characterization. More sophisticated analysis methodology for nodal assessment using histogram or voxel-wise analysis should be investigated in the future (Fig. 12.7).

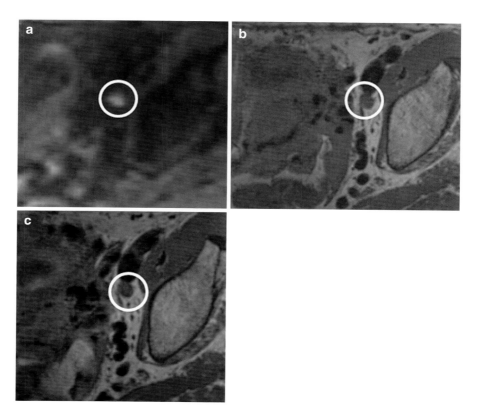

Fig. 12.11. Combined approach using DW-MRI together with lymphotrophic USPIO enhancement in a 74-year-old female patient with bladder cancer. (**a**) Hyperintense structure on the DW-MRI image ($b = 1,000\,s/mm^2$) after USPIO (24–36 h after i.v. administration) corresponds to a lymph node on the (**b**) T2-weighted axial reconstruction pre- and (**c**) post-USPIO. Lymph node revealed minor cortical uptake of USPIO and showed little signal decrease on (**c**) compared to (**b**). Signal decrease is a sign of normal lymph node function with macrophage activity (benign), while the malignant lymph nodes remain isointense. The DW-MRI image (**a**) in this case was already highly suspicious, as all benign lymph nodes have vanished on the DW-MRI images due to the effects of iron in normal nodal tissue on high b-value images. Histopathology confirmed a metastasis of $2 \times 2\,mm$ (true-positive)

Combining two or more techniques, for example PET and DW-MRI or lymph node targeted contrast agents with DW-MRI is likely to evolve and hold substantial promise. As has been reported recently (THOENY et al. 2009), the use of lymphotrophic contrast agents like superparamagnetic iron oxide nanoparticles (USPIO) together with DW-MRI, allow the two techniques to be used in synergy for the detection of suspicious lymph nodes. The novel imaging approach allows identification of malignant nodes by identifying lymph nodes that remain bright following USPIO contrast administration (Fig. 12.11). One requirement of this technique is the confident exclusion of other structures that may mimic the appearance of lymph nodes, including small vascular structures. Once a lymph node is identified, the T2 signal decrease post-USPIO helps to differentiate malignant from benign lymph nodes. The combined approach not only achieves similar or higher diagnostic accuracies on a patient level in the initial cohort of 21 patients (Sens: 73.3%; Spec 86.7%; Accuracy: 83.3%; PPV 65.7%; NPV 90.7%), but even more advantageous is the fact that the time needed for image evaluation reduces from 80 min for the classical reading of USPIO-enhanced MRI without DW-MRI to 13 min using the combined approach.

12.7

Summary and Conclusions

High-quality DW-MRI of lymph nodes can now be performed as part of a primary tumour staging without significantly increasing the imaging time. DW-MRI provides important information non-invasively from a qualitative and functional perspective. This unique modality can help to distinguish benign from malignant lymph nodes, and has achieved promising NPV values. To ensure accurate nodal assessment, it is important to be aware of the potential pitfalls of DW-MR imaging and to review findings in conjunction with morphological sequences for anatomical co-localization and correlation of radiologic findings with histopathology. Increasing familiarity with ADC calculation and post-processing software, including the ability to fuse anatomical and diffusion data, will allow radiologists to gain confidence and thus to provide new information to physicians who are involved in treatment and follow-up of patients with suspected lymph node malignancies (surgery, radiotherapy, chemotherapy). Further, large-scale studies to confirm these initial results are certainly warranted. The introduction of hybrid techniques will further boost the diagnostic accuracy by combining DW-MRI with lymphotrophic contrast media or other imaging methods (PET).

Abbreviations

ADC	Apparent diffusion coefficient
DW-MRI	Diffusion-weighted magnetic resonance imaging
FDG	2-[^{18}F]-fluoro-2-deoxy-D-glucose
NPV	Negative-predictive value
PET	Positron emission tomography
PET-CT	Integrated PET/CT device
PPV	Positive-predictive value
ROC	Receiver operating characteristic
Sens	Sensitivity
Spec	Specificity
USPIO	Ultrasmall superparamagnetic particles of iron oxide

Acknowledgement The authors of this chapter were supported by research grant no. 320000-113512/1 from the Swiss National Foundation for Scientific Research and Harriet C. Thoeny in addition from Carigest SA, Geneva.

References

Abdel Razek AA, Soliman NY, Elkhamary S, Alsharaway MK, Tawfik A (2006) Role of diffusion-weighted MR imaging in cervical lymphadenopathy. Eur Radiol 16:1468–1477

Akduman EI, Momtahen AJ, Balci NC, Mahajann N, Havlioglu N, Wolverson MK (2008) Comparison between malignant and benign abdominal lymph nodes on diffusion-weighted imaging. Acad Radiol 15:641–646

Bellin MF, Lebleu L, Meric JB (2003) Evaluation of retroperitoneal and pelvic lymph node metastases with MRI and MR lymphography. Abdom Imaging 28:155–163

Briganti A (2009) How to improve the ability to detect pelvic lymph node metastases of urologic malignancies. Eur Urol 55:770–772

Choi KD, Jo JW, Park KP, Kim JS, Lee TH, Kim HJ, Jung DS (2007) Diffusion-weighted imaging of intramural hematoma in vertebral artery dissection. J Neurol Sci 253:81–84

Crippa F, Gerali A, Alessi A, Agresti R, Bombardieri E (2004): FDG-PET for axillary lymph node staging in primary breast cancer. Eur J Nucl Med Mol Imaging 31:97–102

de Bondt RB, Hoeberigs MC, Nelemans PJ, Deserno WM, Peutz-Kootstra C, Kremer B, Beets-Tan RG (2009) Diagnostic accuracy and additional value of diffusion-weighted imaging for discrimination of malignant cervical lymph nodes in head and neck squamous cell carcinoma. Neuroradiology 51:183–192

Escalona S, Blasco JA, Reza MM, Andradas E, Gomez N (2009) A systemic review of FDG-PET in breast cancer. Med Oncol DOI 10.1007/s12032-009-9182-3

Facey K, Bradbury I, Laking G, Payne E (2007) Overview of the clinical effectiveness of positron emission tomography imaging in selected cancers. Health Technol Assess 11:III–IV; XI–267

Fehr MK, Hornung R, Varga Z, Burger D, Hess T, Haller U, Fink D, von Schulthess GK, Steinert HC (2004) Axillary staging using positron emission tomography in breast cancer patients qualifying for sentinel lymph node biopsy. Breast J 10:89–93

Goerres GW, Michel SC, Fehr MK, Kaim AH, Steinert HC, Seifert B, von Schulthess GK, Kubik-Huch RA (2003) Follow-up of women with breast cancer: comparison between MRI and FDG PET. Eur Radiol 13:1635–1644

Hamm B, Caseiro-Alves F, Bellin M-F, Padhani A, Passariello R, Roy C (2007) USPIO-enhanced intravenous MR lymphography for staging pelvic cancers: results of a European multicenter phase III trial including 271 patients. RSNA, Chicago

Harisinghani MG, Barentsz J, Hahn PF, Deserno WM, Tabatabaei S, van de Kaa CH, de la Rosette J, Weissleder R (2003) Noninvasive detection of clinically occult lymph node metastases in prostate cancer. N Engl J Med 19: 2491–2499

Harisinghani MG, Saksena MA, Hahn PF, King B, Kim J, Torabi MT, Weissleder R (2006) Ferumoxtran-10 enhanced MR lymphangiography: does contrast-enhanced imaging alone suffice for accurate lymph node characterization? AJR 186:144–148

Hasegawa I, Boiselle PM, Kuwabara K, Sawafuji M, Sugiura H (2008) Mediastinal lymph nodes in patients with non-small cell lung cancer: preliminary experience with diffusion-weighted MR imaging. J Thorac Imaging 23:157–161

Heesakkers RA, Hövels AM, Jager GJ, van den Bosch HC, Witjes JA, Raat HP, Severens JL, Adang EM, van der Kaa CH, Fütterer JJ, Barentsz J (2008) MRI with a lymph node specific contrast agent as an alternative to CT scan and lymph node dissection in patients with prostate cancer: a prospective multicohort study. Lancet Oncol 9:850–856

Heesakkers RA, Jager GJ, Hövels AM, de Hoop B, van den Bosch HC, Raat F, Witjes JA, Mulders PF, van der Kaa Ch, Barentsz JO (2009) Prostate cancer: detection of lymph node metastases outside the routine surgical area with ferumoxtran-10 enhanced MR imaging. Radiology 251:408–414

Heidenreich A, Varga Z, Von Knobloch R (2002) Extended pelvic lymphadenectomy in patients undergoing radical prostatectomy: high incidence of lymph node metastasis. J Urol 167:1681–1686

Hellwig D, Baum RP, Kirsch C (2009) FDG-PET, PET/CT and conventional nuclear medicine procedures in the evaluation of lung cancer: a systematic review. Nuklearmedizin 48:59–69

Holzapfel K, Duetsch S, Fauser C, Eiber M, Rummeny EJ, Gaa J (2008) Value of diffusion-weighted MR imaging in the differentiation between benign and malignant cervical lymph nodes. Eur J Radiol DOI 10.1016/j.ejrad.2008.09.034

Kim JK, Kim KA, Park BW, Kim N, Cho KS (2008) Feasibility of diffusion-weighted imaging in the differentiation of metastatic from nonmetastatic lymph nodes: early experience. J Magn Reson Imaging 28:714–719

King AD, Tse GM, Ahuja AT, Yuen EH, Vlantis AC, To EW, van Hasselt AC (2004) Necrosis in metastatic neck nodes: diagnostic accuracy of CT, MR imaging, and US. Radiology 230:720–726

King AD, Ahuja AT, Yeung DK, Fong DK, Lee YY, Lei KI, Tse GM (2007) Malignant cervical lymphadenopathy: diagnostic accuracy of diffusion-weighted MR imaging. Radiology 245:806–813

Kodama J, Seki N, Nakamura K, Hongo A, Hiramatsu Y (2007) Prognostic factors in pathologic parametrium-positive patients with stage IB-IIB cervical cancer treated by radical surgery and adjuvant therapy. Gynecol Oncol 105:757–761

Kwee TC, Takahara T, Ochiai R, Nievelstein RAJ, Luijten PR (2008) Diffusion-weighted whole-body imaging with background body signal suppression (DWIBS): features and potential applications in oncology. Eur Radiol 18:1937–1952

Kwee TC, Takahara T, Luijten PR; Nievelstein RAJ (2009) ADC measurements of lymph nodes: inter- and intra-observer reproducibility study and an overview of the literature. Eur J Radiol DOI 10.1016/j.ejrad.2009.03.026

Lin G, Ho KC, Wang JJ, et al (2008) Detection of lymph node metastasis in cervical and uterine cancers by diffusion-weighted magnetic resonance imaging at 3T. J Magn Reson Imaging 28:128–135

Lovrics PJ, Chen V, Coates G, Cornacchi SD, Goldsmith CH, Law C, Levine MN, Sanders K, Tandan VR (2004) A prospective evaluation of positron emission tomography scanning, sentinel lymph node biopsy, and standard axillary dissection for axillary staging in patients with early stage breast cancer. Ann Surg Oncol 11:846–853

Lutman CV, Havrilesky LJ, Cragun JM, Secord AA, Calingaert B, Berchuck A, Clarke-Pearson DL, Soper JT (2006) Pelvic lymph node count is an important prognostic variable for FIGO stage I and II endometrial carcinoma with high-risk histology. Gynecol Oncol 102:92–97

Nakai G, Matsuki M, Inada Y, Tatsugami F, Tanikake M, Narabayashi I, Yamada T (2008) Detection and evaluation of pelvic lymph nodes in patients with gynecologic malignancies using body diffusion-weighted magnetic resonance imaging. J Comput Assist Tomogr 32:764–768

Nomori H, Mori T, Ikeda K, Kawanaka K, Shiraishi S, Katahira K, Yamashita Y (2008) Diffusion-weighted magnetic resonance imaging can be used in place of positron emission tomography for N staging of non-small cell lung cancer with fewer false-positive results. J Thorac Cardiovasc Surg 135:816–822

Ono K, Ochiai R, Yoshida T, Kitagawa M, Omagari J, Kobayashi H, Yamashita Y (2009) Comparison of diffusion-weighted MRI and 2-[fluorine-18]-fluoro-2-deoxy-D-glucose positron emission tomography (FDG-PET) for detecting primary colorectal cancer and regional lymph node metastases. J Magn Reson Imaging 29:336–340

Padhani AR, Liu G, Koh DM, Chenevert TL, Thoeny HC, Takahara T, Dzik-Jurasz A, Ross BD, Van Cauteren M, Collins D, Hammoud DA, Rustin GJ, Taouli B, Choyke PL (2009) Diffusion-weighted magnetic resonance imaging as a cancer biomarker: consensus and recommendations. Neoplasia 11:102–125

Park SO, Kim JK, Kim KA, Park BW, Kim N, Cho G, Choi HJ, Cho KS (2009) Relative apparent diffusion coefficient: determination of reference site and validation of benefit for detecting metastatic lymph nodes in uterine cervical cancer. J Magn Reson Imaging 29:383–390

Rockall AG, Sohaib SA, Harisinghani MG, Babar SA, Singh N, Jeyarajah AR, Oram DH, Jacobs IJ, Shepherd JH, Reznek RH (2005) Diagnostic performance of nanoparticle-enhanced magnetic resonance imaging in the diagnosis of lymph node metastases in patients with endometrial and cervical cancer. J Clin Oncol 23:2813–2821

Sakurada A, Takahara T, Kwee TC, Yamashita T, Nasu S, Horie T, Van Cauteren M, Imai Y (2009) Diagnostic performance of diffusion-weighted magnetic resonance imaging in esophageal cancer. Eur Radiol 19:1461–1469

Schiavina R, Scattoni V, Castellucci P, Picchio M, Corti B, Briganti A, Franceschelli A, Sanguedolce F, Bertaccini A, Farsad M, Giovacchini G, Fanti S, Grigioni WF, Fazio F, Montorsi F, Rigatti P, Martorana G (2008) 11C-choline positron emission tomography/computerized tomography for preoperative lymph node staging in intermediate-risk and high-risk prostate cancer: comparison with clinical staging nomograms. Eur Urol 54:392–401

Silvera S, Oppenheim C, Touzé E, Ducreux D, Page P, Domigo V, Mas JL, Roux FX, Frédy D, Meder JF (2005) Spontaneous intracerebral hematoma on diffusion-weighted images: influence of T2-shine-through and T2-blackout effects. AJNR 26:236–241

Stattaus J, Bockisch A, Forsting M, Müller SP (2005) Value of imaging for lymph node metastases from renal cell, bladder, prostate, penile, and testicular cancers. Urologe A 44:614–624

Sumi M, Sakihama N, Sumi T, Morikawa M, Uetani M, Kabasawa H, Shigeno K, Hayashi K, Takahashi H, Nakamura T (2003) Discrimination of metastatic lymph nodes with diffusion-weighted MR imaging in patients with head and neck cancer. AJNR 24:1627–1634

Sumi M, Van Cauteren M, Nakamura T (2006) MR microimaging of benign and malignant nodes in the neck. AJR 186:749–757

Suoglu Y, Erdamar B, Katircioglu OS, Karatay MC, Sunay T (2002) Extracapsular spread in ipsilateral neck and contralateral neck metastases in laryngeal cancer. Ann Otol Rhinol Laryngol 111:447–454

Takahara T, Imai Y, Yamashita T, Yasuda S, Nasu S, Van Cauteren M (2004) Diffusion weighted whole body imaging with background body signal suppression (DWIBS): technical improvement using free breathing, STIR and high resolution 3D display. Radiat Med 22:275–282

Thoeny HC, De Keyzer F, Oyen RH, Peeters RR (2005) Diffusion-weighted MR imaging of kidneys in healthy volunteers and patients with parenchymal diseases: initial experience. Radiology 235:911–917

Thoeny HC, Triantafyllou M, Birkhaeuser FD, Froehlich JM, Tshering DW, Binser T, Fleischmann A, Vermathen P, Studer UE (2009) Combined ultrasmall superparamagnetic particles of iron oxide-enhanced and diffusion-weighted magnetic resonance imaging reliably detect pelvic lymph node metastases in normal-sized nodes of bladder and prostate cancer patients. Eur Urol 55:761–769

Triantafyllou M, Binser T, Birkhaeuser F, Studer UE, Fleischmann A, von Gunten M, Froehlich JM, Vermathen P, Thoeny HC (2009) Diffusion-weighted MRI to detect pelvic lymph node metastases in patients with bladder or prostate cancer: comparison with histopathology as gold standard. In: Proceedings of the ISMRM, Hawaii

Vandecaveye V, De Keyzer F, Hermans R (2008) Diffusion-weighted magnetic resonance imaging in neck lymph adenopathy. Cancer Imaging 8:173–180

Vandecaveye V, De Keyzer F, Poorten VV, Dirix P, Verbeken E, Nuyts S, Hermans R (2009) Head and neck squamous cell carcinoma: value of diffusion-weighted MR imaging for nodal staging. Radiology 251:134–146

Vermeersch H, Loose D, Ham H, Otte A, Van de Wiele C (2003) Nuclear medicine imaging for the assessment of primary and recurrent head and neck carcinoma using routinely available tracers. Eur J Nucl Med Mol Imaging 30:1689–1700

Wahl RL, Siegel BA, Coleman RE, Gatsonis CG; PET Study Group (2004) Prospective multicenter study of axillary nodal staging by positron emission tomography in breast cancer: a report of the staging breast cancer with PET Study Group. J Clin Oncol 22:277–285

White ML, Zhang Y, Robinson RA (2006) Evaluating tumours and tumourlike lesions of the nasal cavity, the paranasal sinuses, and the adjacent skull base with diffusion-weighted MRI. J Comput Assist Tomogr 30:490–495

Whittaker CS, Coady A, Culver L, Rustin G, Padwick M, Padhani AR (2009) Diffusion-weighted MR imaging of female pelvic tumours: a pictorial review. Radiographics 29:759–774

Xue HD, Li S, Sun F, Sun HY, Jin ZY, Yang JX, Yu M (2008) Clinical application of body diffusion weighted MR imaging in the diagnosis and preoperative N staging of cervical cancer. Chin Med Sci J 23:133–137

Evaluation of Malignant Bone

Disease Using DW-MRI

K. Nakanishi and A. Gutzeit

SUMMARY

The bones are frequently involved as a site of metastatic disease in patients with cancer. Accurate determination of the presence, location and extent of bone involvement is of therapeutic and prognostic importance. Diffusion-weighted MR imaging performed regionally or as whole-body imaging has been shown to have a high diagnostic accuracy for the identification of bone metastases when combined with conventional MR imaging. Both qualitative and quantitative DW-MRI have also been found to be of value for distinguishing between benign and malignant causes of vertebral fractures. There is also promise in the application of quantitative ADC for evaluating treatment response of malignant bone diseases, as current imaging criteria are inadequate in assessing treatment changes of bone lesions to therapy.

K. Nakanishi, MD, PhD
Department of Diagnostic Radiology, Osaka Medical Center for Cancer and Cardiovascular Diseases, Nakamichi, Higashinari-Ku, 537-8511 Osaka, Japan
A. Gutzeit, MD
Department of Diagnostic and Interventional Radiology, Kantonsspital Winterthur, Brauerstrasse 15, Postfach 834, CH-8401 Winterthur, Switzerland

13.1

Introduction

DW-MRI is widely used for imaging of the central nervous system, especially for the diagnosis of acute stroke, although its use in the body has been limited because of several artefacts due to cardiac motion, respiration and limited signal-to-noise ratio (ICHIKAWA and ARAKI 1999; GUO et al. 2002; HUISMAN 2003; TAKAHARA et al. 2004). However, advances in MR imaging technologies have enabled reliable acquisition of DW-MR images in the body using relatively high *b*-values (e.g. $b = 1,000\,s/mm^2$) (ICHIKAWA and ARAKI 1999). By applying the diffusion-weighted whole-body imaging with background signal suppression (DWIBS) technique, whole-body DW-MR images can be acquired within a reasonable scan time for disease evaluation. When these images are displayed using an inverted grey scale, they superficially resemble images acquired using 18-fluorodeoxyglucose positron emission tomography (PET) imaging (TAKAHARA et al. 2004) and have been shown to be helpful for tumour assessment (see Chap. 14).

MR imaging results in intrinsically high image contrast between soft tissues and bones (SUGIMOTO et al. 1988; JACOBSSON et al. 1991; IMAMURA et al. 2000; NAKANISHI et al. 2005, 2007). With increasing age, the normal cellular marrow is replaced by fat, thus modifying the signal characteriztics of the bone marrow on MR imaging. However, the fat-replaced bone marrow provides a high signal intensity background to facilitate the detection of hypointense disease on conventional T1-weighted MR imaging. There is also emerging data that support the use of DW-MRI (NONOMURA et al. 2001) for the detection and characterization of bone involvement in patients with cancer, as well as for assessing tumour response to treatment. The evaluation of tumour response to treatment of bone disease is particularly challenging because to date, there is no reliable imaging technique that can be applied to quantify the degree of treatment change. As emphasized in previous chapters, assessment of bone disease should not be made in isolation using DW-MRI, but should be combined with conventional imaging (including radiographs, CT and conventional MR imaging) for the best assessment to be made.

In this chapter, we will survey the range of malignant conditions that may be encountered in the bones of oncological patients. Conventional and DW-MRI imaging techniques that can be applied for the detection and characterization of bone involvement will be discussed. The emphasis of discussion will be on the evaluation of metastatic bone disease and in the systemic workup of patients with underlying cancer to determine the extent of disease involvement. We will also survey the imaging criteria that have been developed for the assessment of tumour response to treatment in bones, and highlight the potential of DW-MRI as an imaging technique that can be used to monitor treatment change. Last but not least, we will review some benign bone conditions, which may mimic malignant bone diseases on DW-MRI.

Malignant Conditions of the Bones

Bone tumours can generally be divided into two groups: benign and malignant bone tumours. Malignant bone tumours can in turn be subdivided into primary malignant bone tumours and bone metastases.

When a focal bone lesion is encountered, knowledge of the age of the patient and the location of disease are helpful for image interpretation. Imaging features which are useful for lesion characterization include the nature of the tumour matrix, the zone of transition of the lesion and adjacent bone or soft tissue changes. One of the key features in radiological assessment is identifying the presence and nature of any associated periosteal reaction, which may be characterized as interrupted or non-interrupted, the former being typical of malignant bone diseases. When all these factors are considered, it is possible in most cases to make a relatively specific radiological diagnosis before definitive histological confirmation becomes available (MILLER 2008).

Bone metastases are the most common malignant bone tumours and for this reason should always be considered in the differential diagnoses of suspicious lesions, especially in the elderly. In patients with cancer, the development of metastatic bone involvement represents disseminated disease which carries a poor prognosis. As such, accurate determination of the presence and extent of bone metastases is important. Bone metastases commonly arise from tumours of the lung, breast, prostate and thyroid, and usually affect vertebrae of the spine, skull and proximal long bones. Not uncommonly, bone metastases may be complicated by a pathological fracture, which may make it difficult to identify the malignant disease in the presence of substantial secondary changes. The bones can also be affected by haematological malignancies including lymphomas. Leukaemia and multiple myeloma frequently infiltrate the bone marrow, and involvement may be focal or diffuse (BAUR-MELNYK et al. 2008a, b). Non-invasive imaging techniques are viewed upon as important tools to assess prognosis of the disease and for planning treatment strategies in patients with haematological malignancies (LECOUVET 1998). However, the lack of existing standards for assessing bone involvement in malignant bone disease remains an unresolved radiological issue.

Conventional Imaging for the Detection of Bone Involvement in Cancer

In clinical practice, the first step taken to diagnose bone disease is usually by conventional radiography. The main disadvantage of this technique is the low sensitivity. Bone metastasis is only visible at the earliest when there has been a loss of the bone mineral content of 50% or more (RUBENS 1998) (Fig. 13.1). For this reason, additional imaging such as CT, radionuclide bone scans, [18]FDG-PET or MR imaging are frequently employed.

CT is highly sensitive for identifying cortical destruction, pathological fractures, and periosteal

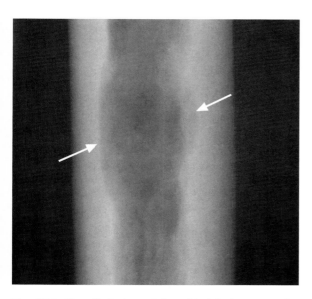

Fig. 13.1. Magnified view of the mid right humerus of a 68-year-old man with multiple myeloma shows endosteal scalloping of the inner bony cortex due to myelomatous disease infiltration (*arrows*). However, the radiograph is relatively insensitive to pathological processes and the radiograph may be normal even in the presence of significant disease infiltration

changes. Other advantages of CT include its wide availability and quick examination time. By performing high-resolution imaging, it is possible to perform 3D and multiplanar image reconstructions to provide the surgeon with spatially relevant information for surgical planning. However, the main drawbacks of CT are its low sensitivity for small volume disease affecting the bones and the relatively high radiation exposure (MAHNER et al. 2008).

The sensitivity of radionuclide bone scintigraphy is dependent on the osteoblastic activity associated with the pathological process. The technique is very sensitive for bone metastases, especially for osteoblastic disease arising from breast and prostate cancers (HRICAK et al. 2007). The key disadvantage is its lower sensitivity for lytic bone disease (e.g. metastases from renal cell and bladder carcinoma) and bone marrow infiltration (e.g. leukaemia and multiple myeloma). For example, the sensitivity of bone scintigraphy for detecting myeloma deposits is only 40–60%, this being the reason that the technique is not used for routine disease staging (WINTERBOTTOM et al. 2009). A further limitation of bone scintigraphy is the potential false-positives that can arise from healing fractures or degenerative changes.

[18]FDG-PET is more sensitive than bone scan for detecting bone malignancies because tumours show higher tracer uptake as a result of increased metabolism (CHERAN et al. 2004). Although [18]FDG-PET is more specific, issues remain with regards to small lesions (<1 cm), radiation burden with repeated scans and poor visualization of tumours with low metabolic activity (e.g. prostate carcinoma, renal cell carcinoma, bronchoalveolar cell carcinoma).

MR imaging has been shown to be a highly sensitive technique for the detection of bone diseases, such as bone metastases. Conventional MR imaging includes T1-weighted, T2-weighted and STIR imaging as well as contrast-enhanced T1-weighted sequences. Specialized imaging protocols combining these techniques have been used with reportedly good results. With the introduction of whole-body MR imaging using multi-channel receiver coils, this has enabled imaging of the body from head to toe. Whole-body MR imaging has been adopted for the evaluation of bone and bone marrow diseases and several studies have confirmed that the diagnostic accuracy using MR imaging is higher than radionuclide bone scintigraphy and CT for the detection of bone metastases and primary tumours (EUSTACE et al. 1997; COSTELLOE et al. 2009).

13.4

Considerations for Conventional MR Imaging and DW-MRI

Diffusion-weighted MR imaging is a promising new tool for the detection and evaluation of malignant bone diseases. However, the technique should not be used in isolation. High-quality morphological imaging (especially T1-weighted imaging) is also necessary to aid interpretation of observed changes within the bones and for precise anatomical localization of the lesion. To date, there have been few larger-scale studies comparing the diagnostic accuracy of DW-MRI alone or in combination with conventional morphological imaging for the assessment of malignant bone diseases. It will be important that further studies are undertaken in the future.

13.4.1
Conventional MR Imaging

When using conventional MR imaging to assess bone disease, evaluation is usually made using T1-weighted and short-tau inversion recovery (STIR) imaging. This combination of sequences has been shown to be effective for the detection of focal bone diseases (YASUMOTO et al. 2002; SCHMIDT et al. 2009). Imaging should be performed in two orthogonal planes to provide accurate information on the exact anatomical localization and extension of the lesion. Compared with DW-MRI, conventional T1-weighted and STIR images are usually acquired at higher spatial resolution, which provides better anatomical delineation of disease. In particular, T1-weighted imaging is useful for identifying foci of sclerotic bone disease, as these lesions are relatively signal suppressed on STIR and high b-value DW-MR imaging. Thus, combining T1-weighted imaging with STIR and DW-MR imaging can be helpful towards evaluating the osteolytic vs. osteosclerotic disease fractions, thereby providing useful information which may reflect on the underlying tumour biology.

Conventional T1-weighted and STIR imaging can be incorporated into a whole-body imaging protocol for disease assessment. This is typically achieved by performing T1-weighted fast spin-echo (SE) and STIR imaging in the sagittal and coronal planes at multiple anatomical stations in the body. Such imaging implementation is well described in the published literature (EUSTACE et al. 1997; SCHMIDT et al. 2009). One suggested imaging protocol is outlined below:

- *T1-weighted sagittal images of the spine.* Five image sections of T1-weighted fast spin-echo images of the spine are acquired in the sagittal plane using three imaging stations [TR/TE, 400/13 ms. Echo train length (ETL) 4, section thickness 7, 300 mm field of view (FOV), scan matrix = 352 × 264, imaging time 4 min 33 s].
- *T1-weighted coronal images of the whole body.* 32 fast spin-echo T1-weighted images of the whole body acquired coronally using six imaging stations [TR/TE100/4.6 ms, ETL 128, 7 mm section thickness, 300 mm FOV, scan matrix = 240 × 180, imaging time 6 min 24 s].
- *STIR sagittal images of the spine.* Five STIR sagittal image sections of the whole spine acquired using three imaging stations [TR/TE/TI 2,500/70/170 ms, ETL 15, section thickness 7, 300 mm FOV, scan matrix 288 × 316, imaging time 6 min 15 s].
- *STIR coronal images of whole body.* 32 STIR images of the whole body acquired coronally at six imaging stations [TR/TE/TI 1,350/40/165 ms, ETL 65, section thickness 7, 300 mm FOV, scan matrix = 320 × 185, imaging time 6 min 24 s].

With technological advancement, it is now possible to perform high spatial resolution T1-weighted imaging using a 3D volume interpolated technique (THOMSON et al. 2008). One variant of this approach is to apply a fat–water separation sequence, such as one employing a 2-point DIXON technique, which would enable fat-only and water-only images to be generated. The water-only images resemble fat-suppressed images and can be helpful for lesion identification (SUAREZ et al. 2009; VANEL et al. 2009) (Fig. 13.2). 3D volume interpolated imaging may also be acquired before and after contrast administration (THOMSON et al. 2008).

13.4.2
Diffusion-Weighted MR Imaging (DW-MRI)

13.4.2.1
Regional DW-MRI

DW-MRI is usually performed in the body across a target region of interest using a free-breathing single-shot echo-planar imaging technique. Imaging is typically performed in the axial plane. The choice and number of b-values included in the measurement depends in part on whether the images are to be used for qualitative or quantitative assessment.

Fig. 13.2. Coronal water-only images derived using a 2-point DIXON technique (**a**) before and (**b**) after intravenous gadolinium-DTPA contrast administration. Such images can be rapidly acquired in breath-hold to provide good radiological contrast for the assessment of bones and soft tissues in the body

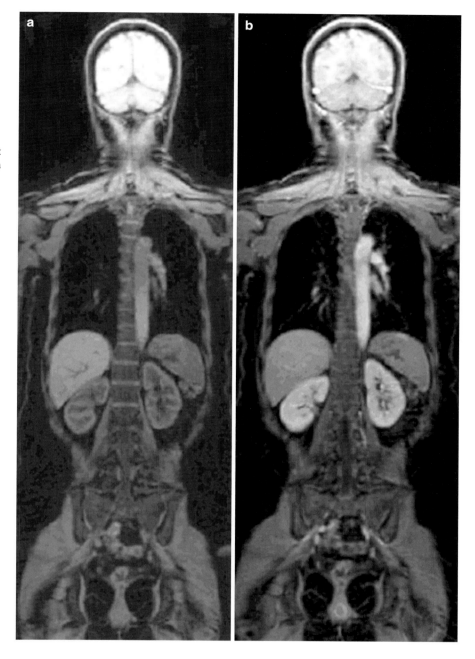

For qualitative assessment, a single high b-value (e.g. 600–1,000 s/mm^2) may suffice. The choice of the higher b-value may in part be limited by the scanner capability, which determines the image quality and signal-to-noise ratio. Generally, using a higher b-value would result in better background signal suppression, optimal for detecting tissues with reduced water diffusivity. Sometimes, the quality of DW-MR images of the lower thoracic and lumbar spine may be poor as a result of respiratory motion. If this occurs, it has been shown that the application of navigator-tracked respiratory-triggered DW-MRI can significantly improve the image quality (SPUENTRUP et al. 2003). For quantitative ADC calculations, three or more b-values would provide a more accurate fit of DW-MRI data, resulting in a more precise ADC estimate. Imaging using different b-values and the evaluation of quantitative ADC data were discussed in Chaps. 1–3.

In the appendicular skeleton, it is possible to apply alternative image acquisition schemes for DW-MRI. In one report (ONER et al. 2007), the application of a non-Carr-Purcell-Meiboom-Gill, single-shot, fast spin-echo sequence was found to result in images with a higher contrast-to-noise ratio compared with EPI technique. In the spine, it has also been shown that a steady-state free precession (SSFP) technique can be used for the assessment of vertebral pathologies (BAUR et al. 2001a, b, 2002a, b; RAYA et al. 2006) by visual and semi-quantitative analysis of the measured signal intensities. However, ADC quantification using the SSFP technique is much more challenging.

13.4.2.2
Diffusion-Weighted Whole-Body Imaging with Background Signal Suppression (DWIBS)

For whole-body imaging, DW-MRI is performed using single-shot STIR-EPI sequences (TR 6243/TE 59/TI 180 ms) using b-values of 0 and 600–1,000 s/mm^2. Thin image partition of 4–5 mm is typically used, with 1 mm of overlap. Images are acquired axially during free breathing and are performed at multiple imaging stations from the neck down to at least the pelvis. Where a receiver coil with a large field is available and if the patient is not too large or tall, imaging coverage may be achieved in just two stations on some MR imaging systems. Otherwise, imaging at four to five anatomical stations may be necessary, depending on the extent of coverage desired. Employing an imaging field of view (FOV) of 450 mm at each imaging station and an imaging matrix of 112 × 112, imaging at each station can be achieved in approximately 5 min.

Once the images are acquired, radial maximum intensity projections (MIPs) of the inverted grey-scale high b-value images may be processed and viewed on a workstation (see Chap. 14).

13.5
DW-MRI for the Detection and Characterization of Bone Involvement in Cancer

13.5.1
Normal Appearance of Bones on DW-MRI

Optimal interpretation of DW-MRI relies on knowledge of the normal appearances of bones on imaging.

It must be remembered that bones are dynamic tissues that consist of a mineralized structure in which non-mineralized mesenchymal, haematopoietic and other connective tissue elements are distributed. In young adults, haematopoietically active red marrow is found predominantly in the pelvis and in the proximal long bones (VANDE BERG et al. 1998). However, with increasing age, red marrow tissue is progressively replaced by fat, such that macroscopically it appears yellow in colour and is therefore known as "yellow marrow". In adults, about 50% marrow tissue is yellow marrow and this is predominantly located in the appendicular skeleton. The remaining 50% consists of red marrow found mainly within the axial skeletal and proximal long bones. In the elderly, the proportion of yellow marrow can further increase. Yellow marrow is composed of 95% fat cells, whereas red marrow is composed of 60% haematopoietic cells and 40% fat cells (VANDE BERG et al. 1998). Using MR imaging, the marrow elements of bony tissues are well demonstrated. On T1-weighted imaging, red marrow appears intermediate signal intensity compared with the high signal intensity of yellow marrow. One useful fact to remember is that the pattern of distribution of red marrow in the body tends to be symmetrical across vertebrae and from one side of the body to the other (DAFFNER et al. 1986; WEINREB 1990; VANDE BERG et al. 1998), a feature which may help to distinguish red marrow from disease infiltration.

Not surprisingly, there is considerable variation in the appearances of the bones and bone marrow on DW-MRI although the full range of imaging findings has not been fully documented. However, it is clear that the appearances of bones on DW-MRI vary with age as a result of fatty involution, and the DW-MRI appearance alters in tandem with the imaging findings on T1-weighted and STIR imaging. Fatty yellow marrow shows high signal intensity on T1-weighted imaging, and signal attenuation on high b-value DW-MRI because of the fat-suppression pulse that is applied with the EPI diffusion-weighted measurement. The limited mobility of protons associated with fat also means that normal yellow marrow returns lower ADC values compared with hypercellular or disease-infiltrated bone marrow (NONOMURA et al. 2001). However, nulling of the fat signal by fat suppression may result in greater errors in the calculated ADC of normal bone marrow, because of the diminished accuracy of measuring signal attenuation from protons associated with the fatty tissues.

Regional variations in ADC values of normal bone marrow in non-oncological adult patients aged between 28 and 82 years have been reported (ZHANG et al. 2008). It was found that the mean ADC value of lumber vertebral bodies (0.62×10^{-3} mm²/s) was significantly higher than that measured from the left ilium (0.40×10^{-3} mm²/s) or the left femur (0.36×10^{-3} mm²/s), reflecting the greater degree of fatty involution in the long bones and pelvis of adults (ZHANG et al. 2008). In addition, osteoporosis which may result in increased fat deposition in bones has been found to be associated with a decrease in bone ADC values (YEUNG et al. 2004). However, in another study, no relationship was found between the ADC values of vertebral bodies and the bone density determined by dual X-ray absorptiometry (GRIFFITH et al. 2006).

On DWIBS imaging, the normal fat-replaced bone marrow is signal-suppressed on the high *b*-value images (BAUR et al. 2001a, b). From the discussion above, it would be clear that in younger patients with haematopoietically active red marrow, the distribution of red marrow can be observed using DWIBS as these relatively cellular areas would be reflected in a high signal intensity. As in Fig.13.3 residual red marrow in the metaphyses of long bones in the younger individual demonstrate higher signal intensity compared with the bone marrow findings in the older man.

13.5.2
DW-MRI Detection of Metastatic Bone Disease

There are emerging studies demonstrating the value of DW-MRI for the detection of metastatic disease compared with conventional MR imaging and radionuclide studies (NAKANISHI et al. 2005; KOMORI et al. 2007; LICHY et al. 2007; MOON et al. 2007; NAKANISHI et al. 2007; NEMETH et al. 2007; LUBOLDT et al. 2008; OHNO et al. 2008; TAKANO et al. 2008; XU et al. 2008; LAURENT et al. 2009). In one of the largest studies to date, Ohno et al. (2008) evaluated 203 patients with non-small-cell lung cancers. Forty patients were found to have stage IV disease of which 11 had metastases only to bones. Interestingly, the addition of DW-MRI to conventional T1-weighted and STIR imaging resulted in a similar diagnostic accuracy and inter-observer agreement compared with ¹⁸FDG–PET–CT (OHNO et al. 2008). Using DW-MRI alone was significantly less accurate on a per-patient and per-lesion basis compared with ¹⁸FDG-PET–CT alone or the combination of DW-MRI with T1-weighted and STIR imaging. In another study, it was shown that DW-MRI was equal, if not superior to STIR and T1-weighted SE sequences, but as effective as ¹¹C-choline PET-CT for the detection of bone metastases in patients with prostate cancer (LUBOLDT et al.

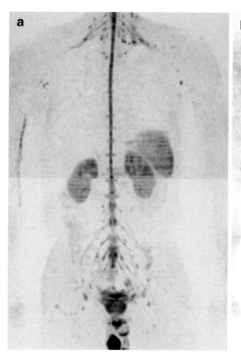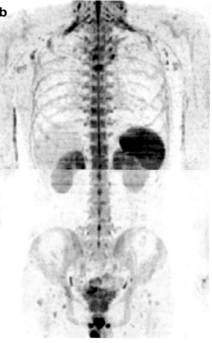

Fig. 13.3. Normal findings on DWIBS using a STIR EPI DW-MRI technique in (**a**) a 45-year-old man and (**b**) a 35-year-old man. These DW-MR images at a *b*-value of 600 s/mm² are displayed using an inverted grey scale. Note that in the older man (**a**), the signal intensity of the normal bone marrow is suppressed, although the spinal cord, nerve roots, kidneys, spleen and testes return low signal intensity on the inverted grey-scale images. However, in the younger man (**b**), there is relatively more signal returned from the red marrow within the bones especially in the axial skeleton

2008). Initial experience in 35 patients with metastatic melanoma showed that DWIBS was superior to [18]FDG-PET–CT for the detection of metastatic disease including bones (Laurent et al. 2009).

In our experience, we have assessed the diagnostic value of DW-MRI for detecting bony metastasis compared with conventional whole-body MR imaging and bone scintigraphy (Nakanishi et al. 2007). We found that the mean sensitivity and positive predictive value (PPV) of the combination DW-MRI with conventional MR imaging were 96% and 98%, respectively, which were superior to conventional MR sequences alone (88% and 98%) or bone scintigraphy alone (96% and 94%). Based on current evidence, DW-MRI and DWIBS appear to be highly promising for detecting metastatic disease to the bone, but the technique should be combined with conventional imaging for the best diagnosis to be made. An example of DWIBS in a patient with multiple bone metastases from prostate cancer is shown in Fig.13.4. The MIP images show the metastatic rib lesions clearly, which in this case, also correlate well with the bone scintigram appearance.

One of the key reasons why conventional imaging should not be ignored is because osteoblastic metastases may be missed on DW-MRI. Osteoblastic metastases may arise from prostate, breast, medulloblastoma, neuroendocrine and gastric cancers. Dense osteoblastic lesions often appear dark on the high b-value DW-MR images and may be difficult to distinguish from the signal suppressed fatty marrow (Fig. 13.5) (Hacklander et al. 2006). Osteoblastic metastases are better visualized on T1-weighted imaging, the corresponding CT imaging or by their increased tracer uptake on bone scintigraphy.

The advantages of DW-MRI over bone scintigraphy include the fact that osteolytic bone lesions may not be tracer-avid and hence may not be visible on scintigraphy (Fig. 13.6). Moreover, DW-MRI is useful for depicting lesions in the anterior ilium which may be less well seen on bone scintigraphy due to the position of the lesion in relation to the isotope camera (Fig. 13.7). There is a limit to the metabolic dimension of lesions that can be confidently detected using bone scintigraphy or [18]FDG-PET–CT. Bone lesions measuring less than 1 cm in diameter may be missed if they are not intensely tracer-avid. In our experience, small lesions measuring 1 cm or less are frequently better visualized on DW-MRI. In addition, DW-MRI or DWIBS may help to detect

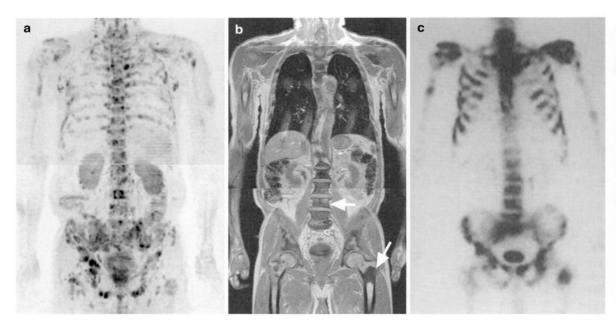

Fig. 13.4. Images of a 69-year-old man with multiple bone metastases from prostate carcinoma. (**a**) Maximum intensity projection of the inverted grey-scale $b = 600 \, \text{s/mm}^2$ image shows multiple metastases in the bones depicted as low intensity lesions. (**b**) An image section from the whole-body T1-weighted acquisition shows very low intensity foci along the spine and within the left proximal femur, suggestive of osteoblastic metastases (*arrows*). (**c**) Bone scintigraphy confirms increased tracer uptake within the metastases. In this case, note the correspondence of imaging findings between DW-MRI, T1-weighted imaging and bone scintigraphy

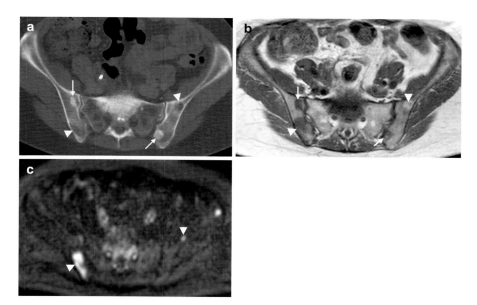

Fig. 13.5. Axial images of a 56-year-old woman with metastatic breast cancer. (**a**) CT imaging of the pelvis shows sclerotic (*arrows*) and lytic (*arrowheads*) bone metastases. (**b**) The sclerotic metastases return low signal intensity on T1-weighted imaging (*arrows*), although the lytic metastases (*arrowheads*) show more variable T1 signal intensity. (**c**) DW-MRI at $b = 1,000\,\text{s/mm}^2$ demonstrates the high signal intensity from the lytic metastases (arrowheads) but the sclerotic bone metastases are signal-suppressed (Courtesy Dr. Koh, Royal Marsden Hospital, UK)

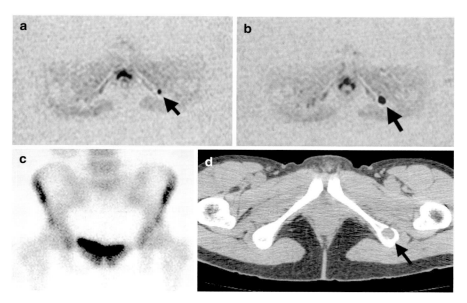

Fig. 13.6. Solitary metastatic lesion. Images of a 54-year-old woman with leiomyosarcoma of the uterus. (**a**) Focus of impeded diffusion in the left inferior pubic ramus (*arrow*) was missed on the initial reading of the inverted grey-scale DW-MR image at a b-value of $600\,\text{s/mm}^2$. (**b**) Repeat imaging 3 months later showed that the disease in the left pubic ramus has enlarged consistent with a metastasis (*arrow*). (**c**) The lesion was not visible on bone scintigraphy (**d**) CT imaging revealed an osteolytic lesion corresponding to the DW-MRI abnormality associated with cortical destruction (*arrow*)

Fig. 13.7. Solitary metastasis. Images of a 68-year-old woman with breast carcinoma. (**a**) On the $b = 600\,s/mm^2$ inverted grey-scale coronal maximum intensity projection image, an area of decreased signal intensity is seen within the left ilium (*arrow*). (**b**) The corresponding area appears bright on the short-tau inversion recovery fat-suppressed image (*arrow*). (**c**) However, no significant tracer uptake was observed on bone scintigraphy. (**d**) Radiography reveals lucency and irregularity in the left ilium (*arrow*) which corroborate with the diagnosis of bone metastasis

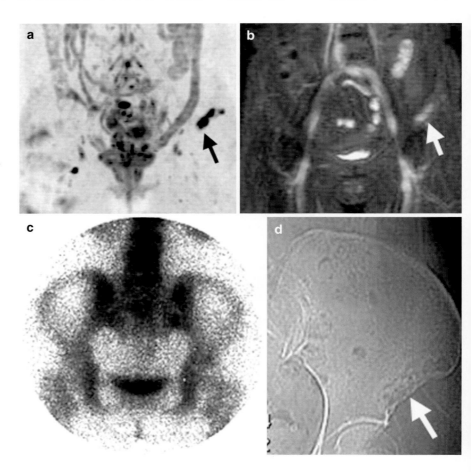

unsuspected sites of extra-skeletal disease, such as in the lungs, breast, liver or lymph nodes (Fig. 13.8).

13.5.3
DW-MRI for Distinguishing Between Benign and Malignant Causes of Vertebral Collapse

Bone metastases in vertebral bodies occur in up to 10% of patients with primary neoplasms. A common result of such metastases is the collapse or fracture of the vertebral body. In oncological patients, it is often challenging to distinguish between a benign and a malignant vertebral body fracture. It has been estimated that up to one-third of vertebral fractures in patients with known malignancies are benign (FORNASIER et al. 1978). Differentiating benign from malignant causes of a vertebral fracture is important because different therapeutic management is undertaken for each.

Using conventional MR imaging and CT, it is frequently difficult – if not impossible – to determine whether a collapsed vertebral body is the result of a metastatic or benign process. A few radiological signs have been proposed to be helpful in this regard. Bauer et al. (2002a, b) described the "fluid sign" on MR imaging which was more frequently observed in benign osteoporotic fractures (40%) compared with malignant vertebral fractures (6%). This sign was observed as high signal intensity fluid on STIR imaging, often in a linear configuration adjacent to vertebral endplates (BAUR et al. 2002a, b) and associated with high signal changes reflecting marrow oedema within the collapsed vertebral body. Another sign which was first observed on CT imaging in benign vertebral body fractures was the intravertebral "vacuum sign", which referred to linear gas densities within the vertebral body (BHALLA et al. 1998). This phenomenon can be observed in approximately 10% of osteoporotic fractures (PAPPOU et al. 2008). A study in 180 patients with radiological–pathological comparison showed a strong correlation between osteonecrosis and presence of the vacuum sign. The vacuum sign was found to have 85% sensitivity, 99%

Fig. 13.8. DW-MR images of a 34-year-old man with an alveolar soft part sarcoma (ASPS) with spinal and pulmonary metastases. (a) On the sagittal reformat of the DW-MR images at a *b*-value of 600 s/mm², there is a low signal intensity metastasis arising from posterior elements of the lower cervical spine (*arrow*). (b) The coronal maximum intensity projection DW-MR image (inverted grey scale) shows numerous low intensity metastases within the lungs (*arrows*). (c) Axial DW-MR image through the upper abdomen reveals a mass inseparable from the head of the pancreas, consistent with a further site of metastasis

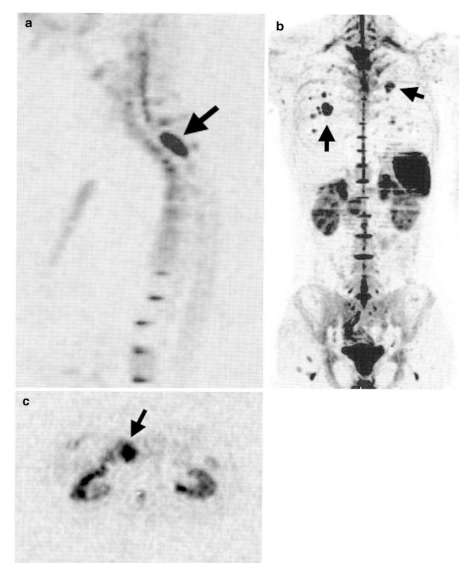

specificity and 91% positive predictive value for vertebral osteonecrosis (LIBICHER et al. 2007).

In 1998, Bauer et al. (1998) showed the feasibility of using the signal intensity of vertebral collapse on DW-MRI to discriminate between benign and malignant fractures. It was observed that malignant fractures were hyperintense compared with normal vertebrae (Fig. 13.9), but benign fractures appeared hypointense or isointense to normal vertebrae on DW-MRI (Fig. 13.10). This difference in MR appearance was ascribed to impeded water diffusion in the hypercellular tumour. However, in a subsequent study, Castillo et al. (2000) reported high signal intensity in both benign and malignant vertebral fractures. However, in that study, a relatively low *b*-value (*b* = 165 s/mm²) was employed making the measurements sensitive to T2-shine-through effects. Further work by Baur et al. found that by increasing the diffusion-weighting of their SSFP imaging sequence it was possible to reduce the incidence of false-positive hyperintense osteoporotic fractures (BAUR et al. 2001a, b) and later achieved a high sensitivity and specificity for the diagnosis of malignant vertebral fractures (BAUR et al. 2002a, b). Another study also independently showed the utility of signal suppression on DW-MRI as a basis for discriminating benign

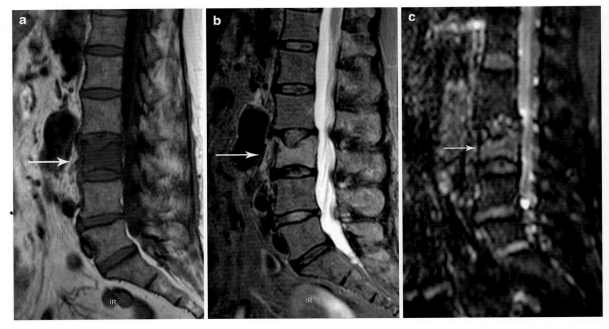

Fig. 13.9. Malignant vertebral fracture. An elderly man with metastatic disease to L3 vertebral body. (a) T1-weighted MR imaging demonstrates hypointensity within the L3 vertebral body (*arrow*) with loss of vertebral height. (b) The vertebral body appears mildly hyperintense on short-tau inversion recovery imaging (*arrow*). (c) Sagittal reformat of DW-MR image at a *b*-value of 1,000 s/mm² shows impeded diffusion within the verterbral body (*arrow*) consistent with malignant disease

from malignant vertebral fractures (SPUENTRUP et al. 2001).

As the measured signal intensity on DW-MRI is influenced by tissue diffusivity and T2-relaxation time, other authors have suggested that the ADC calculation may be a more robust method to discriminate between benign and malignant vertebral fractures. A summary of these findings is presented in Table 13.1. A few important points can be suggested from these observations:

1. There was substantial variation in the reported ADC values of benign and malignant vertebral lesions which reflected differences in the MR techniques applied and the choice of *b*-values.
2. The ADC values of normal bone marrow varied widely between studies. This could reflect physiological differences between studies, but could also be accounted for by measurement errors as a result of SNR variations, the choice of *b*-values or as a consequence of applying fat suppression to quantify diffusivity of fat-containing tissues. Nevertheless, the ADC of normal bone marrow appears to be relatively low in many of the recently published studies (CHAN et al. 2002; MAEDA et al. 2003; GRIFFITH et al. 2006).
3. Malignant vertebral fracture or malignant marrow infiltration returned lower ADC values compared with benign vertebral fractures. However, the optimal ADC threshold value to apply to determine benignity has not been established. This is likely to vary with the imaging technique, as well as the number and choice of *b*-values applied for the DW-MRI study.
4. Infectious spondylosis resulted in low ADC values that were indistinguishable from those of malignant vertebral involvement. Hence, ADC values may not be appropriate for differentiating between malignant and infective conditions.

Despite these cautionary notes, in a well-conducted DW-MRI study performed using a wide range of *b*-values, a hypointense signal observed within a fractured vertebra on high DW-MRI at high *b*-values in combination with an increased ADC would be suggestive of a benign lesion.

Fig. 13.10. Benign vertebral fracture. A middle-aged man with benign vertebral body fracture at T8. (**a**) T1-weighted MR imaging demonstrates hypointensity within the T8 vertebral body (*arrow*) associated with anterior wedging of the vertebral body. (**b**) The vertebral body appears isointense to other vertebral bodies on short-tau inversion recovery imaging (*arrow*). (**c**) Sagittal reformat of DW-MR images at a *b*-value of 1,000 s/mm^2 showed no abnormal increased signal intensity within the verterbral body (*arrow*) consistent with a benign process

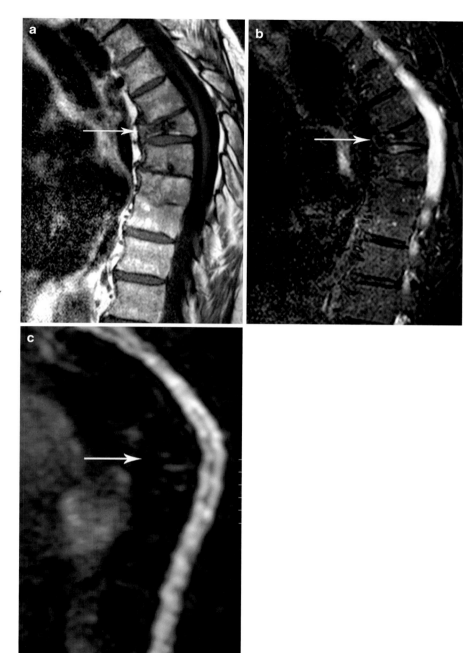

13.5.4
DW-MRI for the Evaluation of Marrow Involvement by Haematological Malignancies

DW-MRI has also been used to demonstrate sites of marrow infiltration in haematological malignancies. For example, DW-MRI has been used to identify areas of marrow infiltration by leukaemia (BALLON et al. 2000). Although there have been reports detailing the improved diagnostic efficacy of whole-body MR imaging using conventional MR techniques for the assessment of patient with multiple myeloma (MULLIGAN et al. 2007; LICHY et al. 2008; DINTER et al. 2009), the role of DW-MRI for the assessment of disease in patients with multiple myeloma has not been established. However, based on our personal

Table 13.1. ADCs of normal vertebrae, benign fracture and malignant vertebral involvement reported in the published literature

	IMAGING STUDIES						
	(HERNETH et al. 2000)	(CHAN et al. 2002)	(HERNETH et al. 2002)	(ZHOU et al. 2002)	(MAEDA et al. 2003)	(GRIFFITH et al. 2006)	(BALLIU et al. 2009)
NUMBER OF PATIENTS	5	32	22	27	64	110	45
Imaging technique	Navigator triggered EPI	Single-shot EPI	Navigator triggered EPI	Single-shot EPI	Line scan DW-MRI	Single-shot EPI	Single-shot EPI
b-Values (s/mm^2)	440, 880	200, 500, 800, 1,000	440, 880	0, 150, 250	5, 1,000	0. 100, 200, 300, 400, 500	0. 500
Mean ADC values ($\times 10^{-3}$ mm^2/s) $\pm$ standard deviation							
Normal vertebrae	1.3 ± 0.23	0.23 ± 0.05	1.66 ± 0.38	0.3–0.7	0.18 ± 0.09	0.43 ± 0.12	
Malignant fracture[*]/ infiltration[**]	0.39 ± 0.11[**]	0.82 ± 0.20[*]	0.71 ± 0.27[*] 0.69 ± 0.24[**]	0.19 ± 0.03[*]	0.92 ± 0.2[*] 0.83 ± 0.17[**]		0.9 ± 1.3[**]
Benign fracture		1.94 ± 0.35	1.61 ± 0.37	0.32 ± 0.05	1.21 ± 0.17		1.9 ± 0.39 (benign oedema)
Others		0.98 ± 0.21 (tuberculous spondylitis)					0.96 ± 0.49 (infectious spondylitis)

experience, it would appear that DW-MRI is also a potentially useful technique for evaluating the degree of marrow involvement by the disease. In an example of a patient with multiple myeloma (Fig. 13.11), DWIBS was used to highlight the anatomical distribution of bone disease in the body. The technique could also prove helpful in elucidating sites of extra-osseous soft-tissue disease in patients with haematological malignancies.

13.6

Assessment of Treatment Response in Malignant Bone Disease

Assessment of the extent of response to treatment, during and after a specific therapy is crucial in clinical evaluation of cancer therapeutics. To unify the criteria of tumour response, the Response Evaluation Criteria in Solid Tumours (RECIST) were introduced in 2000, which were recently updated in version 1.1 (EISENHAUER et al. 2009). Although bone is a common site for metastatic disease, no consensus has

been reached regarding the assessment of treatment response although several suggestions have been made (BAUERLE et al. 2009).

In the original RECIST criteria, bone involvement was not considered to be a site of measurable disease. However, in the recently revised RECIST guidelines (version 1.1) (EISENHAUER et al. 2009), osteolytic lesions or mixed osteolytic/osteoblastic lesions with identifiable soft tissue components are now considered measurable by CT and MR imaging. Osteoblastic lesions, however, are still deemed immeasurable. Furthermore, bone scintigraphy, conventional radiographs and [18]FDG-PET cannot be used to quantify response, although these techniques may be applied to confirm the presence or resolution of lesions. However, size measurement provides a crude index of lesional response to therapy because successful treatment may not reduce lesion size. Hence, size measurement of bone metastases could potentially be confusing as it may not represent true disease response after a specific oncological therapy.

As an alternative to size measurement, Hamaoka et al. (2004) suggested that morphological changes to the appearance of bone metastasis on imaging may be

Fig. 13.11. Multiple myeloma. Images of a 69-year-old man with multiple myeloma with metallic internal fixator in the left humerus. (**a**) Inverted grey-scale coronal maximum intensity projection of the DW-MR image at a *b*-value of 600 s/mm^2 shows multiple low-intensity areas in the ribs, right humerus (*arrow*) and shoulder girdle (*arrows*). (**b**) Radiograph of the right humerus reveals multiple osteolytic (punched out) lesions along the humeral shaft scapula (*arrows*) and clavicle

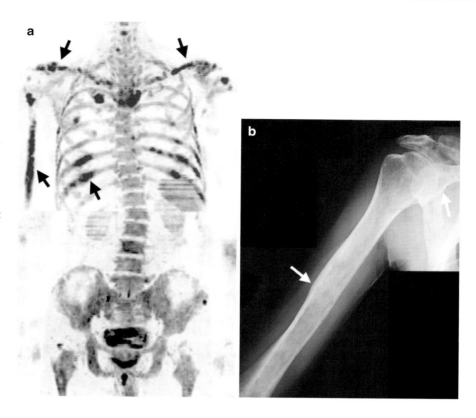

used to gauge disease response. Using this approach, disease response was classified on the basis of disappearance of a lesion or the degree and pattern of calcifications (of an initially osteolytic lesion) after treatment. However, such classification is based on qualitative rather than quantitative assessment, and the criteria are not helpful for assessing osteoblastic disease, except when these lesions completely disappear after treatment.

13.6.1
DW-MRI for Assessing Treatment Response in Bone Malignancies

One of the perceived potentials of using DW-MRI to assess treatment response in bone disease is its ability to provide qualitative and quantitative assessment that reflects biological changes in the tumour following specific oncological therapy. Studies in small series have demonstrated increase in the ADC values within bone tumours and/or a decrease in the signal intensity on the high *b*-value DW-MR imaging following successful therapy (Byun et al. 2002; Hayashida et al. 2006a, b).

However, one of the challenges of performing quantitative DW-MRI for ADC measurements in the bone is the relatively poor SNR, which will impact on the reliability of the ADC measurements. Moreover, as bone tumours are often inhomogeneous, the mean ADC value will represent a mixture of elements representing different tissue types. Nevertheless, applying DW-MRI to quantify the ADC of malignant bone disease is feasible, particularly for circumscribed metastatic deposits associated with soft-tissue components. In such instances, DW-MRI measurements of the malignant disease could be made with good SNR and relatively free of artefacts. Early experience suggests that quantitative ADC values could be used to evaluate the response of malignant bone disease to treatment, and that ADC increases in tumours reflecting treatment response may be observed without any concomitant alterations on conventional morphological imaging (Fig. 13.12). Clearly, more studies are required to validate and demonstrate the efficacy of the technique in this clinical context.

One further development in using ADC to quantify disease response in bones is the application of the so-called functional diffusion map (Lee et al. 2007). Using this analysis method, ADC changes within the

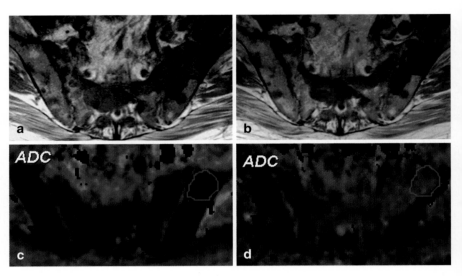

Fig. 13.12. Assessing treatment response of bone disease using DW-MRI. Images of a 72-year-old man with metastatic prostate cancer to bones. Axial T1-weighted imaging of the sacrum (**a**) before and (**b**) after treatment with novel drug (abiraterone) shows no significant difference in the imaging appearance at 28 days after treatment. However, the ADC maps of corresponding area (**c**) before and (**d**) after treatment shows clear increase in the mean ADC value (Pre = 0.69×10^{-3} mm^2/s and Post = 1.52×10^{-3} mm^2/s) within an area of disease (outlined in *red*) in the left ilium indicating drug treatment effects (Courtesy Dr. Koh, Royal Marsden Hospital, UK)

tumour are analysed on a voxel-by-voxel basis and the significance of ADC change is defined by the 5th and 95th percentiles of the pretreatment baseline voxel values. The number and percentage change in voxels above the 95th percentile or below the 5th percentile values after treatment are regarded as significant. Although research is still ongoing, the application of functional diffusion map analysis technique to define tumour response has been shown to correlate with disease survival in patients with cerebral gliomas (HAMSTRA et al. 2008) (see Chap. 10).

13.7
Benign Conditions That May Mimic Malignant Disease on DW-MRI

The high signal intensity observed on a high *b*-value DW-MR image is non-specific and may also result from benign conditions. This is because DW-MRI discriminates on the basis of cellularity, tissue viscosity and structure organization and not necessarily malignancy. For this reason, the readers should be acquainted with a range of benign bone conditions that may mimic malignant bone disease in patients with cancer. A few illustrative examples are presented below.

13.7.1
Osteoarthritis

Osteoarthritis typically occurs as a result of subchondral degeneration. On DW-MRI this condition is observed as mild hyperintensity on DW-MR images at lower *b*-values (e.g. 100 s/mm^2). However, as the *b*-value is increased to about 1,000 s/mm^2, the signal intensity from the degenerate area is usually diminished due to underlying cystic degeneration (Figs. 13.13).

13.7.2
Fracture

Bony fractures may be recognized on DW-MRI. Incidental fractures arising from the thoracic rib cage are not uncommon especially on DWIBS imaging (Fig. 13.14). However, it would be difficult to distinguish between a benign and malignant cause of the rib fracture based on the DW-MR image at a high *b*-value and ADC values alone.

13.7.3
Abscess

Figure 13.15 shows a tuberculous abscess in the soft tissue, which mimics a soft-tissue tumour. When

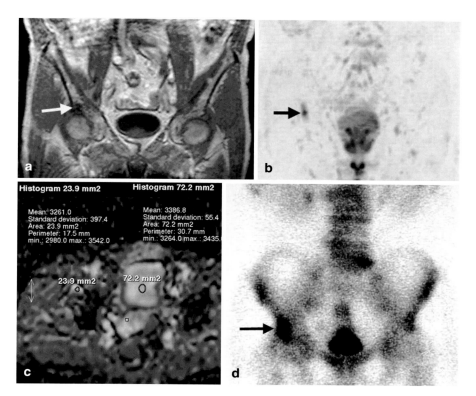

Fig. 13.13. Osteoarthritis. Images of a 69-year-old man with prostate cancer evaluated using whole-body conventional MR imaging and DWIBS techniques. (**a**) A low T1 signal intensity area was detected at the roof of the right acetabulum on T1-weighted coronal imaging (*arrow*). (**b**) This corresponded to an area of decreased signal intensity on the inverted grey-scale coronal maximum intensity projection DWIBS image (*arrow*). (**c**) The mean ADC value of the lesion was high (3.26×10^{-3} mm²/s) and comparable to the ADC value of fluid in the urinary bladder, consistent with a subchondral cyst associated with osteoarthritis. (**d**) However, there was also relative increased tracer uptake in this area on bone scintigraphy, which raised the suspicion for metastasis. Subsequent follow-up imaging showed no confirmatory evidence of metastatic disease

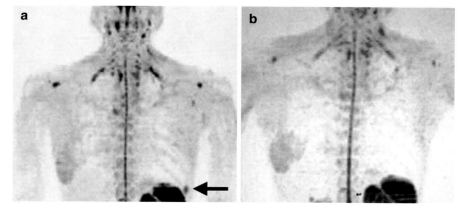

Fig. 13.14. Fracture. Cornonal DW-MR images of a 45-year-old woman with breast cancer who underwent whole-body MR imaging and DWIBS for detecting bone metastases. (**a**) On the inverted grey-scale maximum intensity projection DWIBS image of thorax, there was a solitary low signal intensity focus in the lower left rib (*arrow*). This was interpreted as a rib fracture. (**b**) Follow-up imaging 3 months later showed complete resolution of the abnormality

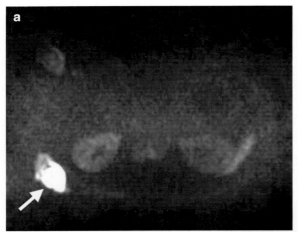

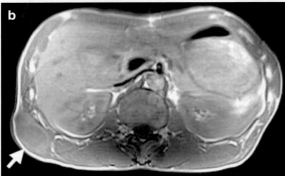

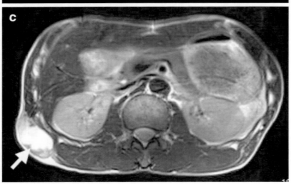

Fig. 13.15. Abscess. Images of a 48-year-old man with soft-tissue swelling in the right flank. (**a**) Axial DW-MR image at a *b*-value of 600 s/mm² showed a high signal intensity mass within the soft tissue of the right flank (*arrow*). (**b**) On T1-weighted imaging, the margins of the mass are mildly hyperintense, although the centre of the mass returns low signal intensity (arrow). (**c**) The mass returned inhomogeneous high signal intensity (*arrow*) on T2-weighted imaging. Pus was aspirated from the lesion and granulomatous inflammation confirmed

associated with bone changes, this appearance could be mistaken as metastatic soft-tissue disease. The composition of pus within an abscess is viscous and rich in protein, thus resulting in high signal intensity on the DW-MR images at high *b*-values and corresponding low ADC value.

13.7.4
Benign Tumour

Benign bone tumours also result in high signal intensity impeded water diffusion related to its underlying cellularity or structural organization (HAYASHIDA et al. 2006a, b).

13.8
Conclusions

In conclusion, DW-MRI is a new imaging tool which can be used to detect and confirm malignant changes in the bones, as well as help distinguish benign from malignant conditions. However, DW-MRI should not be used as a stand-alone technique and should be combined with conventional and cross-sectional imaging techniques for the optimal assessment to be made. The technique is also promising for the assessment of therapeutic response in malignant bone diseases, which may prove useful for assessing the efficacy of therapies in the future.

References

Balliu E, Vilanova JC, Pelaez I, et al (2009) Diagnostic value of apparent diffusion coefficients to differentiate benign from malignant vertebral bone marrow lesions. Eur J Radiol 69:560–6

Ballon D, Dyke J, Schwartz LH, et al (2000) Bone marrow segmentation in leukemia using diffusion and T(2) weighted echo planar magnetic resonance imaging. NMR Biomed 13:321–8

Bauerle T, Semmler W (2009) Imaging response to systemic therapy for bone metastases. Eur Radiol 2009 May 26. [Epub ahead of print]

Baur-Melnyk A, Buhmann S, Becker C, et al (2008a) Whole-body MRI versus whole-body MDCT for staging of multiple myeloma. AJR Am J Roentgenol 190:1097–104

Baur-Melnyk A, Reiser M (2008b) Oncohaematologic disorders affecting the skeleton in the elderly. Radiol Clin North Am 46:785–98

Baur A, Huber A, Durr HR, et al (2002a) [Differentiation of benign osteoporotic and neoplastic vertebral compression fractures with a diffusion-weighted, steady-state free precession sequence]. Rofo Fortschr Geb Rontgenstr Neuen Bildgeb Verfahr 174:70–5

Baur A, Huber A, Ertl-Wagner B, et al (2001a) Diagnostic value of increased diffusion weighting of a steady-state free precession sequence for differentiating acute benign osteoporotic fractures from pathologic vertebral compression fractures. AJNR Am J Neuroradiol 22:366–72

Baur A, Stabler A, Arbogast S, et al (2002b) Acute osteoporotic and neoplastic vertebral compression fractures: fluid sign at MR imaging. Radiology 225:730–5

Baur A, Stabler A, Bruning R, et al (1998) Diffusion-weighted MR imaging of bone marrow: differentiation of benign versus pathologic compression fractures. Radiology 207:349–56

Baur A, Stabler A, Huber A, et al (2001b) Diffusion-weighted magnetic resonance imaging of spinal bone marrow. Semin Musculoskelet Radiol 5:35–42

Bhalla S, Reinus WR (1998) The linear intravertebral vacuum: a sign of benign vertebral collapse. AJR Am J Roentgenol 170:1563–9

Byun WM, Shin SO, Chang Y, et al (2002) Diffusion-weighted MR imaging of metastatic disease of the spine: assessment of response to therapy. AJNR Am J Neuroradiol 23:906–12

Castillo M, Arbelaez A, Smith JK, et al (2000) Diffusion-weighted MR imaging offers no advantage over routine noncontrast MR imaging in the detection of vertebral metastases. AJNR Am J Neuroradiol 21:948–53

Chan JH, Peh WC, Tsui EY, et al (2002) Acute vertebral body compression fractures: discrimination between benign and malignant causes using apparent diffusion coefficients. Br J Radiol 75:207–14

Cheran SK, Herndon JE II, Patz EF Jr (2004) Comparison of whole-body FDG-PET to bone scan for detection of bone metastases in patients with a new diagnosis of lung cancer. Lung Cancer 44:317–25

Costelloe CM, Rohren EM, Madewell JE, et al (2009) Imaging bone metastases in breast cancer: techniques and recommendations for diagnosis. Lancet Oncol 10:606–14

Daffner RH, Lupetin AR, Dash N, et al (1986) MRI in the detection of malignant infiltration of bone marrow. AJR Am J Roentgenol 146:353–8

Dinter DJ, Neff WK, Klaus J, et al (2009) Comparison of whole-body MR imaging and conventional X-ray examination in patients with multiple myeloma and implications for therapy. Ann Hematol 88:457–64

Eisenhauer EA, Therasse P, Bogaerts J, et al (2009) New response evaluation criteria in solid tumours: revised RECIST guideline (version 1.1). Eur J Cancer 45:228–47

Eustace S, Tello R, DeCarvalho V, et al (1997) A comparison of whole-body turboSTIR MR imaging and planar 99mTc-methylene diphosphonate scintigraphy in the examination of patients with suspected skeletal metastases. AJR Am J Roentgenol 169:1655–61

Fornasier VL, Czitrom AA (1978) Collapsed vertebrae: a review of 659 autopsies. Clin Orthop Relat Res (131):261–5

Griffith JF, Yeung DK, Antonio GE, et al (2006) Vertebral marrow fat content and diffusion and perfusion indexes in women with varying bone density: MR evaluation. Radiology 241:831–8

Guo Y, Cai YQ, Cai ZL, et al (2002) Differentiation of clinically benign and malignant breast lesions using diffusion-weighted imaging. J Magn Reson Imaging 16:172–8

Hacklander T, Scharwachter C, Golz R, et al (2006) [Value of diffusion-weighted imaging for diagnosing vertebral metastases due to prostate cancer in comparison to other primary tumors]. Rofo 178:416–24

Hamaoka T, Madewell JE, Podoloff DA, et al (2004) Bone imaging in metastatic breast cancer. J Clin Oncol 22:2942–53

Hamstra DA, Galban CJ, Meyer CR, et al (2008) Functional diffusion map as an early imaging biomarker for high-grade glioma: correlation with conventional radiologic response and overall survival. J Clin Oncol 26:3387–94

Hayashida Y, Hirai T, Yakushiji T, et al (2006a) Evaluation of diffusion-weighted imaging for the differential diagnosis of poorly contrast-enhanced and T2-prolonged bone masses: initial experience. J Magn Reson Imaging 23:377–82

Hayashida Y, Yakushiji T, Awai K, et al (2006b) Monitoring therapeutic responses of primary bone tumors by diffusion-weighted image: initial results. Eur Radiol 16:2637–43

Herneth AM, Naude J, Philipp M, et al (2000) [The value of diffusion-weighted MRT in assessing the bone marrow changes in vertebral metastases]. Radiologe 40:731–6

Herneth AM, Philipp MO, Naude J, et al (2002) Vertebral metastases: assessment with apparent diffusion coefficient. Radiology 225:889–94

Hricak H, Choyke PL, Eberhardt SC, et al (2007) Imaging prostate cancer: a multidisciplinary perspective. Radiology 243:28–53

Huisman TA (2003) Diffusion-weighted imaging: basic concepts and application in cerebral stroke and head trauma. Eur Radiol 13:2283–97

Ichikawa T, Araki T (1999) Fast magnetic resonance imaging of liver. Eur J Radiol 29:186–210

Imamura F, Kuriyama K, Seto T, et al (2000) Detection of bone marrow metastases of small cell lung cancer with magnetic resonance imaging: early diagnosis before destruction of osseous structure and implications for staging. Lung Cancer 27:189–97

Jacobsson H, Goransson H (1991) Radiological detection of bone and bone marrow metastases. Med Oncol Tumor Pharmacother 8:253–60

Komori T, Narabayashi I, Matsumura K, et al (2007) 2-[Fluorine-18]-fluoro-2-deoxy-D-glucose positron emission tomography/computed tomography versus whole-body diffusion-weighted MRI for detection of malignant lesions: initial experience. Ann Nucl Med 21:209–15

Laurent V, Trausch G, Bruot O, et al (2009) Comparative study of two whole-body imaging techniques in the case of melanoma metastases: advantages of multi-contrast MRI examination including a diffusion-weighted sequence in comparison with PET-CT. Eur J Radiol 2009 Jun 2. [Epub ahead of print]

Lecouvet F (1998) Morphologic and quantitative MRI assessment of bone marrow in multiple myeloma and chronic lymphocytic leukemia: clinical and prognostic value. J Belge Radiol 81:301

Lee KC, Bradley DA, Hussain M, et al (2007) A feasibility study evaluating the functional diffusion map as a predictive imaging biomarker for detection of treatment response in a patient with metastatic prostate cancer to the bone. Neoplasia 9:1003–11

Libicher M, Appelt A, Berger I, et al (2007) The intravertebral vacuum phenomen as specific sign of osteonecrosis in vertebral compression fractures: results from a radiological and histological study. Eur Radiol 17:2248–52

Lichy MP, Aschoff P, Plathow C, et al (2007) Tumor detection by diffusion-weighted MRI and ADC-mapping–initial clinical experiences in comparison to PET-CT. Invest Radiol 42: 605–13

Lichy MP, Mueller-Horvat C, Jellus V, et al (2008) Image quality improvement of composed whole-spine MR images by applying a modified homomorphic filter–first results in cases of multiple myeloma. Eur Radiol 18:2274–82

Luboldt W, Kufer R, Blumstein N, et al (2008) Prostate carcinoma: diffusion-weighted imaging as potential alternative to conventional MR and 11C-choline PET/CT for detection of bone metastases. Radiology 249:1017–25

Maeda M, Sakuma H, Maier SE, et al (2003) Quantitative assessment of diffusion abnormalities in benign and malignant vertebral compression fractures by line scan diffusion-weighted imaging. AJR Am J Roentgenol 181:1203–9

Mahner S, Schirrmacher S, Brenner W, et al (2008) Comparison between positron emission tomography using 2-[fluorine-18] fluoro-2-deoxy-D-glucose, conventional imaging and computed tomography for staging of breast cancer. Ann Oncol 19:1249–54

Miller TT (2008) Bone tumors and tumorlike conditions: analysis with conventional radiography. Radiology 246:662–74

Moon WJ, Lee MH, Chung EC (2007) Diffusion-weighted imaging with sensitivity encoding (SENSE) for detecting cranial bone marrow metastases: comparison with T1-weighted images. Korean J Radiol 8:185–91

Mulligan ME, Badros AZ (2007) PET/CT and MR imaging in myeloma. Skeletal Radiol 36:5–16

Nakanishi K, Kobayashi M, Nakaguchi K, et al (2007) Whole-body MRI for detecting metastatic bone tumor: diagnostic value of diffusion-weighted images. Magn Reson Med Sci 6:147–55

Nakanishi K, Kobayashi M, Takahashi S, et al (2005) Whole body MRI for detecting metastatic bone tumor: comparison with bone scintigrams. Magn Reson Med Sci 4:11–7

Nemeth AJ, Henson JW, Mullins ME, et al (2007) Improved detection of skull metastasis with diffusion-weighted MR imaging. AJNR Am J Neuroradiol 28:1088–92

Nonomura Y, Yasumoto M, Yoshimura R, et al (2001) Relationship between bone marrow cellularity and apparent diffusion coefficient. J Magn Reson Imaging 13:757–60

Ohno Y, Koyama H, Onishi Y, et al (2008) Non-small cell lung cancer: whole-body MR examination for M-stage assessment–utility for whole-body diffusion-weighted imaging compared with integrated FDG PET/CT. Radiology 248: 643–54

Oner AY, Aggunlu L, Akpek S, et al (2007) Diffusion-weighted imaging of the appendicular skeleton with a non-Carr-Purcell-Meiboom-Gill single-shot fast spin-echo sequence. AJR Am J Roentgenol 189:1494–501

Pappou IP, Papadopoulos EC, Swanson AN, et al (2008) Osteoporotic vertebral fractures and collapse with intravertebral vacuum sign (Kummel's disease). Orthopedics 31:61–6

Raya JG, Dietrich O, Reiser MF, et al (2006) Methods and applications of diffusion imaging of vertebral bone marrow. J Magn Reson Imaging 24:1207–20

Rubens RD (1998) Bone metastases–the clinical problem. Eur J Cancer 34:210–3

Schmidt GP, Reiser MF, Baur-Melnyk A (2009) Whole-body MRI for the staging and follow-up of patients with metastasis. Eur J Radiol 70:393–400

Spuentrup E, Buecker A, Adam G, et al (2001) Diffusion-weighted MR imaging for differentiation of benign fracture edema and tumor infiltration of the vertebral body. AJR Am J Roentgenol 176:351–8

Spuentrup E, Buecker A, Koelker C, et al (2003) Respiratory motion artifact suppression in diffusion-weighted MR imaging of the spine. Eur Radiol 13:330–6

Suarez SV, Amadon A, Giacomini E, et al (2009) Brain activation by short-term nicotine exposure in anesthetized wild-type and beta2-nicotinic receptors knockout mice: a BOLD fMRI study. Psychopharmacology (Berl) 202:599–610

Sugimoto E, Tamagawa M, Okawara K, et al (1988) [Radiologic detection of metastatic bone tumors]. Gan No Rinsho 34:1491–7

Takahara T, Imai Y, Yamashita T, et al (2004) Diffusion weighted whole body imaging with background body signal suppression (DWIBS): technical improvement using free breathing, STIR and high resolution 3D display. Radiat Med 22:275–82

Takano A, Oriuchi N, Tsushima Y, et al (2008) Detection of metastatic lesions from malignant pheochromocytoma and paraganglioma with diffusion-weighted magnetic resonance imaging: comparison with 18F-FDG positron emission tomography and 123I-MIBG scintigraphy. Ann Nucl Med 22:395–401

Thomson V, Pialat JB, Gay F, et al (2008) Whole-body MRI for metastases screening: a preliminary study using 3D VIBE sequences with automatic subtraction between noncontrast and contrast enhanced images. Am J Clin Oncol 31: 285–92

Vande Berg BC, Malghem J, Lecouvet FE, et al (1998) Magnetic resonance imaging of normal bone marrow. Eur Radiol 8:1327–34

Vanel D, Casadei R, Alberghini M, et al (2009) MR imaging of bone metastases and choice of sequence: spin echo, in-phase gradient echo, diffusion, and contrast medium. Semin Musculoskelet Radiol 13:97–103

Weinreb JC (1990) MR imaging of bone marrow: a map could help. Radiology 177:23–4

Winterbottom AP, Shaw AS (2009) Imaging patients with myeloma. Clin Radiol 64:1–11

Xu X, Ma L, Zhang JS, et al (2008) Feasibility of whole body diffusion weighted imaging in detecting bone metastasis on 3.0T MR scanner. Chin Med Sci J 23:151–7

Yasumoto M, Nonomura Y, Yoshimura R, et al (2002) MR detection of iliac bone marrow involvement by malignant lymphoma with various MR sequences including diffusion-weighted echo-planar imaging. Skeletal Radiol 31: 263–9

Yeung DK, Wong SY, Griffith JF, et al (2004) Bone marrow diffusion in osteoporosis: evaluation with quantitative MR diffusion imaging. J Magn Reson Imaging 19:222–8

Zhang CY, Rong R, Wang XY (2008) Age-related changes of bone marrow of normal adult man on diffusion weighted imaging. Chin Med Sci J 23:162–5

Zhou XJ, Leeds NE, McKinnon GC, et al (2002) Characterization of benign and metastatic vertebral compression fractures with quantitative diffusion MR imaging. AJNR Am J Neuroradiol 23:165–70

Diffusion-Weighted Whole-Body Imaging with Background Body Signal Suppression (DWIBS)

Taro Takahara and Thomas C. Kwee

SUMMARY

In applying diffusion-weighted whole-body imaging with background body signal suppression (DWIBS) technique, DW-MR images are acquired during free breathing, which results in images with high signal-to-noise ratio using relatively thin image sections (4–5 mm). Image acquisition during free breathing is possible because bulk tissue motion, including respiratory motion, may be considered as types of coherent motion, which do not result in significant signal loss unlike intravoxel incoherent motion, which reflects random water motion at a cellular level. The concept of DWIBS allows handling of the acquired images as a volumetric dataset and it exploits both prolonged T2 relaxation time and impeded diffusion that the majority of solid lesions (both benign and malignant) exhibit as mechanisms for image contrast, which is used for clinical evaluation of diseases.

14.1

Introduction

Imaging plays a pivotal role in the non-invasive evaluation of human diseases. Establishing the correct diagnosis and accurate assessment of disease extent allow appropriate treatment planning and disease prognostication. Furthermore, imaging may be applied to monitor treatment response and determine disease persistence or recurrence after therapy.

Computed tomography (CT) now dominates cross-sectional imaging of human diseases in clinical

Taro Takahara, MD, PhD
Thomas C. Kwee, MD
Department of Radiology, Radiotherapy, and Nuclear Medicine, University Medical Center Utrecht, Heidelberglaan 100, 3508 GA, Utrecht, The Netherlands

practice. However, CT is limited in some instances because of a lack of morphological alterations and/or abnormal contrast enhancement of diseased tissues. As a result, small and non-enhancing lesions residing within anatomically normal appearing structures can be missed. In addition, functional or metabolic changes induced by disease may not be visible on CT. Some of the limitations of CT have been addressed by combining nuclear medicine imaging (such as single photon emission computed tomography [SPECT] and positron emission tomography [PET]) with CT (TOWNSEND 2008). However, the major disadvantages of SPECT/CT and PET/CT include high costs, relatively long patient preparation time and exposure of patients to ionizing radiation. Interestingly, MR imaging is not limited by these disadvantages and may be viewed as an alternative or complementary technique to SPECT/CT and PET/CT. Furthermore, a large number of anatomical and functional MR imaging sequences can be combined and employed to aid disease assessment.

With regard to functional MR imaging, there is now substantial interest in applying DW-MRI in the body for tumour assessment (KOH and COLLINS 2007). In the mid-1990s, single-shot echo-planar imaging (EPI) based DW-MRI was established as a technique to evaluate the brain, particularly for the diagnosis of acute ischaemic stroke (SCHAEFER et al. 2000). However, the technique could not be practically extended to extracranial sites because of magnetic susceptibility artefacts and severe image distortions (ICHIKAWA et al. 1998, 1999) associated with the use of EPI measurements in the body. However, the introduction of parallel imaging techniques such as sensitivity encoding (SENSE) (PRUESSMANN et al. 1999), the development of stronger magnetic gradients and the advent of multichannel receiver coils have all helped to overcome these problems. DW-MR images of acceptable to good quality, can now be attained in the body even at relatively high diffusion-weighting or b-values (e.g. $b = 1,000 \, s/mm^2$). However, despite these technical innovations, early approaches to perform DW-MRI in the body regarded breath-hold or respiratory triggered acquisitions as necessary to overcome respiratory induced motion of the abdominal or pelvic viscera. In 2004, Takahara et al. (2004) proposed a unique concept of DW-MRI termed diffusion-weighted whole-body imaging with background body signal suppression, which was abbreviated as DWIBS. This technique intentionally acquires images in free breathing rather than during breath-holding or using respiratory triggering to visualize the viscera. The feasibility and

success of this free breathing approach could not be initially explained but was later clarified by understanding the relationship between motion probing gradients (MPGs) and the type (coherence) of motion.

In this chapter, the principles of DWIBS are first discussed. The technique and instrumentation needed to perform DWIBS in the body is then reviewed, together with practical tips to help optimize image display and interpretation. Last but not the least, the current and emerging applications of DWIBS for the assessment of patients with cancer are surveyed.

14.2
Concept of DWIBS

Using conventional T2-weighted MR imaging, the T2 contrast is usually preserved when images are acquired during free breathing, even though imaging in breath-hold or by respiratory triggering is often preferred because the images have less image blurring.

An analogous comparison can be made with DW-MRI measurements. It was generally thought that the diffusion-weighted contrast would be lost if DW-MRI was performed in free breathing, because respiratory motion (of the order of centimetres) is substantially larger compared with water diffusion distances in tissues (of the order of several micrometres). Thus, it was presumed that DW-MRI performed in free breathing would lead to substantial signal loss; as such breath-hold imaging or respiratory triggering would be necessary to prevent spin dephasing and signal loss as a result of respiratory movement.

When breath-hold DW-MRI is performed, due to the necessarily short image acquisition time, only a limited number of image sections of relatively large (7–10 mm) section thickness can be acquired. As these images are typically obtained using single-shot EPI technique, the image signal-to-noise ratio (SNR) is low and lesion conspicuity may be diminished. By comparison, respiratory triggered scanning improves SNR, but at the expense of an approximately threefold increase in scanning time. Hence, using respiratory triggering would make performing whole-body scanning very time consuming and practically unacceptable. As described previously, the concept of DWIBS was then proposed as a viable method to acquire high quality DW-MR images in free-breathing (TAKAHARA et al. 2004). It was observed that the SNR of images acquired using free breathing DW-MRI technique were considerably better than those obtained by

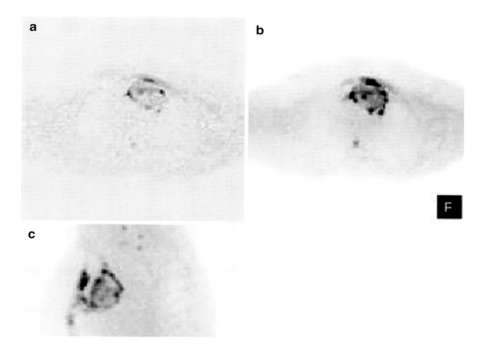

Fig. 14.1. Comparison between breath-hold and free breathing DW-MRI (DWIBS) in a 23-year-old man with thymoma (reprinted from TAKAHARA et al. (2004), with permission). (a) A 9 mm-thick axial image from a 25 s scan using breath-holding. (b) An 8 mm-thick reconstructed axial image calculated from 4 mm thick axial source images from a 430 s scan under free breathing. (c) A 5-mm thick sagittal reconstructed image from the dataset acquired in (b). Note that the signal-to-noise ratio of the free breathing scan (b) was superior to that of the breath-hold scan (a). High resolution sagittal reformatted image was also obtained (c)

breath-hold scanning (Fig. 14.1) [In this chapter, all DW-MRI and DWIBS images presented were acquired at a *b*-value of 1,000 s/mm^2 and displayed using inverted greyscale]. These observations contradicted the earlier assumptions about signal loss related to respiratory motion. Hence, by using free-breathing DW-MRI acquisitions, it was possible to significantly improve image quality, since the image acquisition was no longer time limited (as in breathhold scanning) and nor was it restricted to a particular phase of the breathing cycle (as in respiratory triggered scanning).

Free-breathing DW-MRI is now widely used in the body and represents a very efficient image acquisition technique, which can be used to accommodate a larger number of *b*-values and obtain thinner image sections, as a result of using multiple signal-averaging. The resultant thinner image sections also enable the dataset to be manipulated like an image volume, enabling 3D image displays using tools such as maximum intensity projections (MIPs), volume rendering (VR) and multi-planar reformats (MPR) (Fig. 14.2).

14.3

Reasons for the Feasibility of Free Breathing Imaging Acquisition in Body DW-MRI

The sensitivity of DW-MRI to microscopic diffusion (in the order of several micrometres) of water protons is maintained even during free breathing. To understand the feasibility of free breathing for DWIBS and body DW-MRI, two types of motion should be distinguished: intravoxel "incoherent" motion and intravoxel "coherent" motion. Intravoxel "incoherent" motion refers to the incoherent random movement of water molecules within a voxel (i.e. diffusion). Intravoxel "coherent" motion refers to the coherent motion of water molecules within a voxel. Since the two MPGs in a diffusion-weighted imaging sequence are separated by a very small time interval (typically of the order of 50 ms), much of the phasic respiratory movement can be regarded as coherent motion within the respiratory cycle. Thus,

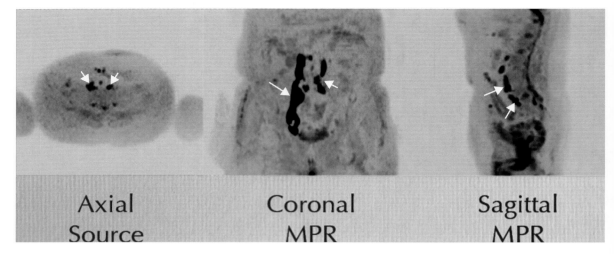

Fig. 14.2. DW-MR images in a 79-year-old man with mantle cell lymphoma. Axial 4 mm thick source image with coronally and sagittally reformatted DWIBS images. Note that high quality multi-planar reformatted (MPR) images were obtained as a result of thin image sections (4 mm) used at image acquisition. Although the applied slice thickness of 4 mm was still substantially thicker than those obtained using multislice CT, the very high contrast between the lesion and surrounding tissue enables multiplanar evaluation. In this example, the paraortic lymphadenopathy (*arrows*)showing impeded diffusion was well demonstrated on the MPR images

for the duration during which the two MPGs are applied, significant signal attenuation arises mainly from the intravoxel "incoherent" motion (i.e. diffusion), whereas the signal is largely unaffected by intravoxel "coherent" motion of phasic respiration. In other words, the acquired phase shift due to coherent motion is equal in each phase-encoding step and therefore, does not significantly result in signal attenuation. This theory was supported by a phantom experiment by MURO et al. (2005). In that study, the ADC measurements obtained from bottles filled with different types of homogeneous fluids that were moving in the MR scanner were not significantly different from the ADC measurements in the comparison non-moving (stationary) bottles (Fig. 14.3).

Thus, DW-MRI and T2-weighted imaging can both be acquired in the presence of respiratory motion in the body. This is because diffusion-weighted contrast is maintained during free breathing, although the use of breath-holding or respiratory triggering can reduce image blurring. However, because DW-MRI images have intrinsically less SNR compared with T2-weighted imaging, it is generally advantageous to perform DW-MRI in free breathing to increase the number of signal averages acquired. This improves the image SNR and allows thinner image partitions, even though there may be some image blurring.

14.4
Important Parameter Settings and Coil Selection for DWIBS

Imaging parameters for different clinical settings are listed in Table 14.1.

14.4.1
Imaging Plane

It is currently recommended to obtain axial image sections using DWIBS (with the phase-encoding in the anterior–posterior direction), in order to minimize the field of view (FOV) and to reduce image distortion. Because DWIBS allows thin axial image sections (e.g. 4 mm) to be acquired, high quality reformatted images may be created in any prescribed plane (Fig. 14.2).

14.4.2
Fat Suppression

DWIBS is combined with either a short inversion time inversion recovery (STIR) pre-pulse or a frequency-selective (chemical shift selective (CHESS)) pre-pulse for fat suppression. Theoretically, STIR will result in a better fat suppression over an extended or larger

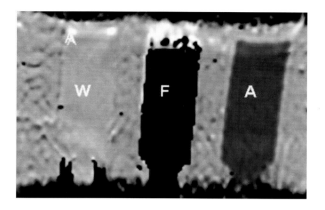

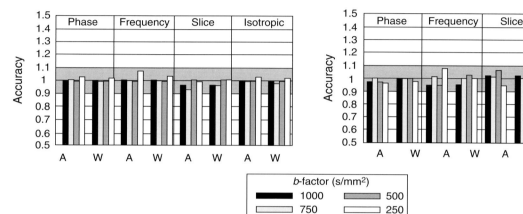

Fig. 14.3. Effect of motion on apparent diffusion coefficient (ADC) measurements. ADC map of phantoms containing water (*W* left), fat (*F* middle), and detergent (*A* right) embedded in agar. The phantom was scanned moving along the axis of the magnetic resonance scanner simulating respiration. Graphs show the calculated ADC values measured when the phantom was moving at a speed of 10 mm/s (*lower left*) and 20 mm/s (*lower right*) in the different directions of motion-probing gradients and *b*-values compared with measurements taken when stationary. Note that the errors for ADC measurement were less than 0.1. This suggests that coherent motion may not affect the ADC measurements (Reprinted from Muro et al. (2005) with permissions)

imaging field of view compared with CHESS, because the technique is less sensitive to magnetic field inhomogeneities. Therefore, STIR can be applied virtually anywhere in the body (Fig. 14.4). In addition, STIR may also be useful in suppressing the background signal arising from bowel loops which may have a short T1 value similar to fat (Fig. 14.5).

One of the main disadvantages of STIR compared with CHESS is that it results in lower image SNR because of the partial loss of proton signal due to the inversion pulse. Hence, to maximize SNR, and since intra-abdominal organs are not associated with significant magnetic field inhomogeneities, CHESS could be used instead of STIR to increase image SNR and reduce acquisition time, when only

a small region of the body is evaluated. However, for DW-MRI of contiguous imaging stations across the whole body, STIR is often preferred because there may be substantial magnetic field inhomogeneities at the root of the neck, shoulders, lungs, breasts and lower extremities, so that a more uniform fat suppression is achieved. However, it may be possible to optimize a whole-body examination by performing imaging at each anatomical station with the most appropriate fat suppression technique (either STIR or CHESS). On selected MR imaging systems, it is possible to combine fat suppression schemes for whole body imaging acquisition, e.g. using STIR in the neck but CHESS for the other parts of the body (Fig. 14.6).

Table 14.1. Suggested imaging parameters for performing DWIBS examinations. [Imaging parameters presented are optimized for a Philips 1.5 T MR system]

Fat suppression technique	STIR		CHESS		CHESS isotropic voxel
Coil	SENSE body 4 elements	XL Torso 32 elements	SENSE body 4 elements	XL Torso 32 elements	Cardiac 5 elements
Field of view (cm)	40	40	40	40	28
Rectangular FOV (%)	75	70	70	70	85
Acquisition matrix	160	160	160	160	112
Scan percentage	80	80	80	80	100
SENSE factor	2	2	2	2	2
Number of slices	60	50 × 2	60	50 × 2	60
Slice thickness/gap (mm)	4/0	4/0	4/0	4/0	2.5/0
Number of scan package	1	1	1	1	1
Scan coverage (cm)	24	40	24	40	15
TR (ms)	9,380	7,192	8,257	8,426	9,377
TI (ms)	180	180	N/A	N/A	N/A
TE (ms)	72	57	72	49	70
Half scan factor	0.63	0.622	0.63	0.622	0.6
b Factor	0, 1,000	0, 1,000	0, 1,000	0, 1,000	800
Number of excitations for $b = 0$	3	2	2	1	0
Number of excitations for high b-value	9	6	6	3	8
Scan time	5:10	2:38 × 2	3:02	1.49 × 2	5:18

14.4.3
b-Value

The b-value determines the degree of background signal suppression in the body, and as such, using higher b-values in the range of 800–1,000 s/mm² would generally result in better signal suppression of the background to facilitate lesion detection. However, the choice of b-values is influenced by the properties of the organ under evaluation, which include the native tissue T2-relaxation time and the range of ADC values of the pathological tissue that is likely to be encountered. This is further discussed in Chaps. 2 and 3. It should, however, be noted that the same b-value when combined with STIR for imaging can result in better lesion-to-background ratio because of more effective background signal suppression compared with CHESS imaging (Fig. 14.7).

14.4.4
Repetition Time

Another important imaging parameter to consider in DWIBS is the repetition time (TR). It should be apparent that the TR used for DWIBS would be longer than that prescribed for conventional DW-MRI over a limited anatomical region. This is because in order to achieve sufficient anatomical coverage, the number of image sections acquired for DWIBS (typically 60–80 image sections per imaging station) is three or four times higher compared with targeted DW-MRI focused upon a specific area or organ (typically 15 or 20 image sections). In conventional DW-MRI, the typical TR used is in the region of about 3,000 ms or less. However, since most malignant lesions have both a prolonged T1 and T2 relaxation time compared with the normal surrounding tissues, the use of a shorter TR may result in poorer signal

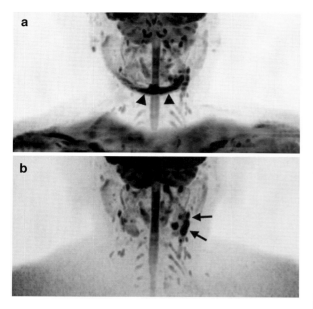

Fig. 14.4. Comparison of different fat suppression techniques for DWIBS in a 28-year-old man with swollen lymph nodes (pathology unknown) (Reprinted from TAKAHARA et al. 2004 with permission). (**a**) Coronally reformatted maximum intensity projection DWIBS image obtained with a CHESS pre-pulse shows insufficient fat suppression around the jaw and clavicle resulting in artefacts (*arrowheads*). (**b**) By comparison, coronally reformatted maximum intensity projection DWIBS images obtained with a STIR pre-pulse showed improved fat suppression. Swollen lymph nodes around the left submandibular gland (*arrow*) were well visualized without significant artefacts

gain from malignant lesions because of their slow T1 recovery, thus resulting in poorer SNR and contrast-to-noise ratios (CNR). Although an operator may choose to increase the TR during a conventional DW-MRI acquisition with a view to improving the CNR, the longer TR would lead to longer scan time and less efficient signal acquisitions. By contrast, DWIBS routinely employs TR values of 5,000 ms or more as and when images are acquired in an inter-leaved slice order, which provides an efficient means of acquiring high quality data. Thus, DWIBS is a technique that results in time-efficient signal gain, and equally important, may result in better contrast between lesions and the adjacent normal tissues due to the full T1 signal recovery between acquisitions. When performing DWIBS in the body with STIR fat suppression, the image acquisition time is typically 5–7 min for each 25 cm area of coverage, using a b-value of 1,000 s/mm^2.

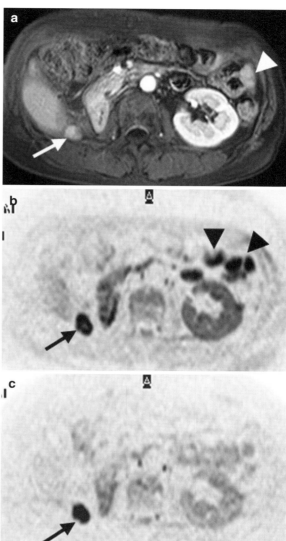

Fig. 14.5. Comparison of different fat suppression techniques for DWIBS with respect to suppression of bowel signal. Images in a 66-year-old woman with peritoneal dissemination from ovarian cancer. (**a**) Axial contrast-enhanced T1-weighted image with fat suppression, (**b**) inverted grey-scale axial DWIBS image obtained with a CHESS pre-pulse and (**c**) inverted greyscale axial DWIBS image obtained with a STIR pre-pulse. A peritoneal metastasis was seen near the hepatic angle (**a–c**, *arrow*). However, on (**a**) fat-suppressed T1-weighted imaging and (**b**) DWIBS obtained with a CHESS pre-pulse, the jejunal bowel loops mimicked metastatic disease (*arrowheads*). Note that by using (**c**) DWIBS with a STIR pre-pulse, the bowel contents with a short T1 relaxation time showed better signal suppression and could be differentiated from metastatic peritoneal disease

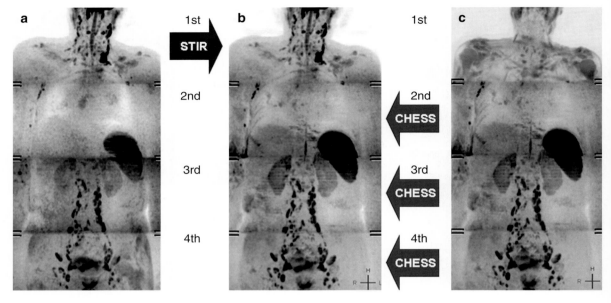

Fig. 14.6. Coronal reformatted DWIBS images using different fat suppression techniques. (**a**) DWIBS performed using only STIR fat suppression and (**c**) DWIBS performed using only CHESS pre-pulse fat suppression at four contiguous imaging stations (first to fourth). Note that using STIR fat suppression resulted in better image quality in the neck, while better SNR and image quality was achieved by using CHESS fat saturation in the rest of the body. (**b**) By combining imaging acquired using STIR fat suppression in the neck with imaging obtained using CHESS technique elsewhere in the body, the best image quality across all imaging stations was achieved, accompanied by a reduction in scan time compared with STIR DW-MRI alone

14.4.5
Coil Selection

When performing DWIBS, either a built-in receiver coil within the bore of the magnet or a surface receiver coil may be employed. The advantages of using a built-in body receiver coil include patient comfort and a larger volume of imaging coverage. However, built-in coils have poorer CNR and SNR compared with surface coils, which may thus compromise lesion detection (Lɪ et al. 2007). When surface receiver coils are used, one approach to achieve whole body imaging is to use a so-called whole-body surface coil design. A whole-body surface coil design combines multiple seamlessly integrated coil elements and independent radiofrequency channels, which offers large anatomical coverage (in the order of 200 cm) and faster image acquisition without time loss, as a result of patient or coil repositioning. However, it is also possible to perform a time-efficient whole-body examination using only one surface coil with more limited coverage, provided it is compatible with parallel imaging (Fig. 14.8). In order to achieve this, an additional table platform would need to be mounted on top of the original MR patient examination table. Spacers are placed between the two table platforms to create a space, within which the surface coil is allowed to be moved from one anatomical position to another. As a result, the patient can remain in the same position, and by repeated repositioning of the surface receiver coil at different anatomical position, whole body DW-MRI data can be acquired. By applying such a coil moving technique, the 3D alignment between anatomical imaging stations is preserved without a significant increase in imaging time (<1 min per station).

14.5
Workflow and Post-Processing

14.5.1
Workflow

A typical workflow for performing DWIBS examination is presented in Fig. 14.9, which comprises seven steps:

Fig. 14.7. The effects of different fat suppression techniques on visibility of liver metastases. DW-MR images of a 66-year-old woman with multiple liver metastases from pancreatic cancer. (**a**) Contiguous 4 -mm-thick inverted greyscale axial source DW-MR images obtained using a CHESS fat-suppression pre-pulse and respiratory triggering. (**b**) Contiguous 4 mm thick inverted greyscale axial source DW-MR images obtained with a STIR pre-pulse under free breathing. The image acquisition time was comparable in each case. However, note that the background liver signal was less using the STIR pre-pulse with better visualization of the small metastatic lesions

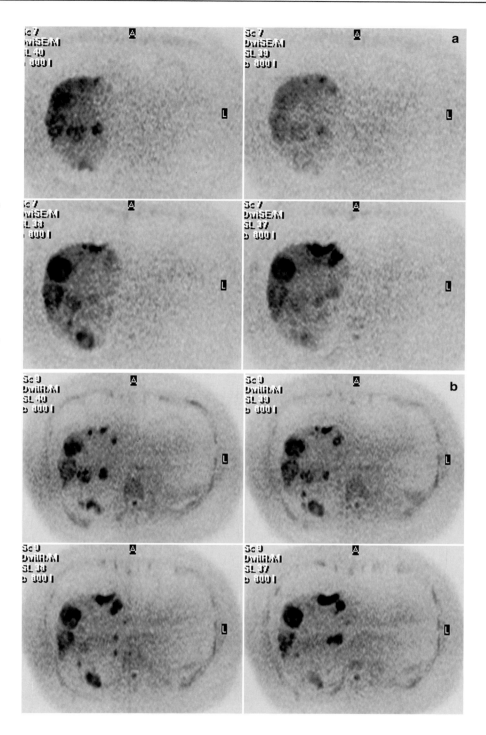

1. Estimating the anticipated distribution of disease in the body
2. Setting the scanning area: In DWIBS, the scanning area should be maximized for the coil coverage used (e.g. 24 cm coverage with 4 mm × 60 image sections; 40 cm coverage with 5 mm × 80 image sections).
3. Performing image acquisition under free breathing and using the highest possible number of excitations for a given imaging time.

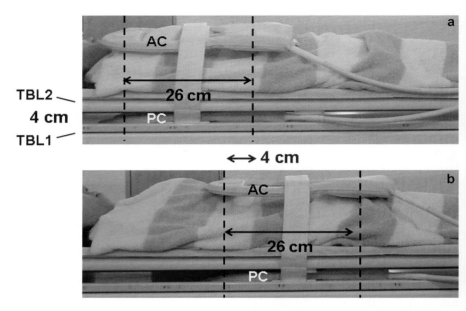

Fig. 14.8. DWIBS imaging using a single sliding surface coil. (**a**) Table preparation. An additional table platform is mounted on the original table, with a 4 cm gap between the two table platforms. In this way, both the anterior and posterior part of the surface coil can move freely in the head–foot direction of the magnet, allowing wide anatomical coverage without the need for patient repositioning. (Equipment shown Gyroscan Achieva 1.5 T system with a 4-element SENSE-body coil, Philips Healthcare, Best, The Netherlands). Typically, an overlap of 4 cm is used between imaging stations. Using an 8 or 16 element coil usually allows 26 to 40 cm coverage at each imaging station

4. Inspecting for the quality of the acquired dataset (e.g. for the presence of ghosting artefacts or poor fat suppression which will degrade the quality of MIP images).
5. Inverting the greyscale of the *b*-value images so that they resemble the greyscale display of nuclear medicine/PET images
6. Producing orthogonal MIP images.
7. Reformatting axial source images into the coronal and/or sagittal plane.

The imaging performed at multiple anatomical positions can be merged to produce a whole body image, using dedicated softwares which are already available on some of the MR imaging platforms (Fig. 14.10).

14.5.2
Post-Processing

14.5.2.1
Maximum Intensity Projection (MIP)

As DWIBS images have excellent lesion-to-background contrast, performing MIP of the acquired images is very helpful for lesion visualization. The MIP images can be used for rapid assessment of lesion extent and distribution, particularly where lesions are widely scattered or are serpingenous in morphology (Figs. 14.11 and 14.12).

14.5.2.2
Volume Rendering (VR)

Similarly, because of the high lesion-to-background contrast ratio of DWIBS images, lesion segmentation may be achieved by using volume rendering (VR) of the DWIBS images. Performing the VR procedure on DWIBS images is easier than performing on CT images, because the background structures are relatively suppressed on DWIBS compared with CT, and therefore the volume of interest is less affected by overlying tissue structures. Although DWIBS images usually lack anatomical details, the position of the skin surface is usually well demonstrated on VR of DWIBS images (Fig. 14.13). It is also possible to display only selected lesions on a MIP image by manual removal of unwanted overlying structures in the VR mode (Fig. 14.14). Although clinically helpful, a validation

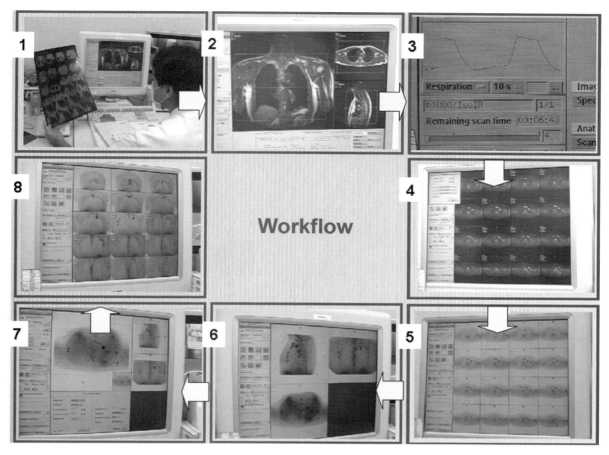

Fig. 14.9. Typical workflow for performing state-of-the-art DWIBS examination. 1: The radiographic technician reviews imaging to determine the sites of abnormality. In this case, a lesion was noted in the left upper lobe of the lung consistent with lung metastasis. 2: A 30 cm scan range was set for evaluation of the entire lung. 3: The respiration profile demonstrates free breathing at image acquisition, rather than using respiratory triggering. The typical scan time of DWIBS using a STIR pre-pulse for fat suppression ranges from 5½ to 7 min for 60 image sections. 4: Display of scan images as a series of contiguous thin image sections. 5: Applying greyscale inversion to the images. 6: Creation of orthogonal multiplanar reformats (MPRs). 7: Plan further MPRs or limited volume maximum intensity projections (MIPs). 8: Coronally reformatted DWIBS images used for disease assessment. The axial source images, MPRs, and MIPs are usually assessed concurrently

study is still needed to demonstrate the diagnostic accuracy of such image rendering technique. VR images may be applied to measure lesion or tumour volumes, which can be used to quantify the total lesion burden, which may prove effective for monitoring tumour response to therapy, compared with uni- or bi-dimensional tumour size measurements (Jaffe 2006).

14.5.2.3
Fusion Images

Suppression of the background signals in body imaging using DWIBS is advantageous for tumour detection. However, effective suppression of the background signal on high *b*-value imaging leads to obscuration of normal anatomical details. Thus, standard T1- and T2-weighted sequences remain indispensable, serving as anatomical references to aid lesion localization. Since DWIBS and conventional MR images can be acquired sequentially without moving the patient, this means that DWIBS images may be fused with conventional MR images (Fig. 14.15) to improve disease assessment. The key benefit of image fusion was recently demonstrated by Tsushima et al. (2007), who showed that using DWIBS/T2-weighted MRI fusion was better than using DWIBS alone, with regards to the sensitivity and specificity, for the visual detection of malignancy in the abdomen. With the

Fig. 14.10. Merging of images acquired at different anatomical stations. (a) *Left column* shows coronal maximum intensity projection images acquired in the chest, abdomen and pelvis. By applying software fusion, the images are collated into a single coronal image display in the *right column* (b) to facilitate viewing and disease assessment

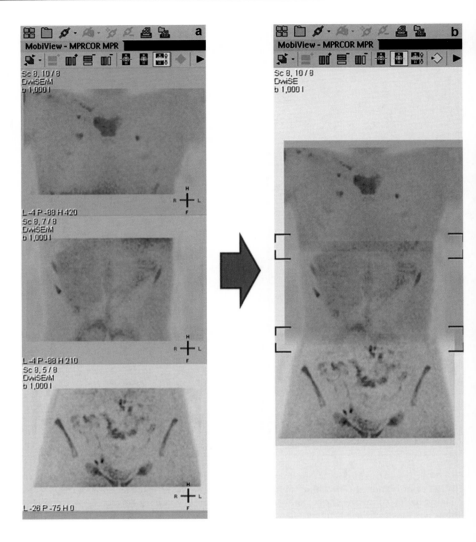

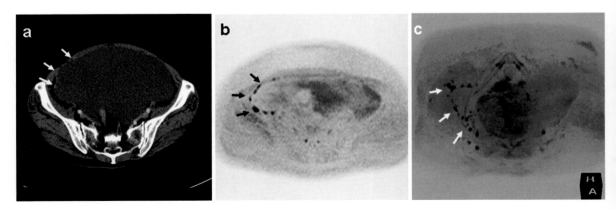

Fig. 14.11. Distribution of peritoneal disease. Images of a 64-year-old woman with ovarian cancer and peritoneal dissemination (reprinted from TAKAHARA et al. 2004, with permission). (a) Contrast-enhanced CT showed multiple small nodules along the peritoneum (*arrows*). (b) Axial DWIBS showed the peritoneal nodules more clearly (*arrows*). (c) Maximum intensity projection DWIBS image from an anterior-superior viewpoint using the axial source dataset showed distribution of metastatic foci along the right abdomen (*arrows*). The primary tumour (black arrow) was also visualized

Fig. 14.12. Recognition of a fibroepithelial polyp in the left ureter. (a) Coronal T2-weighted image showed a dilated left ureter with an intermediate signal intensity mass occupying the lumen (*arrows*). (b) Axial fat-suppressed non-contrast-enhanced T1-weighted image showed a low signal intensity mass in the left lower ureter (*arrow*) surrounded by a crescent of high signal intensity area urine. (c) Axial fat-suppressed T1-weighted image through left renal hilum showed a dilated collecting system (*arrows*)by high intensity presumed haemorrhagic urine. (d) Coronal MIP DWIBS showed a long, serpentine tumour extending along the left ureter (*arrow*). Note that the signal from the haemorrhagic fluid in the kidney on the fat-suppressed T1-weighted imaging was attenuated because of the STIR pre-pulse

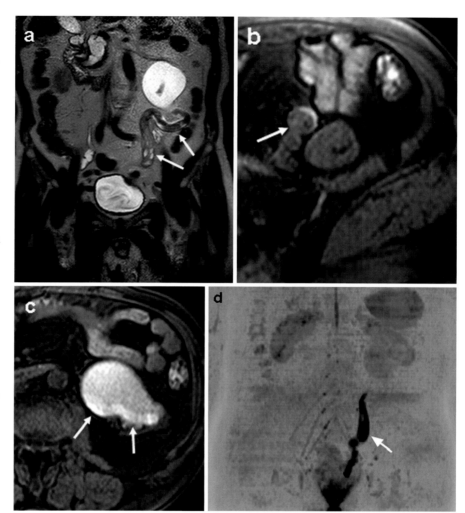

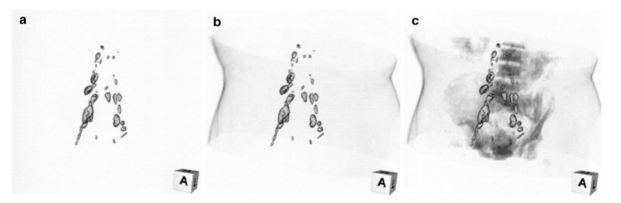

Fig. 14.13. Visualization of the skin line in a case with multiple pelvic lymph node metastases from urinary bladder cancer. (a) Volume rendering (VR) of swollen lymph nodes. (b) Results of fusing VR image of lymph nodes and skin line revealed the distribution of the lymph nodes in relationship to the body contours. (c) The VR image could be further extended to display pelvic bones and lumbosacral vertebrae

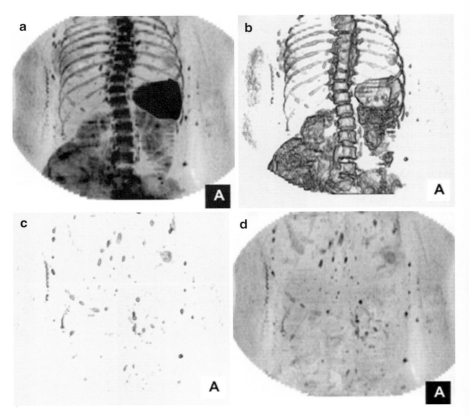

Fig. 14.14. Targeted visualization on maximum intensity projection (MIP) DWIBS image using volume rendering (VR) mask. Images of a man with Type 1 neurofibromatosis. (a) Coronal MIP DWIBS image showed a bulky tumour in the right pelvis and multiple small skin lesions. However, the latter are not well visualized because of the superimposing signal from bones and the pelvic tumour. (b) VR image was created for 3D visualization. (c) Manipulated VR image after removal of bone structures and the spleen. Such segmentation is usually not difficult because of the excellent lesion-to-background contrast in DWIBS. (d) Coronal MIP DWIBS image after applying VR mask created in (c) allows selective visualization of the subcutaneous neurofibromas

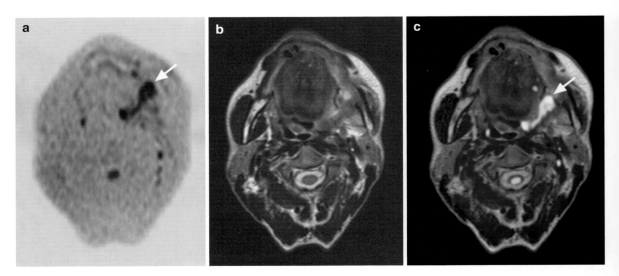

Fig. 14.15. Image fusion of DWIBS and T2-weighted imaging. Images in a 53-year-old man with cancer of the left mandible. (a) Axial DWIBS image, (b) axial T2-weighted image and (c) axial DWIBS/T2-weighted fusion image. The extent and anatomical location of tumour associated with the left mandible (*arrows*) was best seen on the fusion image

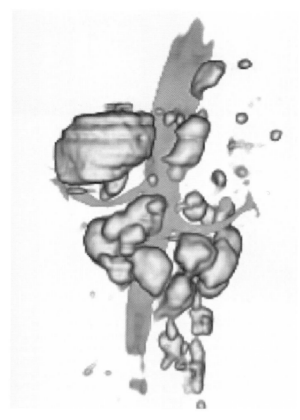

Fig. 14.16. Volume (3D) fusion of DWIBS and non-contrast-enhanced magnetic resonance angiography (MRA). A 64-year-old patient with enlarged lymph nodes from malignant lymphoma. The enlarged lymph nodes in the abdomen were imaged using DWIBS, and the vascular structures (aorta and renal arteries) were imaged using non-contrast-enhanced MRA. Volume rendered images obtained from the DWIBS and MRA dataset were fused three-dimensionally, showing the relationship between lymph nodes to the aorta and the renal arteries (3D fusion software, ZIOSOFT Inc. Tokyo, Japan)

availability of more sophisticated software and workstations, it is also possible to create 3D fusion images (Figs. 14.16 and 14.17). Since DWIBS images may suffer from image distortion as a result of using EPI, a non-rigid registration algorithm may be applied to image fusion (Fig. 14.18).

14.6

DWIBS as a "Signal Intensity-Based" Diagnostic Tool

Although DWIBS is usually performed using two b-values (e.g. 0 and 1,000 s/mm^2) which would allow

for the calculation of the ADC, the main application of this technique is for lesion detection and characterization on the basis of the DW-MRI signal intensity at high b-value, rather than by the assessment of the ADC maps.

To understand the rationale behind this seemingly empirical approach, it is worthwhile to review the historical aspect of MR imaging development. In the early days of MR imaging, many people thought that calculating the absolute T2-relaxation times of lesions were crucial to making a more accurate diagnosis. To calculate tissue T2 relaxation times, it is necessary to perform T2-weighted imaging using at least two different echo times (TEs). However, this approach at least doubled the image acquisition time, and as experience was accrued, it became clear that the discriminatory value of the T2-relaxation time between benign and malignant lesions was not as robust as initially expected (KJAER et al. 1991; GOLDBERG et al.1993; SCHWARTZ et al. 1995; VARGHESE et al. 1997). Furthermore, occasional misregistrations between the two datasets acquired using different TEs could degrade the quality of the T2 parametric map. Thus, using the quantitative T2 values of tissues for disease discrimination is less popular and has not been used in routine clinical practice. Rather, it is the conventional T2-weighted image, which is visually appraised in clinical practice today for the detection and characterization of lesions. T2-weighted images are used on the basis that diseases in the body tend to have longer T2-relaxation times compared with normal tissues.

In an analogous way, DW-MRI can be used as a contrast mechanism to reveal disease foci. If DW-MRI is acquired using two or more b-values, an ADC can be calculated. Most malignant lesions exhibit lower water diffusivity than benign lesions, making ADC measurements a potentially valuable tool for lesion characterization. However, although several studies have reported that the ADCs of malignant lesions are usually lower than those of benign lesions (PARIKH et al. 2008; GOURTSOYIANNI et al. 2008; KIM et al. 2009), there is considerable overlap between the groups. Furthermore, some studies could not discriminate lesions on the basis of the ADC values (KOMORI et al. 2007; HUMPHRIES et al. 2007), cautioning us against the overreliance of any single imaging test for disease evaluation. Furthermore, as discussed earlier, image distortion due to EPI application in DW-MRI and differences in the degree of image distortion between different datasets obtained using different b-values may affect the quality and accuracy of the ADC map.

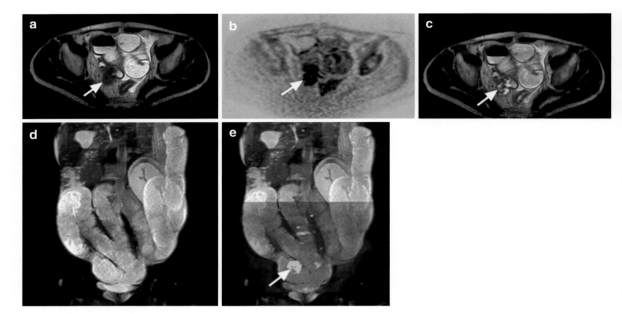

Fig. 14.17. Maximum intensity projection (MIP) fusion for anatomical localization of disease in the abdomen. Images of a 63-year-old man with small bowel obstruction due to metastasis from rectal cancer. (**a**) Axial T2-weighted image, (**b**) axial DWIBS image, (**c**) axial DWIBS/T2-weighted fusion image, (**d**) MIP of coronal fat-suppressed T2-weighted image and (**e**) fusion image of (**d**) and coronal MIP image of DWIBS. On the axial T2-weighted image (**a**), a low signal intensity mass was seen in the terminal ileum (*arrow*) causing small bowel obstruction with free fluid seen surrounding the dilated small bowel. The anatomical location of obstruction was clearly demonstrated on both (**c**) axial DWIBS/T2-weighted fusion and (**e**) coronal MIP DWIBS/T2-weighted fusion images (*arrows*)

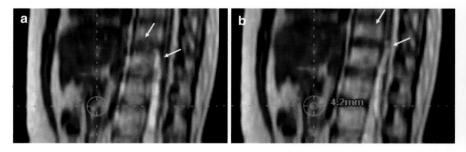

Fig. 14.18. Image fusion using non-rigid registration. (**a**) Sagittal DWIBS/T2-weighted fusion image before applying "automatic deformable" function. (**b**) Sagittal DWIBS/T2-weighted fusion image after applying "automatic deformable" function. Note that the spinal cord (*arrows*) was misregistered in (**a**) due to image distortion, whereas this was corrected in (**b**). In this example, non-rigid registration was performed using Fusion 7D software (CTI-Mirada)

Thus, some parallels could be drawn between the applications of qualitative vs. quantitative DW-MRI with T2-weighted imaging. Like quantitative T2 relaxation times, ADC measurement on its own may be of limited value for discriminating between benign and malignant disease. ADC measurements may eventually prove to be more useful in other areas such as in the (early) evaluation and prediction of tumour response to therapy (Hamstra et al. 2008; Cui et al. 2008). As an adjunct to the quantitative T2 value and ADC calculations, the authors would like to highlight the potential utility of assessing the signal intensity on the high *b*-value DWIBS image. The signal intensity observed on DWIBS is correlated with the T2 relaxation time and inversely correlated with tissue diffusivity, and as such, exploits the additive effect of both contrast mechanisms for the detection and characterization of lesions. In this respect, we may further investigate the most suitable combination of the degree of T2-weighting and diffusion-weighting (i.e. b-value) for lesion evaluation, although currently, only the shortest TE is selected. Also, the most optimal (semi-) quantitative measure of signal intensity in DWIBS remains to be established. In this respect, a lesion-to-spinal cord ratio (LSR) was recently shown to be of value for discriminating between benign and malignant pulmonary lesions (SATOH et al. 2008; UTO et al. 2009). Another approach has been to express the signal intensity of a lesion relative to the averaged background signal intensity.

14.7

Pitfalls in DWIBS

Evaluation of areas close to the heart and the diaphragm may be hampered in DWIBS because of signal loss and artefacts related to incoherent tissue motion (Figs. 14.19 and 14.20).

Although DWIBS offers excellent sensitivity for lesion detection, its specificity is a drawback. It is well known that DW-MRI does not exclusively visualise malignant tumours. Benign pathologies can also demonstrate impeded water diffusion related to their cellular density. Equally important is the fact that not only solid tumours but also viscous fluids can exhibit high signal impeded diffusion at DW-MRI. This is because in a highly viscous environment, the diffusion of water molecules can be impeded, independent of the T2 value or cellular density in the area. This phenomenon may be seen in the normal gallbladder when the subject is fasting. A typical pathological condition in which viscosity may result in impeded diffusion is in an abscess (Fig. 14.21). This knowledge is important when using DWIBS for the post-operative evaluation of rectal carcinoma, as abscess formation may occur as a complication following surgery.

Another potential pitfall of applying DWIBS is that the technique not only visualizes pathological areas with a relatively long T2 relaxation time, impeded water diffusion and/or high viscosity, but also normal anatomical structures. In the body, the normal brain, salivary glands, tonsils, spleen, gallbladder, small intestinal and colonic contents, adrenal glands, prostate,

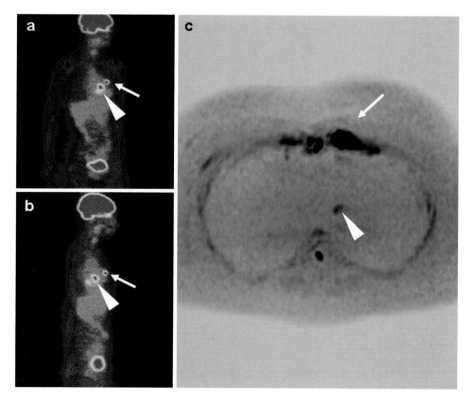

Fig. 14.19. Images of a 58-year-old woman with metastatic mediastinal lymph nodes from lung cancer. (**a & b**) [18]FDG-PET shows metastatic foci in the mediastinum (*arrowhead*) and the chest wall (*arrow*). The former is larger than the latter. (**c**) Axial DWIBS image also shows both lesions, but the lesion in the mediastinum (*arrowhead*) is relatively unclear compared to the lesion in the chest wall (*arrow*), which is likely due to cardiac motion artefacts

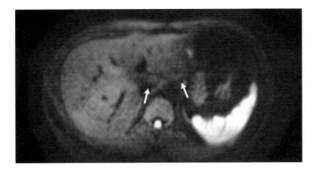

Fig. 14.20. Signal loss in the left lateral segment of the liver in a healthy volunteer. Axial DWIBS image shows signal loss in the left lateral segment of the liver (*arrow*) compared to the right lobe. This artefact is most likely caused by (intravoxel incoherent) cardiac motion

testes, penis, endometrium, ovaries, spinal cord, peripheral nerves, lymph nodes, and bone marrow exhibit varying degrees of high signal intensity at DWIBS. High signal intensities within these organs do not necessarily indicate pathological states, but pathological lesions within these organs may be obscured as a result. The number and signal intensity of normal tissues visualized on DWIBS varies across individuals and is also dependent on the imaging protocol (e.g. more normal tissues with higher signal intensity are observed when applying lower *b*-values). Interestingly, the visibility of the spleen is highly variable and might be dependent on its iron content (which leads to signal loss). Furthermore, the normal bone marrow generally exhibits low signal intensity

Fig. 14.21. Images of a 65-year-old man with infected hydronephrosis. (**a**) Coronal magnetic resonance urography shows severe hydronephrosis on the right side. However, the signal intensity of the dilated ureter and collecting system is lower than that of the urinary bladder and contralateral renal cysts, consistent with reduced T2-relaxivity of the fluid due to pyuria. (**b**) Coronal maximum intensity projection DWIBS image shows increased signal intensity throughout the right urinary tract and the urinary bladder. (**c**) Sagittal T2-weighted image through the bladder shows a fluid-fluid level consisting of high signal intensity serous urine anteriorly and a slightly lower signal intensity layer posteriorly (*arrow*) consistent with pyuria. (**d**) Sagittally reformatted DWIBS image. The posterior layer of fluid in the bladder shows high signal intensity likely related to increased fluid viscosity (due to infection)

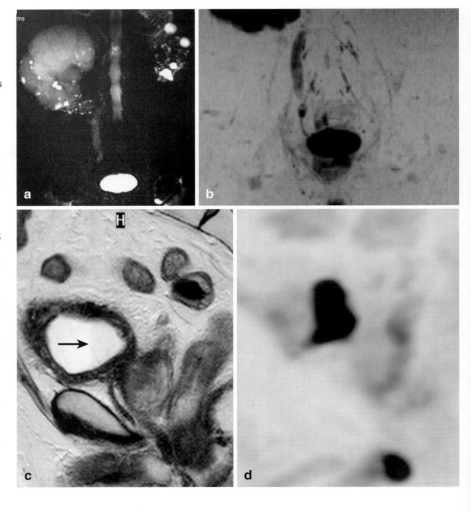

in elderly people, but the bone marrow in young subjects can be of high signal intensity. This is likely related to the fact that the high fat content in the yellow marrow (which accounts for the majority in the elderly) shows lower diffusivity than haemopoeitically active red bone marrow (Baur et al. 2003).

A further pitfall in DWIBS can arise from poor fat suppression. Insufficiently suppressed fat signal may mimic or obscure lesions. In order to minimize diagnostic errors due to poorly suppressed fat, it is important to evaluate acquired DWIBS images in multiple planes. Last but not least, although DWIBS images are suitable for volumetric image processing and MIPs, source images should always be consulted, because subtle lesions may be missed or obscured on the projected images.

Clinical Applications of DWIBS in Oncology

The concept of DWIBS has a wide range of clinical applications, which includes cancer imaging, imaging of infections and inflammations, evaluation of trauma and visualization of peripheral nerves (see Chap. 4). Of these, the most promising application of DWIBS appears to be in oncological imaging.

14.8.1
Tumour Detection and Staging

As DWIBS-based techniques result in images with high lesion-to-background contrast, the technique has been shown to be highly sensitive for the detection of primary tumours (Goshima et al. 2008a; Haider et al. 2007; Ichikawa et al. 2006, 2007; Koh et al. 2008; Matsuki et al. 2007; Ono et al. 2009; Sugita et al. 2009; Tanimoto et al. 2007; Qi et al. 2009) and distant metastases (Fujii et al. 2008; Luboldt et al. 2008; Ohno et al. 2008) throughout the body. Ohno et al. (2008) showed that combining DWIBS with T1-weighted and STIR imaging was as accurate as [18]FDG-PET for the detection of metastatic disease in patients with lung cancers.

Although the spatial resolution of DWIBS is generally lower than that of other MR imaging sequences, studies in patients with urinary bladder cancer (Ek-Assmy et al 2009; Takeuchi et al. 2009; Watanabe et al. 2009) and prostate cancer (Ren et al. 2009) have

shown the utility of DWIBS for primary tumour staging (i.e. T-staging). Once a cancer has been detected, it is also important to accurately assess nodal status (i.e. N-staging), since this has important therapeutic and prognostic implications. Current cross-sectional imaging modalities, however, rely on size and morphological criteria, and thus lack the desired accuracy for characterizing lymph nodes (Torabi et al. 2004). DWIBS may be a valuable tool for the identification and characterization of lymph nodes; normal lymph nodes have a relatively impeded diffusion because of their high cellular density and are well visualized with DWIBS, while surrounding fat tissue is suppressed. Metastatic lymph nodes may have increased cellular density or central necrosis, which restricts or increases diffusion respectively. However, it is still a subject of exploration as to the degree to which it is possible to differentiate healthy lymph nodes or benign lymphadenopathy from malignant lymph nodes using DWIBS by calculating the nodal ADCs (Kwee et al. 2009). Currently, the limited specificity of qualitative DWIBS assessment for nodal characterization may be considered as an important limitation (Fig. 14.22). Nevertheless, DWIBS is an outstanding tool to identify lymph nodes, irrespective of their histological composition (Fig. 14.22). A relatively recent exciting development is the successful use of ultrasmall superparamagnetic iron oxide (USPIO) nanoparticles for the diagnosis of lymph node metastases (Will et al. 2006). However, lymph nodes may not be easily detectable on USPIO-enhanced MR imaging. In this respect, the combination of DWIBS and USPIO-enhanced MR imaging appears to be a very attractive solution (Thoeny et al. 2009).

14.8.2
Monitoring Response to Therapy

Another potential application of DWIBS is for the assessment of radiation and/or chemotherapy. Currently, CT and anatomical MR imaging are the most commonly used techniques for the evaluation of cancer patients post-treatment. Serial measurements of tumour dimensions are made and criteria such as the World Health Organization (WHO) or Response Evaluation Criteria in Solid Tumours (RECIST) are applied to assess therapeutic efficacy (Jaffe 2006). DWIBS may be explored as a technique to enable two dimensional or volumetric tumour measurements. One key advantage of DWIBS is that it is a relatively

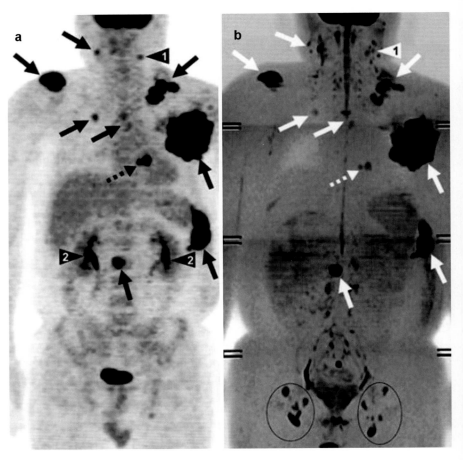

Fig. 14.22. Comparison of ¹⁸FDG-PET and DWIBS images in a 44-year-old man with diffuse large B-cell lymphoma. (**a**) Coronal maximum intensity projection ¹⁸FDG-PET image and (**b**) coronal maximum intensity projection DWIBS image. Both images show cervical, bilateral supra/infraclavicular, mediastinal, left axillary, para-aortic lymph node and splenic involvement (*arrows*) and paracardiac involvement (*dashed arrow*). Note that left-sided cervical lymph nodes shown on DWIBS are not pathologically enlarged, but exhibit significant tracer uptake on ¹⁸FDG-PET (*arrowheads 1*) indicating lymphomatous involvement. On the other hand, the normal-sized bilateral inguinal lymph nodes shown on DWIBS (*encircled*) exhibit no tracer uptake on ¹⁸FDG-PET that would suggest lymphomatous involvement. Thus, specificity of DWIBS for nodal characterization may be limited. Also note physiological tracer accumulation in the urinary tract on ¹⁸FDG-PET (*arrowheads 2*) that may obscure potential lesions in this area, whereas DWIBS does not suffer from this disadvantage (Reprinted from KWEE et al. 2008 with permission)

quick method that can be used to appraise lesion response "at a glance" (Figs. 14.23 and Fig. 14.24).

Furthermore, the technique allows quantification of the total tumour burden by applying appropriate segmentation techniques to allow (automated) total tumour volume measurements (Fig. 14.25) as described previously.

Currently, DWIBS images are usually acquired using a slice thickness of 4 mm, but in the near future it is expected that further improvements in multichannel coils and accelerated parallel imaging will allow acquisition of true isotropic high-resolution volume data sets. Another important advantage of DWIBS is that it does not require administration of any contrast agents. For this reason, the technique may be developed as an alternative to CT in the follow-up of cancer patients, where the administration of contrast is contraindicated (MASUI et al 2005) (Fig. 14.26).

A disadvantage of the current approach of obtaining repetitive tumour size measurements on CT or MR imaging is that it cannot be used to give an early

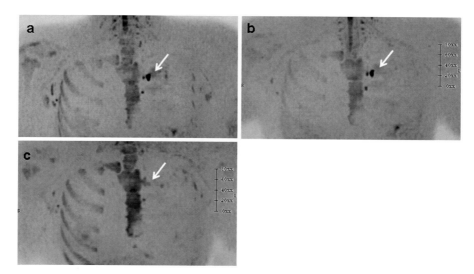

Fig. 14.23. Monitoring the effects of chemotherapy and radiotherapy using DWIBS. DW-MR images of a 39-year-old woman with metastatic parasternal lymph nodes after left mastectomy. (a) Coronal maximum intensity projection DWIBS image shows parasternal lymph node metastasis (*arrow*). Chemotherapy was initiated after this examination. Note that the left-sided ribs are not well visualized due to previous history of radiation therapy. (b) Follow-up examination 3 months after initiation of therapy. Although a parasternal lymph node can still be seen (*arrow*), signal intensity of the ribs is suppressed, probably due to chemotherapy-induced suppression of red bone marrow. (c) Follow-up examination 6 months after initiation of therapy. The parasternal lymph node has almost disappeared (*arrow*). Signal intensity of ribs has normalized except for the left-sided ribs which had undergone previous radiation therapy

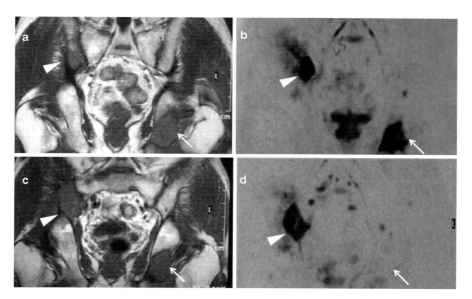

Fig. 14.24. DWIBS pre and post-irradiation in a 58-year-old man with multiple pelvic bone metastases from renal cell carcinoma. (a) Coronal T1-weighted image and (b) coronally reformatted DWIBS image before irradiation. (c) Coronal T1-weighted image and (d) coronally reformatted DWIBS image after irradiation to the disease in the left ischium (*arrows*). There was also disease in the right ilium (*arrow-heads*) which was not treated. After irradiation, the treated disease in the left ischium showed marginal changes on T1-weighted imaging but there was complete disappearance of the lesion on DWIBS, suggesting treatment response. Note, however, the enlargement of untreated lesion in the right ilium (*arrowheads*)

Fig. 14.25. Follow-up examination after chemotherapy in a 73-year-old man with a gastrointestinal stromal tumour of the rectum. Axial DW-MRI of the pelvis at site of disease (**a**) at initiation of chemotherapy and (**b**) at 3 months follow-up. Coronal volume rendered (VR) image through the area (**c**) at initiation of chemotherapy and (**d**) at 3 months follow up. Follow-up examination at 3 months showed significant tumour growth with more than four times increase in tumour volume. Tumour volume assessment may prove to be more accurate than unidimensional tumour measurements for treatment response evaluation. However, DW-MR images are prone to image distortion and development of good distortion correction techniques will be important

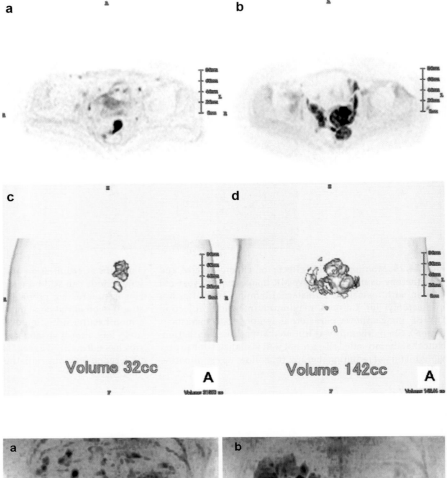

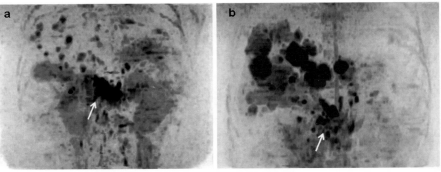

Fig. 14.26. DWIBS in a 65-year-old man with aggressive pancreatic cancer. (**a**) Coronal maximum intensity projection (MIP) DWIBS image showed advanced pancreatic tumour (*arrow*) and multiple liver metastases. (**b**) Coronal MIP DWIBS 4 months later. There was considerable enlargement of the liver metastases but no significant change to the primary tumour (*arrow*). As these images can be rapidly acquired, MIP images can be used to quickly survey the disease state "at a glance"

assessment of the effectiveness of radiation and/or chemotherapy. Early identification of patients who are likely to show a poor response to a certain treatment can be of great advantage: it provides the opportunity to adjust individual treatment regimes more rapidly, thus sparing patients unnecessary morbidity, expense and delay in receiving effective treatments.

PET is a promising functional imaging modality for the early assessment of response to therapy for a variety of tumours (WEBER 2005), but DWIBS, which is much less expensive and does not require any patient preparation may also be of value. Similar to PET, DWIBS is able to detect functional changes in areas involved with tumour before structural changes become visible. In addition, the recently described parametric response map of diffusion allows calculation and visualization of tumour ADC changes during treatment and takes into account spatial heterogeneity of tumour response. The technique has been shown to be of value for predicting treatment response in patients with brain tumours (HAMSTRA et al. 2008), and its feasibility for evaluating treatment response of metastatic bone disease from prostate cancer has been presented (LEE et al. 2007). Extracranial application of parametric response mapping of diffusion using DWIBS would be very attractive, but is technically challenging and requires further investigation.

14.8.3
Detection of Tumour Persistence or Recurrence

Differentiating persistent or recurrent tumour from non-tumoural post-therapeutic change is of importance for patient management, but is often difficult with CT or anatomical MR imaging. Functional imaging techniques, such as PET may allow better differentiation. The less expensive DWIBS may also be of value (Figs. 14.27 and Fig. 14.28). It can be hypothesized that persistent or recurrent tumour tissue will show a more impeded diffusion than treatment-related changes, because of higher cellular density in the former. However, whether or not it is possible to differentiate persistent or recurrent tumour tissue from non-tumoural post-therapeutic changes using DWIBS still has to be determined because available literature on this topic is inconclusive (GOSHIMA et al. 2008b, NISHIE et al. 2008).

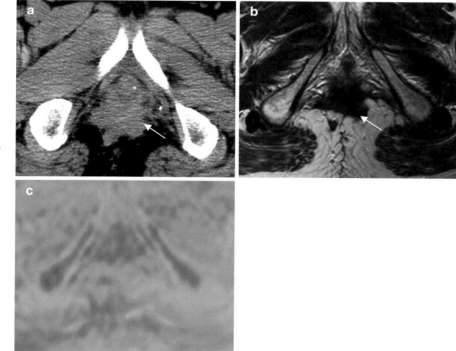

Fig. 14.27. Post-operative fibrosis in 76-year-old man. (**a**) Non-contrast-enhanced CT shows irregular shaped mass posterior to the rectum (*arrow*). (**b**) T2-weighted image shows low intensity in the corresponding area (*arrow*) consistent with fibrosis rather than local recurrence of the carcinoma. (**c**) DW-MR image ($b = 1,000\,\text{s/mm}^2$) shows no high signal intensity. This finding increases the certainty of the diagnosis of post-operative fibrosis (Courtesy: K. KATAHIRA, Kumamoto Chuo Hospital, Japan)

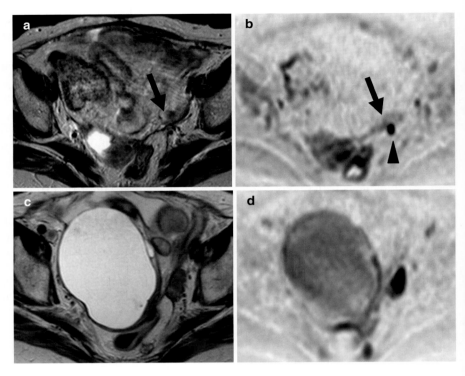

Fig. 14.28. Metastasis from carcinoma of the sigmoid colon in a 78-year-old woman. (**a**) Initial post-operative T2-weighted image shows an irregular shaped intermediate signal intensity area in the left pelvis (*arrow*). (**b**) DW-MR image (*b* = 1,000 s/ mm²) displayed in inverted greyscale obtained at the same time shows only faint low signal intensity (*arrow*) consistent with fibrosis. However, an *oval shaped* low signal intensity lesion (*arrowhead*) is also demonstrated suspicious for metastasis (**c**) T2-weighted image and (**d**) DW-MR image obtained 5 months later. Both images show significant increase in size of the mass confirming nodal metastasis. Although metastatic disease was not diagnosed on the initial imaging, the possibility was suggested by DW-MRI (Courtesy: K. Katahira, Kumamoto Chuo Hospital, Japan)

References

Baur A, Dietrich O, Reiser M (2003) Diffusion-weighted imaging of bone marrow: current status. Eur Radiol 13: 1699–708

Cui Y, Zhang XP, Sun YS, Tang L, Shen L (2008) Apparent diffusion coefficient: potential imaging biomarker for prediction and early detection of response to chemotherapy in hepatic metastases. Radiology 248:894–900

El-Assmy A, Abou-El-Ghar ME, Mosbah A, et al (2009) Bladder tumour staging: comparison of diffusion- and T2-weighted MR imaging. Eur Radiol 19:1575–81

Fujii S, Matsusue E, Kanasaki Y, et al (2008) Detection of peritoneal dissemination in gynecological malignancy: evaluation by diffusion-weighted MR imaging. Eur Radiol 18: 18–23

Goldberg MA, Hahn PF, Saini S, et al (1993) Value of T1 and T2 relaxation times from echoplanar MR imaging in the characterization of focal hepatic lesions. AJR Am J Roentgenol 160:1011–17

Goshima S, Kanematsu M, Kondo H, et al (2008a) Diffusion-weighted imaging of the liver: optimizing b value for the detection and characterization of benign and malignant hepatic lesions. J Magn Reson Imaging 28:691–7

Goshima S, Kanematsu M, Kondo H, et al (2008b) Evaluating local hepatocellular carcinoma recurrence post-transcatheter arterial chemoembolization: is diffusion-weighted MRI reliable as an indicator? J Magn Reson Imaging 27:834–9

Gourtsoyianni S, Papanikolaou N, Yarmenitis S, Maris T, Karantanas A, Gourtsoyiannis N (2008) Respiratory gated diffusion-weighted imaging of the liver: value of apparent diffusion coefficient measurements in the differentiation between most commonly encountered benign and malignant focal liver lesions. Eur Radiol 18:486–92

Haider MA, van der Kwast TH, Tanguay J, et al (2007) Combined T2-weighted and diffusion-weighted MRI for localization of prostate cancer. AJR Am J Roentgenol 189:323–8

Hamstra DA, Galbán CJ, Meyer CR, et al (2008) Functional diffusion map as an early imaging biomarker for high-grade glioma: correlation with conventional radiologic response and overall survival. J Clin Oncol 26:3387–94

Humphries PD, Sebire NJ, Siegel MJ, Olsen ØE (2007) Tumours in pediatric patients at diffusion-weighted MR imaging: apparent diffusion coefficient and tumour cellularity. Radiology 245:848–54

Ichikawa T, Haradome H, Hachiya J, Nitatori T, Araki T (1998) Diffusion-weighted MR imaging with a single-shot echoplanar sequence: detection and characterization of focal hepatic lesions. AJR Am J Roentgenol 170:397–402

Ichikawa T, Haradome H, Hachiya J, Nitatori T, Araki T (1999) Diffusion-weighted MR imaging with single-shot echo-planar imaging in the upper abdomen: preliminary clinical experience in 61 patients. Abdom Imaging 24:456–61

Ichikawa T, Erturk SM, Motosugi U, et al (2006) High-B-value diffusion-weighted MRI in colorectal cancer. AJR Am J Roentgenol 187:181–4

Ichikawa T, Erturk SM, Motosugi U, et al (2007) High-b value diffusion-weighted MRI for detecting pancreatic adenocarcinoma: preliminary results. AJR Am J Roentgenol 188:409–14

Jaffe CC (2006) Measures of response: RECIST, WHO, and new alternatives. J Clin Oncol 24:3245–51

Kim S, Jain M, Harris AB, et al (2009) T1 hyperintense renal lesions: characterization with diffusion-weighted MR imaging versus contrast-enhanced MR imaging. Radiology 25:796–807

Kjaer L, Thomsen C, Gjerris F, Mosdal B, Henriksen O (1991) Tissue characterization of intracranial tumours by MR imaging. In vivo evaluation of T1- and T2-relaxation behavior at 1.5 T. Acta Radiol 32:498–504

Koh DM, Collins DJ (2007) Diffusion-weighted MRI in the body: applications and challenges in oncology. AJR Am J Roentgenol 188:1622–35

Koh DM, Brown G, Riddell AM, et al (2008) Detection of colorectal hepatic metastases using MnDPDP MR imaging and diffusion-weighted imaging (DWI) alone and in combination. Eur Radiol 18:903–10

Komori T, Narabayashi I, Matsumura K, et al (2007) 2-[Fluorine-18]-fluoro-2-deoxy-D-glucose positron emission tomography/computed tomography versus whole-body diffusion-weighted MRI for detection of malignant lesions: initial experience. Ann Nucl Med 21:209–15

Kwee TC, Takahara T, Luijten PR, Nievelstein RA (2009) ADC measurements of lymph nodes: Inter- and intra- observer reproducibility study and an overview of the literature. Eur J Radiol doi:10.1016/j.ejrad.2009.03.026

Lee KC, Bradley DA, Hussain M, et al (2007) A feasibility study evaluating the functional diffusion map as a predictive imaging biomarker for detection of treatment response in a patient with metastatic prostate cancer to the bone. Neoplasia 9:1003–11

Li S, Sun F, Jin ZY, Xue HD, Li ML (2007) Whole-body diffusion-weighted imaging: technical improvement and preliminary results. J Magn Reson Imaging 26:1139–44

Luboldt W, Küfer R, Blumstein N, et al (2008) Prostate carcinoma: diffusion-weighted imaging as potential alternative to conventional MR and 11C-choline PET/CT for detection of bone metastases. Radiology 249:1017–25

Masui T, Katayama M, Kobayashi S, Sakahara H. (2005) Intravenous injection of high and medium concentrations of computed tomography contrast media and related heat sensation, local pain, and adverse reactions. J Comput Assist Tomogr 29:704–8

Matsuki M, Inada Y, Tatsugami F, Tanikake M, Narabayashi I, Katsuoka Y (2007) Diffusion-weighted MR imaging for urinary bladder carcinoma: initial results. Eur Radiol 17:201–4

Muro I, Takahara T, Horie T, et al (2005) Influence of respiratory motion in body diffusion weighted imaging under free breathing (examination of a moving phantom). Nippon Hoshasen Gijutsu Gakkai Zasshi 61:1551–8

Nishie A, Stolpen AH, Obuchi M, Kuehn DM, Dagit A, Andresen K (2008) Evaluation of locally recurrent pelvic malignancy: performance of T2- and diffusion-weighted MRI with image fusion. J Magn Reson Imaging 28:705–13

Ohno Y, Koyama H, Onishi Y, et al (2008) Non-small cell lung cancer: whole-body MR examination for M-stage assessment–utility for whole-body diffusion-weighted imaging compared with integrated FDG PET/CT. Radiology 248:643–54

Ono K, Ochiai R, Yoshida T, et al (2009) Comparison of diffusion-weighted MRI and 2-[fluorine-18]-fluoro-2-deoxy-D-glucose positron emission tomography (FDG-PET) for detecting primary colorectal cancer and regional lymph node metastases. J Magn Reson Imaging 29:336–40

Parikh T, Drew SJ, Lee VS, et al (2008) Focal liver lesion detection and characterization with diffusion-weighted imaging: comparison with standard breath-hold T2-weighted imaging. Radiology 246:812–22

Pruessmann KP, Weiger M, Scheidegger MB, Boesiger P (1999) SENSE: sensitivity encoding for fast MRI. Magn Reson Med 42:952–62

Qi LP, Zhang XP, Tang L, Li J, Sun YS, Zhu GY (2009) Using diffusion-weighted MR imaging for tumour detection in the collapsed lung: a preliminary study. Eur Radiol 19:333–41

Ren J, Huan Y, Wang H, et al (2009) Seminal vesicle invasion in prostate cancer: prediction with combined T2-weighted and diffusion-weighted MR imaging. Eur Radiol doi: 10.1007/s00330-009-1428-0

Satoh S, Kitazume Y, Ohdama S, Kimula Y, Taura S, Endo Y (2008) Can malignant and benign pulmonary nodules be differentiated with diffusion-weighted MRI? AJR Am J Roentgenol 191:464–70

Schaefer PW, Grant PE, Gonzalez RG (2000) Diffusion-weighted MR imaging of the brain. Radiology 217:331–45

Schwartz LH, Panicek DM, Koutcher JA, Heelan RT, Bains MS, Burt M (1995) Echoplanar MR imaging for characterization of adrenal masses in patients with malignant neoplasms: preliminary evaluation of calculated T2 relaxation values. AJR Am J Roentgenol 164:911–5

Sugita R, Yamazaki T, Furuta A, Itoh K, Fujita N, Takahashi S (2009) High b-value diffusion-weighted MRI for detecting gallbladder carcinoma: preliminary study and results. Eur Radiol 19:1794–8

Takahara T, Imai Y, Yamashita T, Yasuda S, Nasu S, Van Cauteren M (2004) Diffusion weighted whole body imaging with background body signal suppression (DWIBS): technical improvement using free breathing, STIR and high resolution 3D display. Radiat Med 22:275–82

Takeuchi M, Sasaki S, Ito M, et al (2009) Urinary bladder cancer: diffusion-weighted MR imaging–accuracy for diagnosing T stage and estimating histologic grade. Radiology 251:112–21

Tanimoto A, Nakashima J, Kohno H, Shinmoto H, Kuribayashi S (2007) Prostate cancer screening: the clinical value of diffusion-weighted imaging and dynamic MR imaging in combination with T2-weighted imaging. J Magn Reson Imaging 25:146–52

Thoeny HC, Triantafyllou M, Birkhaeuser FD, et al (2009) Combined ultrasmall superparamagnetic particles of iron oxide-enhanced and diffusion-weighted magnetic resonance imaging reliably detect pelvic lymph node metastases in normal-sized nodes of bladder and prostate cancer patients. Eur Urol 55:761–9

Townsend DW (2008) Multimodality imaging of structure and function. Phys Med Biol 53:R1–39

Tsushima Y, Takano A, Taketomi-Takahashi A, Endo K (2007) Body diffusion-weighted MR imaging using high b-value for malignant tumour screening: usefulness and necessity of referring to T2-weighted images and creating fusion images. Acad Radiol 14:643–50

Torabi M, Aquino SL, Harisinghani MG (2004) Current concepts in lymph node imaging. J Nucl Med 45:1509–18

Uto T, Takehara Y, Nakamura Y, et al (2009) Higher sensitivity and specificity for diffusion-weighted imaging of malignant lung lesions without apparent diffusion coefficient quantification. Radiology 252:247–54

Varghese JC, Hahn PF, Papanicolaou N, Mayo-Smith WW, Gaa JA, Lee MJ (1997) MR differentiation of phaeochromocytoma from other adrenal lesions based on qualitative analysis of T2 relaxation times. Clin Radiol 52:603–6

Watanabe H, Kanematsu M, Kondo H, et al (2009) Preoperative T staging of urinary bladder cancer: does diffusion-weighted MRI have supplementary value? AJR Am J Roentgenol 192:1361–6

Weber WA (2005) Use of PET for monitoring cancer therapy and for predicting outcome. J Nucl Med 46:983–95

Will O, Purkayastha S, Chan C, et al (2006) Diagnostic precision of nanoparticle-enhanced MRI for lymph-node metastases: a meta-analysis. Lancet Oncol 7:52–60

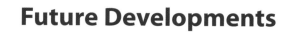

Future Developments

Multifunctional MR Imaging Assessments:
A Look into the Future

Anwar Padhani

CONTENTS

SUMMARY

There is an increased opportunity to perform MR imaging using functional imaging techniques at a variety of organ sites, in a relatively short examination time acceptable to patients. These techniques yield quantitative information which reflects on specific aspects of the underlying tumour or tissue biology. Many of these techniques are used to provide unique information as surrogate biomarkers for tumour behaviour, including response of tumours to treatment. The multi-parametric approach combines the information from different functional imaging techniques, which goes beyond what can be achieved using any single functional technique, thus allowing an improved understanding of the biological processes, and the biological responses to therapeutic interventions. Multi-parametric MR imaging has many potential clinical roles. It is useful for pharmaceutical drug development and for predicting therapeutic efficacy.

Anwar Padhani, MBBS, FRCP, FRCR
Paul Strickland Scanner Centre, Mount Vernon Hospital, Rickmansworth Road, Northwood, Middlesex HA6 2RN, United Kingdom

15.1

Introduction

To date, imaging innovations are focused on improving spatial resolution and data acquisition speeds to achieve excellence in anatomical resolution. Recognizing that this approach has intrinsic limitations (i.e. we need more than just sharper pictures), increasing importance has been placed on "functional" imaging techniques that depict physiological processes within tumours and tissues in vivo without tissue disruption. Thus, we have seen the clinical deployment of a variety of radionuclide imaging probes, perfusion CT and microbubble-enhanced ultrasound.

MR imaging techniques such as diffusion-weighted MR imaging (DW-MRI), dynamic contrast-enhanced MR imaging (DCE-MRI), dynamic susceptibility contrast-enhanced MR imaging (DSC-MRI), blood oxygenation level dependent MR imaging (BOLD-MRI) and proton MR spectroscopic imaging (^{1}H-MRSI) have also become available for clinical use, although they are most widely applied in research settings. Although these techniques have been used to evaluate non-malignant conditions, this chapter is focused on discussing these techniques in oncological practice. Functional MR imaging techniques yield qualitative image contrast and quantitative biomarker data that is spatially resolved and so can be fused onto the morphological/anatomical images. Table 15.1 summarizes these functional MR imaging techniques and the quantitative information that can be derived for each. The principal considerations in this chapter will be the new opportunities brought on by the improved ability of MR imaging to acquire *multiple*, *quantitative* and *biologically relevant* parameters, in a spatial and time resolved way (ZERHOUNI 2008).

The ability to perform multi-parametric MR imaging in the clinical setting has resulted from developments in a number of areas. First, technological advancements within MR imaging which allow multifunctional data to be acquired in a time window which is acceptable to patients and so can be repeated. Second, advances in computing power and software for image analysis allow derivation of quantitative biologically relevant biomarker data, which can be mapped spatially onto the corresponding anatomical images. Third, progress in information technologies enables the integration of quantitative imaging features with other biological data using bioinformatics approaches. The specifics of any individual functional MR imaging technique or multi-parametric enabling technologies will not be discussed; interested readers are invited to review reference works shown in Table 15.1. Instead, this chapter will focus on discussing the potential utility of multi-parametric MR imaging to inform our understanding of biological processes and the biological responses to therapeutic interventions, and will also consider in brief what needs to be done to demonstrate objectively that benefits do accrue from the adoption of such multi-parametric imaging approaches.

15.2
Uses of Multifunctional MR Imaging

Functional imaging techniques can non-invasively depict the molecular processes or pathophysiological functions of tumours, peri-tumoural regions and organ structures. In so doing, it is possible to map spatially, the distribution of biologically important micro-environmental characteristics (such as the levels of oxygenation, cell proliferation and energetics, intra- and extracellular pH), cellular metabolic features, molecular derangement, as well as physiological alterations.

These images reflect the genotypic and phenotypic characteristics of tumours (DIEHN et al. 2008; LENKINSKI et al. 2008; POPE et al. 2008). Functional imaging can therefore be harnessed as a method to spatially depict the hallmarks of cancer, such as self-sufficiency in growth signals, avoidance of immunosurveillance, insensitivity to antigrowth signals, tissue invasion and metastasis, deregulated and limitless tumour cell proliferation, substantiated angiogenesis, evading apoptosis, and the consequences of altered metabolism including altered glycolysis and tumour acidification (KROEMER and POUYSSEGUR 2008). However, it must be remembered that many observations made using functional imaging techniques represent changes that occur downstream to the genetic alterations of cancer. These measurements made on a macroscopic spatial scale using functional MR imaging techniques are used to reflect changes occurring at a cellular or sub-cellular level.

Regardless of the imaging modality, individual functional imaging techniques are often used on their own (usually registered to the morphological imaging) to depict particular molecular alteration, metabolic signature or physiological state. The multi-parametric approach is an extension of this process. By combining the information derived from a number of imaging techniques, it is possible to build a multifaceted model of tumours by accounting for their different pathophysiological properties. It has been shown that using a multi-parametric approach is valuable in a number of broad areas:

1. *Depiction of tumour biology*. Functional imaging is used to demonstrate cellular derangements, metabolic features and other characteristics of the tumour microenvironment. By using a combination of different techniques, it is possible to cross-validate observations, in order to enhance

Table 15.1. Summary of functional MR imaging techniques, the quantitative parameters derived and their biological correlates

Functional imaging technique	Principles of MR measurements	Biological property on which imaging is based	Commonly derived quantitative imaging parameters/ biomarkers	Pathophysiological correlates
Diffusion weighted MRI (DW-MRI) (KOH and COLLINS 2007; THOENY and DE KEYZER 2007; KOH et al. 2008; PATTERSON et al. 2008)	Single-shot echo-planar DW-MRI acquisition. Contrast agent not required.	Diffusivity of water	Apparent diffusion coefficient (ADC)	Tissue architecture: cell density, extracellular space tortuosity, gland formation, cell membrane integrity, necrosis
Diffusion tensor imaging (DTI) (LE BIHAN and VAN ZIJL 2002)	Non-contrast enhanced imaging. Single-shot echo-planar DW-MRI acquisition in 6 or more diffusion gradient encoding directions	Degree of directionality of water movement. Actual direction of water movement.	Relative anisotropy (RA) Fractional anisotropy (RA) Volume Ratio (VR)	Tissue organization and structure
Dynamic contrast-enhanced MRI (DCE-MRI) (CHOYKE et al. 2006; PADHANI and CHOYKE 2006)	T1-weighted MR imaging at high temporal sampling after gadolinium contrast administration. Mathematical modelling of acquired data	Contrast medium uptake rate in tissues, which is influenced by: Transfer rates Extracellular volume Plasma volume fraction	Initial area under gadolinium curve (IAUGC) Transfer and rate constants (K^{trans}, k_{ep}) Leakage space fraction (v_e) Fractional plasma volume (v_p)	Vessel density Vascular permeability Perfusion Extravascular space Plasma volume
Dynamic susceptibility contrast MRI (DSC-MRI) (PADHANI and CHOYKE 2006)	T2*-weighted MR imaging at high temporal sampling to measure first pass of gadolinium contrast through tissue after injection	Blood volume and blood flow	Relative blood volume/ flow (rBV/rBF) Mean transit times (MTT)	Vessel density Blood flow Tumour grade
^{1}H-MR spectroscopic imaging (^{1}H-MRSI) (ALGER 2006; PAYNE and LEACH 2006)	Single voxel or 3D chemical shift imaging. Metabolite assignment based on proton chemical shift effects	Cell membrane turnover/energetics and replacement of normal tissues	Quantified ratios of metabolites including choline, creatine, lipids, citrate, lactate and others depending on echo time	Tumour grade Proliferation index
Blood oxygenation level dependent (BOLD) or intrinsic susceptibility weighted (ISW) MRI (HOWE et al. 2001; ROBINSON 2006)	T2*-weighted imaging performed at different echo times to detect susceptibility effects	Deoxyhaemoglobin shows higher relaxivity than oxyhaemoglobin. Measurement also reflect blood volume, perfusion and Intrinsic composition of tissues	Intrinsic tissue relaxation rates (R2* = 1/T2*)	Ferromagnetic properties of tissues Level of tissue oxygenation

the understanding and interpretation of the imaging findings.

2. *Clinical characterization of disease.* Functional imaging techniques can be applied at all stages of the cancer patient's journey, but especially for lesion characterization and the assessment of therapy response.

3. *Radiotherapy planning.* Multi-parametric MR imaging may be used for radiotherapy planning to improve the conformality of dose prescription

according to underlying biology and to monitor the effects of radiation on tumours and tissues.

4. *Drug development.* In early drug development, functional imaging techniques can provide valuable pharmacodynamic data to clarify the in vivo mechanisms of drugs; and as decision supporting tools for the prioritization of new drug development.

Unfortunately, the range of biological characteristics that can be depicted by clinical MR imaging are still limited compared with positron emission tomography (PET). This principally relates to the higher sensitivity and versatility of PET, as advances in medicinal chemistry has enabled the synthesis of a variety of tracer compounds that are analogues of biologically important molecules, which are used to probe specific cellular events in vivo. In this chapter, the application of multi-parametric MR imaging in each of the four broad areas described above will be discussed, citing examples from the MR imaging literature where possible. The PET literature will also be discussed where appropriate, to illustrate more broadly the benefits that can be accrued from adopting a multi-parametric imaging approach. Although this book is primarily focused on the applications of DW-MRI in the body, the following discussion will take a broader view of all current functional MR imaging techniques, and will also include their utilization in cerebral tumours to highlight the developments in multi-parametric MR imaging.

<h2>15.3</h2>

Depiction of Tumour Biology

Using a multi-parametric MR imaging approach, the depiction of biological processes on MR imaging can be refined, and there is also an opportunity to clarify the relationships between different measured biological characteristics and functions. This could lead to an enhanced understanding of the interplay between these characteristics, the underlying tumour pathophysiology and interpretation of the imaging findings.

15.3.1
Improving the Visualization of Tumour Characteristics

An example of a more refined appreciation of a biological characteristic can be seen when BOLD-MRI

and DSC-MRI are combined to assess the spatial distribution of tissue hypoxia (PADHANI et al. 2007). Tumour hypoxia (defined as tissue $pO_2 < 10\,mmHg$) represents a significant challenge to the curability of human tumours. Hypoxia leads to treatment resistance and enhanced tumour progression (HOCKEL and VAUPEL 2001). The ability to visualize tissue hypoxia using imaging can allow better selection of cancer patients who would benefit from anti-hypoxia directed therapies. Tumour hypoxia can be detected by non-invasive and invasive techniques although their interrelationships remain largely undefined. PET imaging (^{18}F-MISO and ^{64}Cu-ATSM-PET) and BOLD-MRI are the leading imaging contenders for human application, based on their non-invasive nature, ease of use and robustness (TATUM et al. 2006). However unlike PET techniques, BOLD-MRI cannot be used alone to map tissue oxygenation.

The primary source of image contrast in BOLD-MRI is endogenous paramagnetic deoxyhaemoglobin which increases the transverse relaxation rate ($R_2^* = 1/T_2^*$) of water in blood and surrounding tissues. Thus, BOLD-MRI is sensitive to pO_2 within vessels and in tissues adjacent to perfused vessels (HOWE et al. 2001). However, the image contrast observed on BOLD-MRI is dependent on interactions between tissue perfusion, levels of red blood cell oxygenation, as well as on static tissue components (e.g. iron containing myoglobin found in muscles and tissue collagen, in fibrosis).

If BOLD-MRI is to reflect the tissue oxygenation status of a volume of tissue, it is important for red blood cells to (1) be delivered to and (2) reside within the tissue (at least for a time), so that haemoglobin deoxygenation can occur, resulting in an increase in the measured R_2^*. This implies that if blood flow is relatively high and tissue residence time for red cells are relatively low (e.g. in hyperdynamic circulation which limits blood oxygen equilibrium with tissue compartments remote from blood vessels), then R_2^* only reflects tissue blood volumes. These observations mean that it is also necessary to know the distribution of blood volume in tissue, in order to enable correct interpretation of R_2^* images and to infer oxygenation status as shown in Fig. 15.1. If a tissue is perfused but has a high R_2^* in one area/region compared to another area/region in the same tissue (i.e. the static components being the same), then one can infer that the higher R_2^* region is relatively more hypoxic; this hypothesis being supported by preclinical and clinical data (ROBINSON et al. 2003; HOSKIN et al. 2007). Multifunctional MR imaging of a

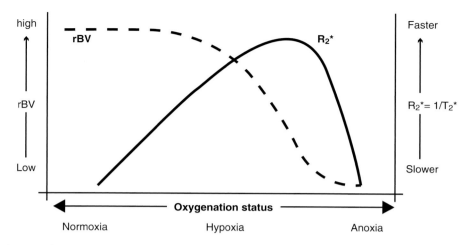

Fig. 15.1. Stylized diagram showing the anticipated change in blood volume and intrinsic susceptibility MR imaging with changes in tissue oxygenation status. To correctly interpret intrinsic susceptibility contrast MR images (R_2^*) to infer oxygenation status, it is necessary to know whether or not tissues are perfused. R_2^* values are increased with increasing tissue hypoxia provided the blood flow continues. When there is no tissue perfusion of blood with erythrocytes to anoxic tissues, then R_2^* values are decreased

patient with multiple liver metastases, which shows the relationship between R2* and tissue perfusion is illustrated in Fig. 15.2. Morphological images as well as the spatial distribution quantitative maps derived from BOLD-MRI, DW-MRI and DCE-MRI are shown for reference. Note the regional differences in the measured R_2^* within the liver and in the metastasis in right hepatic lobe.

15.3.2
Corroborating with and Validating Against Other Functional Imaging Techniques

Multifunctional imaging examinations can be used as a means of validating an emerging imaging biomarker or modification of a quantitative imaging technique against an accepted standard. This may be achieved by ascertaining the strength of relationships between two imaging biomarkers (often one being more established) and exploring the circumstances under which the strength of relationships may be changed.

An example where this type of validation has been done is for the DCE-MRI biomarker transfer constant (K^{trans}). Transfer constant (K^{trans}) represents the inflow constant of a low molecular weight, gadolinium chelate contrast agent into tissues, following intravenous injection. This inflow constant in theory represents both blood flow into the tissue and contrast leakage into the extravascular extracellular space. However, in extracra-

nial tumours, blood flow tends to dominate transfer constant values because of high microvessel permeability and high first pass extraction fraction (TOFTS et al. 1999). In such an instance, the measurement of the transfer constant can be said to be "flow limited", and therefore largely reflects blood flow. Indirect validation of this theory against immuno-histochemical microvessel density measurements and tissue expressions of pro-angiogenic growth factors including vascular endothelial growth factor have been done with mixed results (PADHANI and DZIK-JURASZ 2004). More appropriate validation studies using accepted surrogates of tissue perfusion including ^{14}C-aminoisobutyric acid quantitative autoradiography have also been reported (FERRIER et al. 2007). More recently, in vivo correlative imaging studies have been performed. Thus, transfer constant as a predominant marker of tumour blood flow has now been validated against blood volume/blood flow derived from DSC-MRI studies (Fig. 15.3) (LANKESTER et al. 2007b), ^{15}O-water PET (EBY et al. 2008) and microbubble ultrasound (NIERMANN et al. 2007). These multispectral imaging validation studies have also shown that the relationship is not upheld in every tumour type (e.g. in gliomas because a variably intact blood brain barrier reduces the first pass extraction of the contrast agent (WILKINSON et al. 2006) (Fig. 15.4)). Similarly, the strength of correlation also decreases when therapies that reduce microvessel permeability are used, again because the first pass extraction fraction of small molecular weight contrast agents is reduced (WILKINSON et al. 2006).

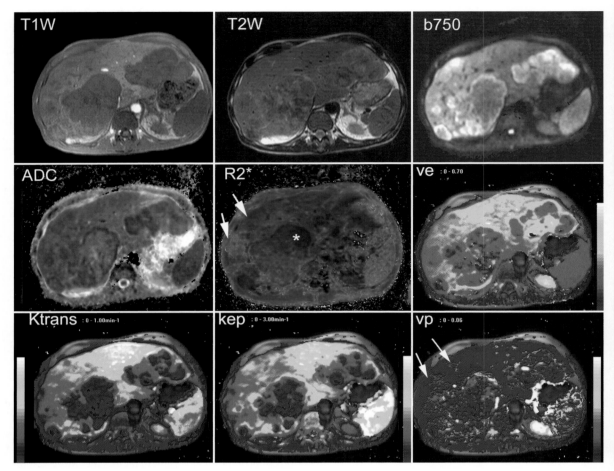

Fig. 15.2. Multifunctional quantitative MR imaging of metastatic liver disease. A 51-year-old man with metastatic rectal cancer. *Top row* images (*left to right*): T1-weighted (T1W), T2-weighted (T2W) and DW-MRI at b = 750 s/mm^2 (*b750*). *Middle row* (*left to right*): Parametric maps of ADC (using b-values 0–750 s/mm^2), R$_2^*$ and leakage space (v_e). *Bottom row* (*left to right*): Maps of transfer constant (K^{trans}), rate constant (k_{ep}) and fraction plasma volume (v_p). The parametric maps of K^{trans}, k_{ep}, v_p and v_e are overlaid on corresponding T1-weighted images. The diffusion images reflect high cellularity at the tumour edges where the $b750$ signal intensity is high and ADC values are lower. The interpretation guideline for R$_2^*$ is shown in Fig. 15.1. On the R$_2^*$ images, there are regional differences in liver R$_2^*$ (*arrows*). Note that there is increased fractional blood volume in areas with increased R$_2^*$ implying that these areas are relatively less well oxygenated. Within the large segment 7 metastasis in the right lobe of liver, there is regional R$_2^*$ variations. More medially, the R$_2^*$ is lower (*) than laterally, with a raised fractional blood volume suggesting better tumour oxygenation compared with area with higher R$_2^*$

Multi-parametric imaging can also be used to assess the validity of a kinetic parameter derived using a technique modification against an existing standard. An example from the DCE-MRI literature is validation of the initial area under the gadolinium concentration curve (IAUGC) as a substitute for transfer constant (K^{trans}). The calculation of the transfer constant requires more complex mathematical modelling which can deter its use at the workbench. Difficulties in deriving transfer constant arise from more complex data acquisition requirements and also from the fact that, the kinetic models used may not exactly fit the DCE-MRI data obtained, because all models make assumptions that may not be valid in a particular tissue or tumour type. By contrast, IAUGC is a semi-quantitative metric that is relatively easy to calculate, as it represents the integral of the area under the gadolinium concentration curve. IAUGC is relatively robust and is able to characterize enhancing regions without the problems associated

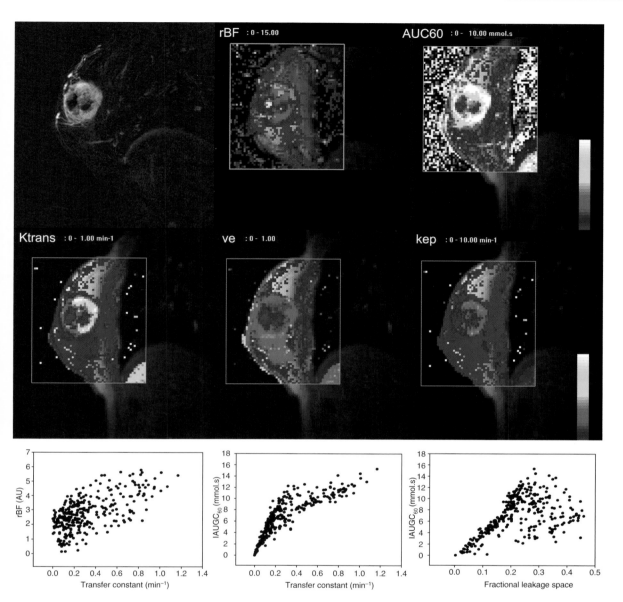

Fig. 15.3. Voxel-by-voxel correlation of DCE-MRI and DSC-MRI in breast cancer. A 45-year-old woman with poorly differentiated infiltrating ductal carcinoma. MR imaging was performed in the sagittal plane. *Top row* images (*left to right*): T1-weighted subtraction sagittal image following IV contrast medium, map of relative blood flow (rBF), map of initial area under the gadolinium contrast medium curve for 60 s (AUC$_{60}$). *Middle row* (*left to right*): Maps of transfer constant (K^{trans}), leakage space (v_e), rate constant (k_{ep}). *Bottom row* (*left to right*) voxel-by-voxel correlations of K^{trans} (*x*-axis) with rBF (*y*-axis), K^{trans} (*x*-axis) with AUC$_{60}$ (*y*-axis) and v_e (*x*-axis) with AUC$_{60}$ (*y*-axis). There is a broad positive linear correlation between K^{trans} and rBF consistent with the assertion that K^{trans} is dominated by blood flow in untreated tumours. The relationships between AUC$_{60}$ and K^{trans} and v_e are more complex with at least two positive linear relationships with K^{trans}. Linear correlations between AUC$_{60}$ and v_e are seen up to a v_e of 20%, after which the relationship is lost. These data show that AUC$_{60}$ does not have a simple relationship with the physiology parameters and depend to some degree, on both transfer constant and leakage space

with model fitting. Hence, if IAUGC is to be used as a practical substitute for transfer constant, then it needs to be validated. The strength of correlations against the transfer constant will depend on the cutoff time used for calculating the IAUGC, with 60 s being recommended by an international consensus panel (Leach et al. 2005). Preclinical and clinical correlations between transfer constant and IAUGC$_{60}$,

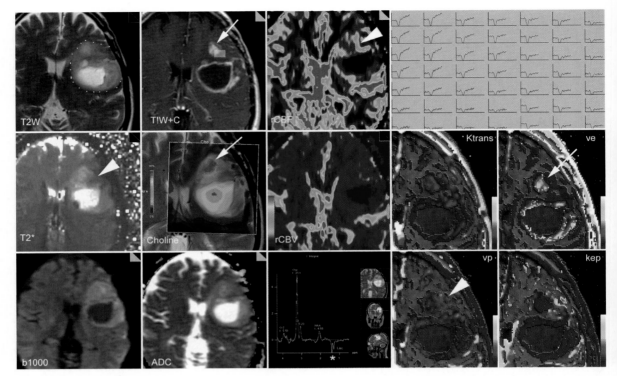

Fig. 15.4. Multi-parametric imaging of brain glioma. A 39-year-old man with a glioblastoma multiforme tumour in the left frontal lobe. *Top row* (*left to right*): T2-weighted (T2W), post-contrast T1-weighted (T1W + C), relative blood flow (rCBF) and DSC curves (ROI) shown is the semi-transparent white box on T1W + C image). *Middle row* (*left to right*): T_2^* map, map of Choline distribution from ^{1}H-MRSI, relative cerebral blood volume (rCBV), transfer constant (K^{trans}), leakage space (v_e). *Bottom row* (*left to right*): DW-MRI using $b = 1,000 \, \text{s/mm}^2$ (b1,000), ADC ($b = 0$–$1,000 \, \text{s/mm}^2$), single voxel 1H-MRS (TE = 135 ms) from region of interest showing high choline concentration, fractional plasma volume (v_p) and rate constant (k_{ep}). The tumour extent is well seen on the T2-weighted image (*white dotted outline*). Blood–brain barrier breakdown has occurred at the edge of the necrotic cavity, and anteriorly, where increased choline (Cho) is seen on MRSI (*arrows*). Note elevated, inverted bifid peak of lactate (*) on the MRS spectra. Lateral to the area with elevated choline levels, there is a region of increased rCBF (also v_p) (*arrowheads*). This area has a fast T_2^* compared to the rest of the tumour (*arrowhead*), suggesting increased blood deoxyhaemoglobin levels. In this example, the spatially registered multi-parametric displays are helpful towards understanding the relationships between important imaging defined biological characteristics in brain tumour

both at the patient and voxel level, have been reported before and after therapy, demonstrating that IAUGC$_{60}$ may be used as a practical substitute for transfer constant (LANKESTER et al. 2005, 2007a, b; THUKRAL et al. 2007). However, readers should remember that IAUGC is a semi-quantitative parameter that does not have a simple relationship to the parameters derived using DCE-MRI (perfusion, permeability and leakage space) (WALKER-SAMUEL et al. 2006), being dependent on both transfer constant and leakage space to varying degrees (Fig. 15.3). On the other hand, transfer constant appears to provide a more direct insight into underlying pathophysiological vascular properties.

15.4

Clinical Characterization of Disease

Morphological MR imaging plays a pivotal role in the management of cancer patients, being used at every stage of the cancer journey from initial diagnosis and lesion characterization, to assessing response to treatment and attempting to gauge the activity of residual disease, as well as for detecting tumour relapse. Whilst clearly important, morphological MR imaging has substantial limitations. Detection of malignant lesions can be difficult, particularly when the disease burden is small, or when the disease is intermixed with normal tissues or benign processes (e.g. malignant tumour foci in coexisting benign nodular prostatic hyperplasia). Lesion characterization can be equally problematic, for example, in differentiating liver metastases from other solid liver lesions or when predicting tumour grade. Moreover, assessments of disease response by tumour size measurements are limited in their utility, particularly for cytostatic molecular–targeted agents. The detection and assessment of residual disease is also problematic for morphology-based imaging. Finally, determining disease relapse in areas of therapy induced scarring can be complicated, requiring serial comparisons to be made with prior examinations (e.g. differentiating tumour recurrence from post-surgical/post-radiotherapy fibrosis). The limitations of morphological-based diagnosis can be successfully addressed using functional imaging techniques, notably [18]FDG-PET, DCE-MRI and DW-MRI. This section will demonstrate that the multi-parametric MR imaging approach can enhance our ability to address limitations inherent in morphological assessments.

15.4.1
Disease Detection and Localization

Improvements in disease detection can be useful for the screening of asymptomatic individuals and can also be helpful for improving the staging accuracy of patients with known cancers. There is a large literature base showing that functional imaging techniques are useful for detecting malignant disease in either asymptomatic subjects (screening) or in those with known malignancy, where disease at distant sites is not suspected.

MR mammography (essentially a DCE-MRI technique) is now recommended for screening pre-menopausal women who are at high genetic risk of breast cancer. Likewise, [18]FDG-PET is the modality of choice for assessing the possibility of distant spread of disease for patients, in whom major surgery is to be undertaken at a variety of anatomical sites including the liver, lung and oesophagus. In the liver, Koh et al. recently compared detection rates of liver metastases in colorectal cancer patients using two MR imaging techniques: MnDPDP (a hepatocyte-specific contrast agent) enhanced MR imaging and DW-MRI. Imaging with targeted contrast agents may also be viewed as a sort of functional imaging as it relies on contrast uptake in specific tissues for disease characterization. Using receiver operating characteristic curves analyses, they found that the combined dataset had higher diagnostic accuracy (Koh et al. 2008). Interestingly, it has also been suggested that the detection of malignant liver lesions on DW-MRI can be improved by the concomitant administration of super paramagnetic iron oxide particles (SPIOs; a liver Kupffer cell-specific contrast agent) (Naganawa et al. 2005); the mechanism of this is likely to be due to susceptibility mediated destruction of signal from the normal liver, thus leaving only metastases (non-Kupffer cell containing) contributing to return signal on DW-MRI. This finding may well explain the findings of Nasu et al. who compared the performance of DW-MRI against SPIOs and showed that combined assessments were more accurate for liver lesion detection, particularly for small lesions (Nasu et al. 2006). A combined approach of ultrasmall SPIO-enhanced MR imaging combined with DW-MRI was also described in a recent study, for improved detection of pelvic lymph-node metastases in normal-sized nodes of patients with bladder and prostate cancer (Thoeny et al. 2009).

Another important clinical area where the multifunctional approach is proving to be of clinical value is the localization of prostate cancer. The importance of locating significant intra-prostatic focal disease lies in two clinical areas. Firstly, it is estimated that as many as 30–50% of men with persistently raised serum prostate specific antigen (PSA) levels and in whom there have been multiple negative biopsies have undiagnosed cancers. Secondly, the usage and future success of local ablative treatments (e.g. radiofrequency or thermal ablation) of prostate cancer is dependent on accurate identification of the dominant intra-prostatic lesion, also known as the index lesion.

A few studies have evaluated the value of ^{1}H-MRSI in patients with elevated PSA levels and previous negative biopsies to localize peripheral zone tumours and have shown that combining MR imaging and ^{1}H-MRSI could potentially help to direct biopsies towards suspicious sites so as to increase the cancer detection rates and thereby limit the total number of biopsies (Amsellem-Ouazana et al. 2005; Prando et al. 2005; Cirillo et al. 2008). Multi-parametric MR imaging can easily be undertaken in the prostate gland (Fig. 15.5) and has been used to improve the detection of prostatic tumours. For example, Futterer et al. showed that it was only when ^{1}H-MRSI and morphological data were combined with DCE-MRI, that lesion localization in the prostate was optimal (Futterer et al. 2006) (Fig. 15.6). Mazaheri et al. suggested combining DW-MRI and ^{1}H-MRSI for lesion localization, but only for the

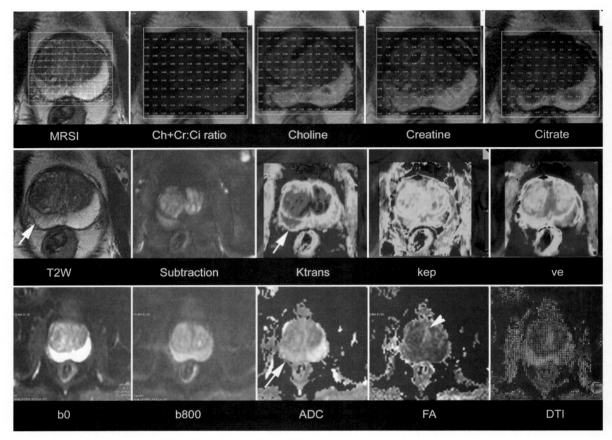

Fig. 15.5. Multifunctional MR imaging of the prostate gland. A 58-year-old man with focal prostatitis in the right peripheral zone (*arrow*) evaluated at 3T without endorectal coil. *Top row* (*left to right*): Multi-voxel MRSI superimposed on T2-weighted imaging and the spatial distribution of important prostate metabolites from ^{1}H-MRSI; choline and citrate over creatine ratio ((Ch + Cr)/Ci ratio), choline, creatine and citrate. *Middle row* (*left to right*): T2-weighted (T2W), post-contrast T1-weighted subtraction (subtraction), transfer constant (K^{trans}), rate constant (k_{ep}), and leakage space (v_e). *Bottom row* (*left to right*): DW-MRI images at $b = 0\,\text{s/mm}^2$ (*b*0), $b = 800\,\text{s/mm}^2$ (*b*800), ADC map, fractional anisotropy (FA) map and diffusion tensor image (DTI) where *red* colour indicates horizontal motion, *green* = anterior–posterior and *blue* = superior–inferior movement of water). Note the relative elevation of citrate in the peripheral zone of the prostate. Although there is slight restriction of water movement in the area of the inflammation on ADC map (*arrow*), there is no significant difference in fractional isotropy. The hypertrophied transition zone show significant increased FA within the fibrous centre (*arrowhead*). Increased transfer constant is seen within the transition zone and in the area of peripheral zone prostatitis. Such spatially registered multi-parametric displays can be helpful for understanding relationships of important biological characteristics in the prostate gland

peripheral zone of the prostate gland (MAZAHERI et al. 2008). In prostate cancers, lesion localization is particularly problematic in the transition zone because benign prostatic hyperplasia shares many of the MR imaging characteristics of cancers (nodule formation, mass effect and hypervascularization). Recent data suggests that using diffusion tensor image (DTI) may also be helpful and that by combining fractional anisotropy (FA) with apparent diffusion coefficient (ADC) values, it is possible to discriminate cancers within the transitional zone (XU et al. 2009).

A number of studies have recently reported that multi-parametric imaging can help to guide prostate biopsies in men with persistently raised serum PSA levels. For example, Hambrock et al. combined DCE-MRI with DW-MRI, and reported that 57% of 63 patients could be diagnosed to have an underlying cancer using this approach, of whom 45% had aggressive disease (Gleason score ≥7) (HAMBROCK et al. 2008).

Fig. 15.6. Prostate lesion localization with multi-parametric MR imaging. A 58-year-old man with raised serum PSA level and negative transrectal ultrasound-guided prostate biopsy. *Top row*: T2-weighted (T2W) and post-contrast subtraction T1-weighted (T1W + C subtraction) images of the prostate show a 8 mm nodule in the left peripheral zone that is avidly enhancing (*arrow*). *Middle row*: DW-MRI at $b = 900$ s/mm^2 (b900) and ADC map calculated using $b = 0$ and 900 s/mm^2 (ADC) shows low ADC values within the nodule (*arrow*). The lesion is not seen on the b900 image because of persistent high signal intensity of the peripheral zone. *Bottom row*: Single and multi-voxel ^{1}H-MRSI spectra (Choline, creatine and citrate) show no significant metabolic changes at the site of abnormality. A Gleason 3-4 tumor was diagnosed at the third prostate biopsy

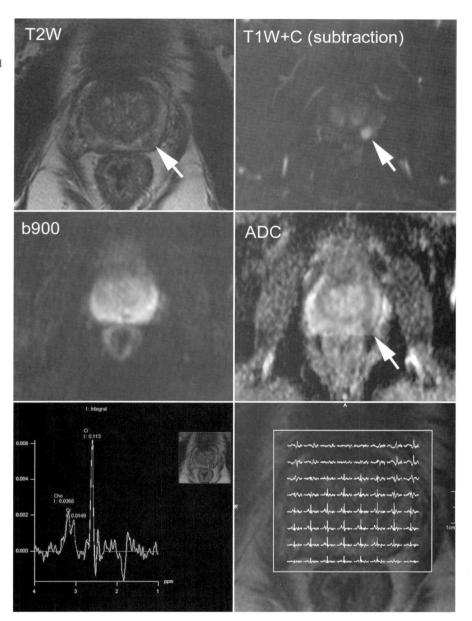

15.4.2
Lesion Characterization

There are many clinical circumstances, when different imaging modalities are used to clarify the nature of an abnormality found by another technique. For example, in the liver, lesion characterization using dynamic contrast enhancement and delayed uptake with a liver specific contrast agent (such as gadoxetic acid) can be combined with DW-MRI. The MR imaging assessment can be extended by the addition of microbubble-enhanced ultrasound or ^{18}FDG-PET

examinations, if there remains doubt about the nature of lesions.

Quantitative multi-parametric approach has been applied for the evaluation of parotid tumours, where the addition of DW-MRI to DCE-MRI assessment aided the distinction between benign and malignant lesions (YABUUCHI et al. 2008). The role that multifunctional imaging has in the characterization of brain lesions and the promise of multi-parametric imaging for evaluating the changing phenotype of prostate cancer will be discussed in this section.

As an overarching observation, readers should note that when multifunctional assessments are used to characterize lesions, results from individual modalities may be discordant. In clinical practice, discordant results are normally dealt with by adopting the majority opinion, taking into account the clinical circumstances. Frequently, it is only by taking several observations over a period of time that the true nature of lesions is revealed. The biological meaning and the clinical importance of discordant results are not completely understood.

15.4.2.1
Cerebral Tumours

There is a long tradition in using multifunctional imaging techniques to evaluate brain diseases, so as to circumvent brain biopsies as far as possible. Techniques such as DW-MRI, DTI, fMRI (using BOLD contrast), DCE-MRI, DSC-MRI and ^{1}H-MRSI are commonly applied in brain tumour imaging (Fig. 15.4). As already noted, these techniques yield a number of quantitative parameters/imaging biomarkers (Table 15.1) that can improve the definition of tumour boundaries, aid tumour characterization, assess tumour response to therapy and distinguish radiation-induced necrosis from tumour recurrence (PROVENZALE et al. 2006).

A major limitation associated with histopathological grading of gliomas is the sampling error associated with stereotactic biopsy. Ideally, the tumour grade of a glioma should reflect the highest grade within the tumour. Therefore, for histopathological assessment to be accurate, it is important to know where the highest tumour grade is likely to be located prior to biopsy. Currently, neurosurgeons rely on histological sampling from areas showing contrast medium enhancement in the tumour, which is often associated with higher tumour grade. However, contrast material enhancement alone is an inaccurate predictor of high tumour grade. Ginsberg et al. (1998) demonstrated that lack of enhancement was not a reliable indicator for a low grade glioma. In another study, all low-grade tumours showed contrast enhancement, but one-fifth of glioblastomas did not show (KNOPP et al. 1999). Not surprisingly, the reliance on contrast enhancement to target brain tumour biopsies results in a grading accuracy rate of between 55 and 85%, which may lead to an inappropriate choice of therapy.

DSC-MRI, DCE-MRI and ^{1}H-MRSI have all been shown to correlate with tumour grade to various extents. Relative cerebral blood volume (rCBV) derived from DSC-MRI appears to have the strongest predictive value for tumour grade (LAW et al. 2003; ZONARI et al. 2007); the biological basis could be explained by higher microvessel density found with increasing tumour grade. rCBV values have been shown to correlate with the mitotic rates, microvessel density, histological grade and choline levels. A number of studies have reported that rCBV cannot reliably distinguish between grade III astrocytomas from grade IV glioblastoma multiforme (GBM). This is likely to be because increasing microvessel leakiness in GBM results in loss of compartmentalization of contrast medium and subsequently underestimates rCBV. Heterogeneity in the spatial distribution of rCBV is also a hallmark for higher tumour grades. Lower rCBV is seen in brain lymphoma and in radiation necrosis (ROLLIN et al. 2006; HU et al. 2008), conditions which may mimic high grade gliomas on morphological imaging. A number of studies have used DCE-MRI for the same purpose, and correlations of transfer constant with tumour grade are present, but in general, less strong compared to rCBV (CHA et al. 2006; LAW et al. 2006a, b). Therefore, the spatial distribution of rBV and transfer constant can be used to guide non-invasive tumour biopsy, both being more reliable than the degree of enhancement observed on static post-contrast scans. ^{1}H-MRSI can also be used to grade astroglial tumours (LAW et al. 2003; ZONARI et al. 2007) and is able to distinguish glial neoplasms from other tumours such as meningiomas (HOWE et al. 2003). Zonari et al. compared the performance of ^{1}H-MRS, DSC-MRI and DW-MRI in the same patients and found in logistic regression analyses, that rCBV, NAA/Cr ratio, and lactate were independent predictors of high grade tumours (ZONARI et al. 2007). ADC values derived from DW-MRI appear less useful compared to DSC-MRI and ^{1}H-MRSI for distinguishing between high- and low-grade neoplasms (ROLLIN et al. 2006; ZONARI et al. 2007), despite strong negative correlations between ADC and choline levels on ^{1}H-MRSI, being demonstrated in several studies (GUPTA et al. 1999; YANG et al. 2002). Based on these imaging findings, many institutions are now beginning to utilize a multifunctional approach for guiding stereotactic brain biopsy.

Low-grade gliomas (grade II) are a heterogeneous group of infiltrative primary brain tumours that grow slowly for several years, but at an unpredictable time, most progress to high-grade gliomas (grade III or GBM), which carry a poor prognosis. Many institutions adopt an expectant, "active surveillance" management policy of regular clinical and imaging examinations in patients, who are not decompensated by tumour. Further biopsy is performed at the first sign of clinical or imaging progression with a view to aggressive therapy. New contrast enhancement appears to be a delayed manifestation of this transformation process. Therefore, additional markers of malignant change that ideally reflect the earlier stages of tumour transformation from a low grade to a high grade phenotype are needed. Recent studies indicate that rCBV derived from DSC-MRI can predict the time of progression of low grade tumours, with tumours showing low rCBV more likely to stay stable over time (Law et al. 2006a, b) (Fig. 15.7). Furthermore, when lesions were evaluated over time, the rCBV of tumours

that remained stable did not change, whereas those patients destined to transform showed increases in rCBV that could be observed 12–18 months prior to clinical and imaging transformation (TOFTS et al. 2007; DANCHAIVIJITR et al. 2008). It remains to be seen whether the multifunctional approach (by adding ¹H-MRSI and DW-MRI) can further improve the predictive performance of rCBV in this regard.

15.4.2.2
Prostate Cancer

An active surveillance policy is also adopted for patients with low risk prostate cancer (low tumour

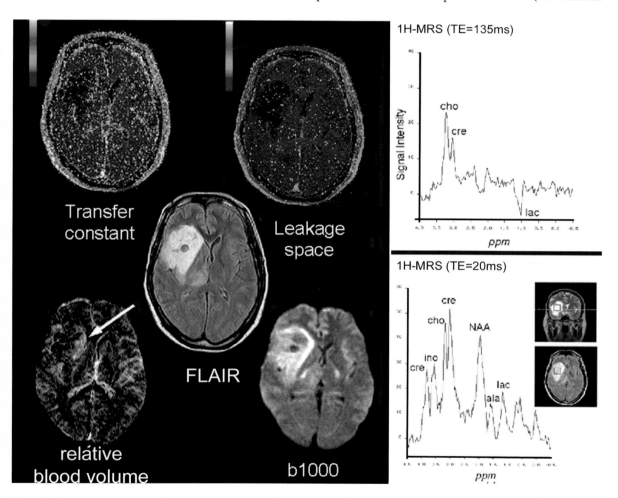

Fig. 15.7. Low grade glioma with high blood volume. Multiparametric MR imaging of a non-enhancing, low grade glioma in a 42-year-old man. No significant enhancement is seen on the maps of the transfer constant (K^{trans}) or leakage space (v_e). There is a region of increased relative blood volume (*arrow*) towards the medial edge of the tumour, coinciding with the area of impeded water diffusion on the $b = 1,000$ s/mm² DW-MRI image (*b*1,000). On single voxel ¹H-MRS (TE = 135 ms), little NAA is detected with a prominent inverted lactate peak within the centre of the tumour on the MRS spectra. About 14 months after the illustrated examination, this glioma transformed to high-grade

burden, Gleason score ≤6; PSA < 10 ng/mL; stage T1–T2a disease) who are suitable for radical treatment, should the disease progress. Importantly, if the tumour does not progress, then overtreatment of these patients can be avoided. Currently, monitoring consists of serum PSA testing, digital rectal examinations (DRE) and repeat biopsy as necessary, although the optimum monitoring protocol has not been established. Unfortunately, because TRUS biopsies are not targeted to tumours within the prostate gland, relying instead, on systematic sampling of the gland by multiple tissue cores, there is always doubt as to how accurately TRUS biopsies reflect the "true" underlying tumour grade and volume. In fact, it is widely recognized that about half of such "low-risk" men actually have a greater volume or a higher grade of cancer, which are missed as a result of inadequate or poor prostate sampling. In order to mitigate the uncertainty introduced by TRUS biopsy, many groups are now applying multifunctional MR imaging (mainly ^{1}H-MRSI, DCE-MRI and DW-MRI) to assess the suitability of patients for active surveillance. The biological basis for using these techniques comes from correlations found between tumour grade and ^{1}H-MRSI (specifically Choline plus Creatine to Citrate ratio) and DW-MRI (the ADC value) (ZAKIAN et al. 2005; TAMADA et al. 2008). In support of this is published data from deSouza et al. who showed significantly higher tumour ADCs in actual low-risk active surveillance patients compared with those with intermediate risk localized prostate cancer at baseline (DESOUZA et al. 2008).

In patients with early stage prostate cancer, using multifunctional assessments could help in the identification of adverse features that may indicate that active surveillance is not an appropriate management option. Adverse features include larger tumour volume, or functional imaging features suggesting high-grade underlying tumour (abnormal spectroscopy or very low ADC value on DW-MRI). However, currently, only anecdotal evidence exists for the efficacy of this approach and a number of studies are ongoing. Interestingly deSouza et al. (2008) have recently shown that even in low risk patients undergoing active surveillance, it is those patients with lower tumour ADC values that progressed; that is, subsequent biopsies showed upward Gleason grade migration, or the patients went on to receive radical treatment (GILES et al. 2009). Interesting data is beginning to emerge in this regard including uncoupling of functional imaging characteristics at baseline (i.e. some imaging features suggesting increased

tumour aggressiveness whereas others do not) with changes towards a more uniform aggressive appearance (Fig. 15.8).

15.4.3
Assessment of Therapy Response

Monitoring tumour changes in response to treatment with multifunctional imaging can provide valuable information on the in vivo mechanism of drug action and patient outcome. A number of studies have employed a multi-parametric MR imaging approach for monitoring the effects of conventional therapies, and it is this aspect that will be considered in this section. Multifunctional approaches for monitoring the effects of radiotherapy and drugs with novel mechanisms of action will be discussed in Sects. 15.5 and 15.6 respectively.

A good example of a study which showed an improved understanding of the biological effects of therapy using multi-parametric MR imaging was reported by Kamel et al. who evaluated serial changes on gadolinium contrast-enhanced MR imaging and DW-MRI in patients with unresectable hepatocellular carcinoma (HCC) after transarterial chemoembolization (TACE) (KAMEL et al. 2009). In this multiple time points observational study, the biological properties assessed were (1) tumour mass (by size changes on morphological imaging), (2) underlying vascular properties of tissues (by qualitative relative arterial and portal phase enhancement assessments) which depend on tissue perfusion, microvessel permeability surface area product and extracellular leakage space, and (3) cellular density and extracellular space tortuosity (by ADC values). Kamel et al. observed that tumour size remained relatively unchanged for up to 4 weeks after chemoembolization, whilst changes in dynamic contrast enhancement and tissue diffusivity had dissimilar time courses. They found that reductions in the degree of enhancement were seen immediately after chemoembolization and were sustained over the observation period. However, increase in ADC values became most apparent after 1–2 weeks, but had returned to the baseline values by 4 weeks.

The biological basis of the observations made by Kamel et al. can be explained if the mechanism of action of the treatment administered is considered. Clearly, the primary insult following TACE is blood supply disruption (MARELLI et al. 2007). Given the delivery mechanism of the therapy and our *a priori*

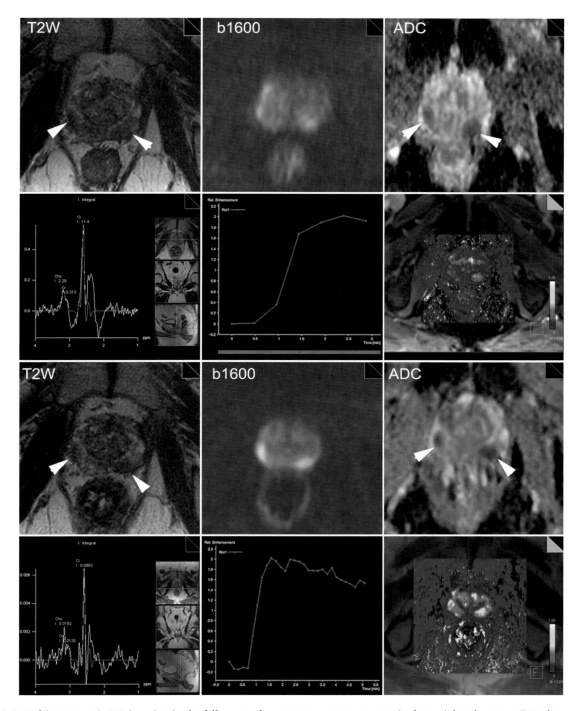

Fig. 15.8. Multi-parametric MR imaging in the follow-up of prostate cancer. A 75-year-old man with bilateral prostate cancers (*arrowheads*) graded Gleason 3 + 3 on active surveillance. *Top two rows* (*left to right*). T2-weighted (T2W), DW-MRI at $b = 1,600 \, s/mm^2$ ($b1,600$), ADC maps from $b = 0$ to $800 \, s/mm^2$ (ADC), ^{1}H-MRS, signal intensity time curves of T1-weighted contrast-enhanced imaging of the left sided tumour and transfer constant (K^{trans}) map ($0–0.3 \, min^{-1}$). *Bottom two rows* are as *top two rows* but 6 months later. The prostate cancers are seen in the peripheral zone on T2W, but are also well shown on the ADC maps (*arrowheads*). Note that at 6 months' follow-up, there is an increase in the upslope of the signal intensity time curve after administration of intravenous contrast (washout also) and increase in transfer constant in tumour areas. However, no changes were perceptible on the ADC map or on ^{1}H-MRS. Increased vascularization in tumours supports an evolving malignant phenotype. Currently, this patient remains on close active surveillance

knowledge that most primary and secondary liver malignancies are predominantly supplied by the hepatic artery, immediate reduction in arterial contrast enhancement would be expected. Kamel et al. also noted that the portal enhancement was also reduced but to a lesser extent than the arterial enhancement. There are also sound biological mechanisms to explain ADC increases after treatment; viz. treatment-induced necrosis and cell death (PATTERSON et al. 2008). The transient period of increased ADC values followed by ADC normalization (KAMEL et al. 2009) could be explained by the removal of dead/dying cells, shifts of extracellular water with tissue compaction, fibrosis and regeneration of native tissues that occurs after successful therapy.

15.4.4
Assessing Residual Disease When Relapse Is Suspected

There are few clinical situations where multifunctional imaging is used to assess the activity of residual disease when tumour recurrence is suspected; in general, functional techniques like DCE-MRI and [18]FDG-PET are used in isolation for this purpose.

As an illustration of ongoing work, we use a multiparametric MR imaging approach to assess the pelvis when recurrent prostate cancer is suspected, as indicated by rising serum PSA levels. In the example shown in Fig. 15.9, both DCE-MRI and DW-MRI were performed and they provide complementary information (both are positive or at the same suspected lesion location). However, there are instances when DW-MRI is less successful and DCE-MRI is relatively more useful, for example, when metallic clips are present in the post-surgical bed or when low-dose brachytherapy seeds are present in the prostate gland (susceptibility effects from these degrade DW-MRI image quality). As a result, DCE-MRI appears to be the MR imaging method of choice for evaluating the pelvis for possible recurrent prostate cancer (HAIDER et al. 2008). Occasionally, discordant results are found when DCE-MRI suggests inactive disease but DW-MRI indicates active tumour (Fig. 15.10); this may occur either because of intrinsic tumour biology (high cellularity but low perfusion) or because of the anti-angiogenic effects of concomitant androgen deprivation therapy (ALONZI et al. 2007).

Another example of using a multifunctional MR imaging approach to evaluate residual disease is in the context of a new enhancing lesion within an irradiated area in a patient previously treated for brain tumour. When this occurs, it may be impossible to differentiate tumour recurrence from radiation necrosis on morphological imaging. In radiation necrosis, the emergence of enhancement can be delayed for months following treatment and can produce dramatic appearances. Radiation necrosis most commonly occurs at the site of the previous tumour, even if only whole-brain irradiation was administered. Additionally, radiation-induced lesions occur within 2 years after radiation therapy, the same period during which tumour recurrence is most frequent. Multifunctional imaging investigations performed in this clinical circumstance showed that high rBV is strongly indicative of tumour recurrence, thus negating the use of ^{201}Tl-SPECT for this purpose (HU et al. 2008). ^{1}H-MRSI has also been used for this purpose with the magnitude of the choline signal providing helpful information. However, because of low spatial resolution, the utility of ^{1}H-MRSI is limited in patients with small enhancing lesions (ROCK et al. 2002). DW-MRI does show some ability in distinguishing between active tumour and radiation necrosis, but appears to be less useful in the most common situation where radiation necrosis is intermixed with active tumour.

15.5
Radiotherapy Planning

Advances in imaging hardware related to radiation delivery have led to improvements in the physical conformality of radiation planning, treatment and delivery, to tumours and organ boundaries using conformal and intensity modulated techniques. The additional ability to combine image-depicted biology with image-guided radiotherapy (IGRT) has opened the way for further refinements of target definition and dose delivery, such that it is now possible to shape dose volume distributions not only to the geometry of targets but also to differences in the radiobiology across tumours (LING et al. 2000). It is possible to define additional "targets-within-targets" or "sub-volumes" of prescribed dose within individual tumours, incorporating functional imaging-

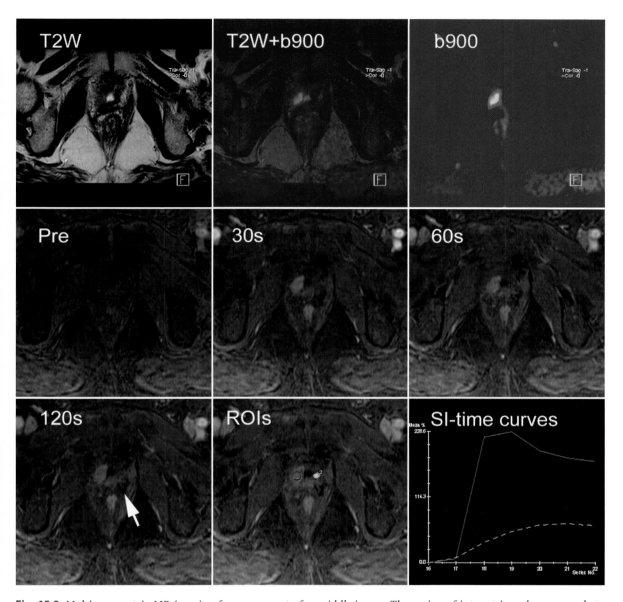

Fig. 15.9. Multi-parametric MR imaging for assessment of tumour relapse after prostatectomy. A 64-year-old man with past history of radical prostatectomy for prostate cancer. *Top row*: T2-weighted imaging (T2W), 50% fusion of T2W with $b = 900\,s/mm^2$ DW-MRI image (*b*900) and the *b*900 DW-MRI image displayed using a colour scale. *Middle* and *lower rows*: serial dynamic contrast-enhanced T1-weighted MR images obtained before (×2) and every 30 s with signal intensity time curves from regions of interest indicated in the *lower row*, *middle* image. The region of interest in *red* corresponds to the red signal intensity time curve, which shows rapid contrast enhancement consistent with tumour relapse. The *yellow* region of interest and signal intensity time curve is from normal peri-urethral tissue. In this case, both DCE-MRI and DW-MRI provide corroborative evidence for disease recurrence at the bladder–urethral junction (high cellularity and perfusion). The *arrow* points to surgical clips in the prostatectomy bed

depicted biological information; this is sometimes called "dose painting by numbers" (Brahme 2003; Bentzen 2005). As a result of these advances, treatments can be given to the optimum dose to an organ or tumour with internal dose modulation, based on an imaging-depicted radiobiologically relevant characteristic such as tumour hypoxia, acidosis or cellular proliferation. Proof of concept CT radiotherapy planning studies have shown that it is theoretically possible to deliver higher doses to more hypoxic

Fig. 15.10. Multiparametric MRI for the assessment of relapsed prostate tumour on hormonal therapy. A 50-year-old man with rising serum PSA levels on androgen deprivation therapy. The T2W image is non-diagnostic showing poor zonal differentiation only. Active disease within the gland is suspected on the basis of the DW-MRI (high signal intensity on $b1,600$ image and low $ADC_{0-1,000}$ values) and ^{1}H-MRSI (high choline peak). However, the signal intensity time curves after contrast medium injection suggest no active disease for bilateral regions of interest (ROIs). Please note that androgen deprivation therapy has an anti-angiogenic effect (therefore changes contrast enhancement) but does not sterilize the cancer within the prostate gland

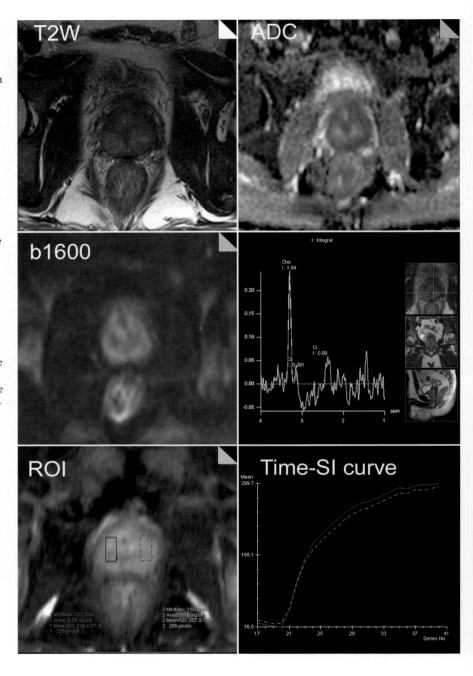

regions of tumours (CHAO et al. 2001); all of this could be done whilst minimizing normal tissue radiation toxicity.

A number of functional imaging techniques are being used to improve the delineation of tumours for radiation planning (^{18}FDG-PET for lung cancer and ^{1}H-MRSI with DCE-MRI for prostate cancer are examples). It is possible to combine two functional techniques (one for delineation and another to depict the spatial distribution of important biological characteristics within tumours) for the same purpose. Thus, ^{18}FDG-PET (for lesion delineation) and ^{64}Cu-ATSM (for hypoxia depiction) can be used together in a dose-painting paradigm. This particular PET approach is not equally applicable to all tumour sites. In prostate cancer, current evidence suggests that ^{11}C-choline PET is not successful for identifying the location of index intra-prostatic lesions particularly for moderate grade tumours (the most common type) and hypoxia depiction is certainly problematic, as benign prostatic hyperplasia is itself hypoxic.

If one were to use BOLD-MRI to map prostate cancer hypoxia, then there is an absolute need to combine BOLD-MRI data with perfusion information in order to generate tumour hypoxia probability maps (see Sect. 15.3.1). However, this combination technique (BOLD-MRI plus perfusion) is not able to localize intraprostatic cancers and it would be necessary to add other methods to delineate the extent of the dominant intraprostatic lesion by techniques such as ¹H-MRSI and DW-MRI (FUTTERER et al. 2006; MAZAHERI et al. 2008) as discussed in Sect. 15.4.1. Thus, for prostate cancer, there is a potential need to perform three to four functional MR imaging techniques if one wants to employ the dose-painting approach, which could make the approach practically unworkable without significant bioinformatics input (see Sect. 15.7).

Furthermore, as we move from the concept of improved precision of energy deposition in tissues to the more relevant biological effects of radiotherapy-triggered events at the molecular level, multifunctional imaging techniques merit consideration as methods for understanding and monitoring radiotherapy effects. This is particularly important with the more complex cocktail regimens such as chemoradiation and combined radiation with novel biological therapies. If studies are well conducted, then multi-parametric functional imaging approaches may be able to tease out those effects due to radiotherapy and any additional effects caused by chemotherapy or novel therapeutics. Unfortunately, there are very few multifunctional imaging studies evaluating the effects of radiation or chemoradiation. An example is the study of Willet et al. who examined the effects of the anti-VEGF antibody bevacizumab on patients with rectal cancer (WILLETT et al. 2004). They found discordant changes on perfusion CT and glucose metabolism (judged on ¹⁸FDG-PET scans). They noted significant reductions in CT perfusion but reported no significant falls in glucose metabolism. Reduction of glucose metabolism was seen only when bevacizumab was given in combination with radiotherapy. These results suggest that bevacizumab and radiotherapy have very different effects and that metabolic disruption is greater after radiation.

Another potential contribution of multifunctional imaging could come from the need to minimize normal tissue toxicity, which in the brain means limiting the radiation dose reaching areas that control vital sensory and motor function. Recent data has shown that fMRI (a specific imaging technique which monitors changes in regional brain vascularity brought on by the performance of a task in an activation paradigm using BOLD-MRI scans) can enable statistical maps to be generated that indicate focal regions of the brain responding significantly to a task. When these fMRI techniques are combined with fibre-tracking techniques using DTI and anatomical images, it becomes possible to show the relationships between tumours and adjacent eloquent areas, as well as involvement of connecting white matter tracts. Employing such techniques has shown significant inter-individual differences in the locations of and involvement by tumour of eloquent tissues and their connecting white matter tracts. It has been repeatedly stated that fMRI (for eloquent areas identification) and DTI (for fibre tracking) should therefore be incorporated into imaging-guided radiotherapy planning of brain tumours.

15.6
Drug Development

Large numbers of new therapeutics are entering development as a result of improved understanding of the molecular and genetic pathways controlling cellular function. Targeted molecular approaches typically seek to inhibit specific phenotypic characteristics that are specific to cancers. As the pharmaceutical industry moves toward increasingly complex multi-targeted therapies, the anticipated effects on tumour tissues de novo have become more difficult to predict. There is growing recognition that biomarkers (including those derived from functional imaging) will play an increasingly important role in the drug development process for a number of reasons. Imaging biomarker changes can be used to confirm mechanisms of action of drugs in vivo. Such pharmacodynamic (PD) data can then be potentially harnessed for making "go–no-go" decisions at early stages of drug development; an important aim of which is to reduce the high cost of pivotal (Phase III) trials for compounds that are unlikely to succeed.

Preclinical and early drug clinical development (Phase I) stages are well suited for the incorporation of multifunctional MR imaging studies. Ideally, preclinical imaging studies should be performed first in order to select imaging techniques and schedules for performing the clinical studies. The limited sample size of Phase I clinical trials also provides the opportunity to rapidly accumulate imaging data across many tumour types and therapies, although this approach needs to be balanced against what can be reasonably concluded from such data, given the limits of small sample size.

There are numerous preclinical examples of functional imaging to evaluate the effects of novel therapeutics. In general, these studies have tended to look at treatment effects using only a single functional imaging modality, such as observing the anti-vascular effects of anti-angiogenic or vascular disruptive agents by DCE-MRI. This approach can be extended using multifunctional imaging approaches in order to more precisely identify areas within tumours that are more responsive to a particular therapeutic approach. An example is the recent study by Berry et al. who evaluated the anti-angiogenic effect of an antibody to VEGF-A in a colorectal xenograft model (BERRY et al. 2008). Whole tumour regions of interest (ROI) are usually employed to see if drug effects are occurring across an entire tumour, but differential changes within the tumour may be masked by using such an approach. Instead, Berry et al. performed a multispectral analysis of co-registered DW-MRI, T2 and proton density images to sub-classify tumour voxels as "necrotic" or "viable". Using DCE-MRI they were able to isolate anti-angiogenic effects in voxels defined as viable. This multi-parametric imaging approach is unique, because it enabled segmentation and measurement of drug effect in tissue classes that were more likely to respond to therapy. By excluding areas of necrosis, a more precise therapeutic assessment could be made, thus addressing the issue of tumour heterogeneity, which can complicate the analysis of DCE-MRI studies (in this context, necrotic voxels are a source of noise in the assessment of therapy response).

There are relatively few studies that have used multifunctional imaging approaches to explore the secondary effects of drugs on the tumour microenvironment or on cellular metabolic disruption. A good example of a multifunctional imaging approach is the preclinical investigations by Beauregard et al. who evaluated the anti-tumour effects of two vascular disruptive agents, noting changes in vascular perfusion (the anticipated primary target) and the tumour energy status (secondary effects resulting from vascular disruption). They used DCE-MRI (with both macromolecular and small molecular weight gadolinium chelates) and phosphorus spec-

troscopy (BEAUREGARD et al. 2001, 2002) to assess the vascular disruptive effects of combretastatin A4 phosphate (CA4P) and dimethylxanthenone-acetic acid (DMXAA) on a variety of tumour models. Antivascular effects were quantified by reductions in perfusion and macromolecular permeability, while the tumour cell energy status was assessed via changes in the ratio of the integrals of the signals, from inorganic phosphate and nucleoside triphosphates. Using these techniques, Beauregard et al. found that there was close concordance between vascular disruption and subsequent changes in cellular energetics. Heterogeneity in response to these drugs was observed in different tumour models and they noted that differential susceptibility to drug was related, at least in part, to tumour macromolecular vascular permeability.

A simplistic review of the Beauregard study could lead to the mistaken assumption that one could use any metabolic imaging test (such as ^{32}P-MRS or ^{18}FDG-PET) as a biomarker to asses the effectiveness of any drug, regardless of the primary mechanism of action. This is an oversimplification that needs to be avoided. We have already noted the spatial and temporal discordance in the changes of imaging biomarkers on multi-parametric imaging. Similarly, uncoupling of functional imaging characteristics has been noted when initially characterizing the disease, and also in those rare clinical scenarios when tumours are actively monitored by serial examinations without therapeutic intervention (for example, in prostate cancers and low-grade gliomas (Fig. 15.8).

In the same way, uncoupling of imaging biomarkers can be observed in therapy assessment settings as discussed above (see Sect. 15.4.3), and also when therapies with novel mechanisms of action are evaluated. For example, findings from a number of studies show that perfusion and glucose metabolism may not change in parallel, in response to anti-angiogenic drugs (HERBST et al. 2002; KURDZIEL et al. 2003; MANKOFF et al. 2003; WILLETT et al. 2004). Decoupling of perfusion and glucose metabolism were shown in a small study by Willett et al. (2004) who examined patients with rectal cancer treated by the anti–VEGF antibody bevacizumab (see Sect. 15.5). Dose-related perfusion–metabolism decoupling was also demonstrated by Herbst et al. (2002) who noted that endostatin (an anti-vascular agent), when given in high doses, resulted in decreased tumour perfusion but increased glucose metabolism. Uncoupling of blood flow and glucose metabolism following anti-angiogenic therapy could result from drug-induced hypoxia and secondary stimulation of glucose metabolism, leading to increased expression of cell surface glucose transporters.

Another good example of multifunctional MR imaging used to assess the sequential tissue effects of anti-angiogenic compounds in humans was published by Batchelor et al. (2007). They evaluated patients with recurrent glioblastoma who were treated with Cediranib, an orally active tyrosine kinase inhibitor of VEGF receptors. Multifunctional MR imaging assessments were undertaken including contrast-enhanced tumour volume, vessel size index, microvessel permeability, extracellular leakage space, water diffusivity and DTI. Using this panel of imaging tests, they were able to show rapid reductions following treatment in transfer constant, extracellular leakage space and water diffusivity which were interpreted as evidence of microvessel normalization. Interestingly, decreases in vessel size index were short-lived despite persistent reductions of transfer constant. Most intriguingly, the enhancing tumour volume which initially decreased, began to expand, despite persistent decreases in microvessel permeability (Fig. 15.11), suggesting that continued tumour growth was not mediated via the VEGF pathway (perhaps via vessel cooption or intussusception (Loges et al. 2009). Intriguingly, the anticipated effects of cell death on DW-MRI were not seen. Tumour cell death via apoptosis should cause increases in ADC values (Patterson et al. 2008) but in fact the reverse was observed (reduced ADC values). The latter finding is likely to be due to water shifts out of tumours caused by reductions of microvessel permeability; a finding supported by reduced leakage space estimates, and one that has been observed at other tumour sites with anti-angiogenic therapy.

These multifunctional imaging observations in drug development reinforces the underlying message of this chapter that it is only by combining biomarker/quantitative data from a number of imaging techniques that one may begin to truly understand how novel therapies affect tumour cells and tissue microenvironments. Such observations can provide unique insights into the mechanism of drug action in vivo, and useful pharmacodynamic information. However, if multifunctional imaging is to take up the unique position of enhancing decision-making at critical milestones in the early phases of the drug development process, then procedural rigour will be needed to establish each biomarker and/or biomarker combination for such a role; this is discussed in the next section.

Challenges for Implementation

From the above discussions, it is clear that we need to think of functional imaging as an important means of biological exploration because of its multidimensional (multispectral, multispatial and temporally resolved) nature. If functional imaging techniques are to evolve successfully into biomarkers that are clinically valuable and important for drug development, then there will need to be agreements on the standards for measurement, analysis and display for the whole spectrum of promising imaging techniques. The current, general lack of such standards is a major impediment to the development and maturation of physiological imaging.

Imaging biomarkers or biomarker combinations need to be validated in the context of well-designed clinical trials, particularly those that are associated with tissue sampling and in studies that incorporate clinical efficacy endpoints (for clinical validation). Initially, it may be better to evaluate imaging methods in conjunction with therapies where the mechanisms of action are well understood, but this should not deter explorations with novel therapeutics or combinations. In this effort, it should not be forgotten that suitable, tissue equivalent phantoms will be required for quality assurance and quality control purposes. Patient reproducibility should be established in as many clinical studies as possible, particularly in multi-centre settings. Heterogeneity in all its aspects should be explored including intra- and inter-patient variability and intra- and inter-lesion variations in response to therapeutic perturbations.

One current concern is the lengthy process of clinical adoption of functional imaging. This, in part, is due to the lack of explicit guidance on the actual qualification steps that are needed to go from biomarker discovery, through the development, to ultimate clinical validation. The lack of explicit guidance/frameworks for development to prompt a coordinated effort is a major contributing cause for the current lack of a strong evidence base and the long timelines for development. Concerted efforts by all stakeholders would hasten research in this area, and would ultimately lead to the evidence that is required for the widespread clinical deployment of such potentially expensive diagnostic technologies.

This chapter has illustrated that it is already possible to acquire spatially matched multi-parametric

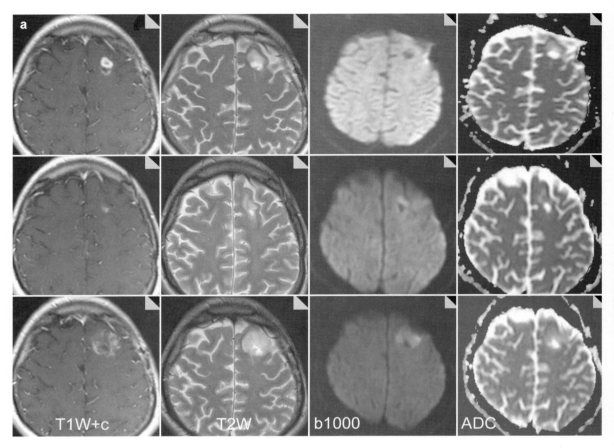

Fig. 15.11. (a) Multi-parametric MR imaging of anti-VEGF antibody therapy. A 35-year-old man with grade III glioma of the left frontal lobe. *Rows*: serial images obtained before, after 10 days and 6 weeks of bevacizumab plus temozolamide. Columns show post-contrast T1-weighted (T1W + c), T2-weighted (T2W), diffusion-weighted (*b*1,000) and ADC maps (*b*0–1,000). Note reduction in enhancement and decrease in tumour size after 10 days. Six weeks after initiating treatment, the tumour has regrown beyond the original size, showing increased enhancement. (**b**) Same patient as in panel (a). *Rows*: serial images obtained before, after 10 days and 6 weeks of bevacizumab plus temozolamide. *Columns* show post-contrast T1-weighted (T1W + c) with rectangular regions of interest (in *red*), relative cerebral blood volume (rCBV) maps, ¹H-MRSI (TE = 135 ms) spectra from tumour area and signal intensity time curve from a DSC-MRI study for voxels within regions of interest shown in *first column*. Increases in choline:NAA ratio suggesting no change in the metabolic signature of the tumour in response to therapy. DSC-MRI curves show late positive enhancement before therapy consistent with loss of compartmentalization (i.e. leakage of contrast into the extravascular space) of the intravenous contrast agent. This effect is largely eliminated after 10 days of therapy consistent with vascular normalization and a reduction in the blood–brain barrier permeability. As the tumour enlarges despite continued therapy, the late positive enhancement is beginning to return. (**c**) Same patient as in panel (a) and panel (b). *Rows*: serial images obtained before, after 10 days and 6 weeks of bevacizumab plus temozolamide. *Columns* show changes in post-contrast T1-weighted (T1W + c); and vascular parameters of transfer constant (K^{trans}), leakage space maps (v_e) and fractional plasma volume (v_p) from the DCE-MRI studies. Note reduction in the transfer constant and leakage space consistent with vascular normalization (*arrows*). Note that at relapse after 6 weeks, even though the tumour size was larger, there was no increase in transfer constant and the degree of enhancement is less intense compared with pretreatment. One possible hypothesis is an evolving tumour phenotype to a more invasive but less angiogenic variant

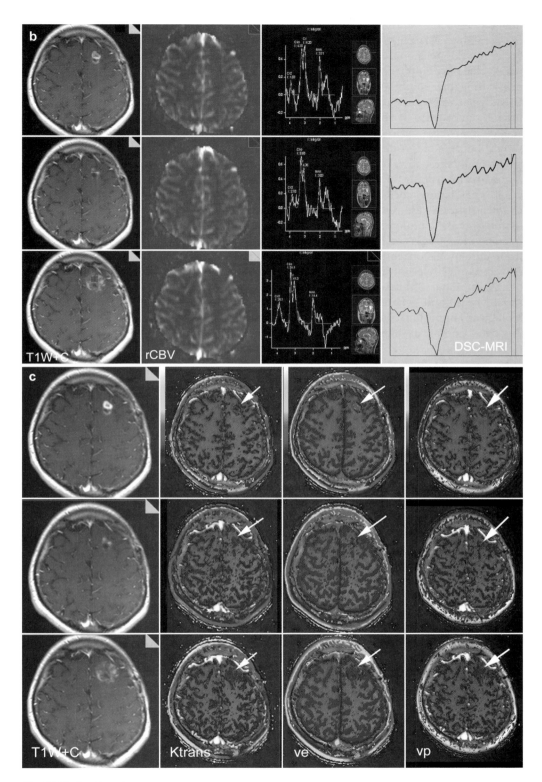

Fig. 15.11. Continued

imaging data at multiple time points over time in potentially every patient. Currently, integration of such multidimensional data represents another major challenge both for the diagnostic and therapeutic imaging communities. Sophisticated, user-friendly software workspaces need to be developed urgently, in order to be able to integrate/cross correlate data analysis procedures. So, for example, it should be possible to define ROI on one modality and to apply these to voxel maps from another technique, and in so doing be able to appreciate voxel-by-voxel correlations between functional imaging characteristics. These computer platforms also need to incorporate bioinformatics approaches, so that imaging biomarkers can be correlated with findings from immunohistochemistry, gene expression profiles and other relevant imaging, tissue and clinical biomarker data. Ultimately, multispectral analyses should be able to generate probability biomaps of biologically important characteristics from the imaging data. Composite biomaps incorporating functional imaging would be invaluable in lesion characterization, therapy planning and for assessing the effects of therapies (McMillan et al. 2007).

15.8

Conclusions

It should be self-evident that there are extraordinary opportunities for multifunctional imaging techniques to evolve into validated and qualified biomarkers that are clinically useful, for pharmaceutical drug development and for predicting therapeutic efficacy. It is difficult to predict the pace at which multifunctional imaging will mature into the roles outlined above. Experience has shown that the rate of development is dependent on a number of factors including evolving clinical demands, ease of use, availability of technology and cost, all driving the pace of change. Nevertheless we can expect (1) fusion of imaging techniques (in hardware and in software) to increasingly yield multidimensional imaging datasets, (2) an increase in quantitative imaging, with these imaging metrics/biomarkers being related mechanistically to the disease processes and (3) progressive requirement of greater use of information technology for the analysis of multilayered datasets (multispectral data processing) and computed aided diagnosis, for imaging diagnoses. In this process, the education of imaging physicians will need to incorporate the fundamentals

of physiology, biochemistry and molecular biology, as well as physical and chemical sciences. Only by leading in these efforts will diagnostic imaging retain ownership of multifunctional imaging in the future.

References

Alger JR (2006) Magnetic resonance spectroscopy in cancer. In: Padhani AR, Choyke P (eds) New techniques in oncologic imaging. Taylor and Francis, Boca Taton, FL, pp 193–211

Alonzi R, Padhani AR, et al (2007) Dynamic contrast enhanced MRI in prostate cancer. Eur J Radiol 63:335–50

Amsellem-Ouazana D, Younes P, et al (2005) Negative prostatic biopsies in patients with a high risk of prostate cancer. Is the combination of endorectal MRI and magnetic resonance spectroscopy imaging (MRSI) a useful tool? A preliminary study. Eur Urol 47:582–6

Batchelor TT, Sorensen AG, et al (2007) AZD2171, a pan-VEGF receptor tyrosine kinase inhibitor, normalizes tumor vasculature and alleviates edema in glioblastoma patients. Cancer Cell 11:83–95

Beauregard DA, Hill SA, et al (2001) The susceptibility of tumors to the antivascular drug combretastatin A4 phosphate correlates with vascular permeability. Cancer Res 61:6811–5

Beauregard DA, Pedley RB, et al (2002) Differential sensitivity of two adenocarcinoma xenografts to the anti-vascular drugs combretastatin A4 phosphate and 5,6-dimethylxanthenone-4-acetic acid, assessed using MRI and MRS. NMR Biomed 15:99–105

Bentzen SM (2005) Theragnostic imaging for radiation oncology: dose-painting by numbers. Lancet Oncol 6:112–7

Berry LR, Barck KH, et al (2008) Quantification of viable tumor microvascular characteristics by multispectral analysis. Magn Reson Med 60:64–72

Brahme A (2003) Biologically optimized 3-dimensional in vivo predictive assay-based radiation therapy using positron emission tomography-computerized tomography imaging. Acta Oncol 42:123–36

Cha S, Yang L, et al (2006) Comparison of microvascular permeability measurements, Ktrans, determined with conventional steady-state T1-weighted and first-pass T2*-weighted MR imaging methods in gliomas and meningiomas. AJNR Am J Neuroradiol 27:409–17

Chao C, Bosch WR, et al (2001). A novel approach to overcome hypoxic tumor resistance: Cu-ATSM-guided intensity-modulated radiation therapy. Int J Radiat Biol Phys 49:1171–82

Choyke PL, Thomassen D, et al (2006) Pharmacokinetic modeling of dynamic contrast enhanced MRI in cancer. In: Padhani AR, Choyke P (eds) New techniques in oncologic imaging. Taylor and Francis, Boca Taton, FL, pp 273–90

Cirillo S, Petracchini M, et al (2008) Value of endorectal MRI and MRS in patients with elevated prostate-specific antigen levels and previous negative biopsies to localize peripheral zone tumours. Clin Radiol 63:871–9

Danchaivijitr N, Waldman AD, et al (2008) Low-grade gliomas: do changes in rCBV measurements at longitudinal perfusion-weighted MR imaging predict malignant transformation? Radiology 247:170–8 deSouza NM, Riches SF, et al (2008). Diffusion-weighted magnetic resonance imaging: a potential non-invasive marker of tumour aggressiveness in localized prostate cancer. Clin Radiol 63:774–82

Diehn M, Nardini C, et al (2008) Identification of noninvasive imaging surrogates for brain tumor gene-expression modules. Proc Natl Acad Sci U S A 105:5213–8

Eby PR, Partridge SC, et al (2008) Metabolic and vascular features of dynamic contrast-enhanced breast magnetic resonance imaging and (15)O-water positron emission tomography blood flow in breast cancer. Acad Radiol 15:1246–54

Ferrier MC, Sarin H, et al (2007) Validation of dynamic contrast-enhanced magnetic resonance imaging-derived vascular permeability measurements using quantitative autoradiography in the RG2 rat brain tumor model. Neoplasia 9: 546–55

Futterer JJ, Heijmink SW, et al (2006) Prostate cancer localization with dynamic contrast-enhanced MR imaging and proton MR spectroscopic imaging. Radiology 24:449–58

Giles LG, Morgan VA, et al (2009) Apparent diffusion coefficient as a predictive biomarker of prostate cancer progression: value of fast and slow diffusion components. In: ISMRM 17th Scientific Meeting and exhibition, Honolulu

Ginsberg LE, Fuller GN, et al (1998) The significance of lack of MR contrast enhancement of supratentorial brain tumors in adults: histopathological evaluation of a series. Surg Neurol 49:436–40

Gupta RK, Sinha U, et al (1999) Inverse correlation between choline magnetic resonance spectroscopy signal intensity and the apparent diffusion coefficient in human glioma. Magn Reson Med 41:2–7

Haider MA, Chung P, et al (2008) Dynamic contrast-enhanced magnetic resonance imaging for localization of recurrent prostate cancer after external beam radiotherapy. Int J Radiat Oncol Biol Phys 70:425–30

Hambrock T, Futterer JJ, et al (2008) Value of 3 tesla multimodality-directed MR-guided biopsy to detect prostate cancer in high risk patients after at least 2 previous negative biopsies. In: RSNA. Chicago, IL, pp 525

Herbst RS, Mullani NA, et al (2002). Development of biologic markers of response and assessment of antiangiogenic activity in a clinical trial of human recombinant endostatin. J Clin Oncol 20:3804–14

Hockel M, Vaupel P (2001) Tumor hypoxia: definitions and current clinical, biologic, and molecular aspects. J Natl Cancer Inst 93:266–76.

Hoskin PJ, Carnell DM, et al (2007) Hypoxia in prostate cancer: correlation of BOLD-MRI with pimonidazole immunohistochemistry-initial observations. Int J Radiat Oncol Biol Phys 68:1065–71

Howe FA, Barton SJ, et al (2003). Metabolic profiles of human brain tumors using quantitative in vivo 1H magnetic resonance spectroscopy. Magn Reson Med 49:223–32

Howe FA, Robinson SP, et al (2001). Issues in flow and oxygenation dependent contrast (FLOOD) imaging of tumours. NMR Biomed 14:497–506

Hu LS, Baxter LC, et al (2008). Relative cerebral blood volume values to differentiate high-grade glioma recurrence from posttreatment radiation effect: direct correlation between image-guided tissue histopathology and localized dynamic susceptibility-weighted contrast-enhanced perfusion MR imaging measurements. AJNR Am J Neuroradiol 30:552

Kamel IR, Liapi E, et al (2009) Unresectable hepatocellular carcinoma: serial early vascular and cellular changes after transarterial chemoembolization as detected with MR imaging. Radiology 250:466–73

Knopp EA, Cha S, et al (1999) Glial neoplasms: dynamic contrast-enhanced T2*-weighted MR imaging. Radiology 211: 791–8

Koh DM, Brown G, et al (2008) Detection of colorectal hepatic metastases using MnDPDP MR imaging and diffusion-weighted imaging (DWI) alone and in combination. Eur Radiol 18:903–10

Koh DM, Collins DJ (2007) Diffusion-weighted MRI in the body: applications and challenges in oncology. AJR Am J Roentgenol 188:1622–35

Koh DM, Takahara T, et al (2008) Practical aspects of assessing tumors using clinical diffusion-weighted imaging in the body. Magn Reson Med Sci 6:211–24

Kroemer G, Pouyssegur J (2008) Tumor cell metabolism: cancer's Achilles' heel. Cancer Cell 13:472–82

Kurdziel KA, Figg WD, et al (2003) Using positron emission tomography 2-deoxy-2-[18F]fluoro-D-glucose, 11CO, and 15O-water for monitoring androgen independent prostate cancer. Mol Imaging Biol 5:86–93

Lankester KJ, Taylor JN, et al (2007b) Dynamic MRI for imaging tumor microvasculature: comparison of susceptibility and relaxivity techniques in pelvic tumors. J Magn Reson Imaging 25:796–805

Lankester KJ, Taylor NJ, et al (2005) Effects of platinum/taxane based chemotherapy on acute perfusion in human pelvic tumours measured by dynamic MRI. Br J Cancer 93: 979–85

Law M, Oh S, et al (2006a) Low-grade gliomas: dynamic susceptibility-weighted contrast-enhanced perfusion MR imaging–prediction of patient clinical response. Radiology 238:658–67

Law M, Yang S, et al (2003) Glioma grading: sensitivity, specificity, and predictive values of perfusion MR imaging and proton MR spectroscopic imaging compared with conventional MR imaging. AJNR Am J Neuroradiol 24:1989–98

Law M, Young R, et al (2006b) Comparing perfusion metrics obtained from a single compartment versus pharmacokinetic modeling methods using dynamic susceptibility contrast-enhanced perfusion MR imaging with glioma grade. AJNR Am J Neuroradiol 27:1975–82

Le Bihan D, van Zijl P (2002) From the diffusion coefficient to the diffusion tensor. NMR Biomed 15:431–4

Leach MO, Brindle KM, et al (2005) The assessment of antiangiogenic and antivascular therapies in early-stage clinical trials using magnetic resonance imaging: issues and recommendations. Br J Cancer 92:1599–610

Lenkinski RE, Bloch BN, et al (2008) An illustration of the potential for mapping MRI/MRS parameters with genetic over-expression profiles in human prostate cancer. MAGMA 2:411–21

Ling CC, Humm J, et al (2000) Towards multidimensional radiotherapy (MD-CRT): biological imaging and biological conformality. Int J Radiat Oncol Biol Phys 47:551–60

Loges S, Mazzone M, et al (2009) Silencing or fueling metastasis with VEGF inhibitors: antiangiogenesis revisited. Cancer Cell 15:167–70

Mankoff DA, Dunnwald LK, et al (2003) Changes in blood flow and metabolism in locally advanced breast cancer treated with neoadjuvant chemotherapy. J Nucl Med 44:1806–14

Marelli L, Stigliano R, et al (2007) Transarterial therapy for hepatocellular carcinoma: which technique is more effective? A systematic review of cohort and randomized studies. Cardiovasc Intervent Radiol 30:6–25

Mazaheri Y, Shukla-Dave A, et al (2008) Prostate cancer: identification with combined diffusion-weighted MR imaging and 3D 1H MR spectroscopic imaging–correlation with pathologic findings. Radiology 240:480–8

McMillan KM, Rogers BP, et al (2007) An objective method for combining multi-parametric MRI datasets to characterize malignant tumors. Med Phys 34:1053–61

Naganawa S, Sato C, et al (2005) Diffusion-weighted images of the liver: comparison of tumor detection before and after contrast enhancement with superparamagnetic iron oxide. J Magn Reson Imaging 21:836–40

Nasu K, Kuroki Y, et al (2006). Hepatic metastases: diffusion-weighted sensitivity-encoding versus SPIO-enhanced MR imaging. Radiology 239(1):122–30

Niermann KJ, Fleischer AC, et al (2007) Measuring tumor perfusion in control and treated murine tumors: correlation of microbubble contrast-enhanced sonography to dynamic contrast-enhanced magnetic resonance imaging and fluorodeoxyglucose positron emission tomography. J Ultrasound Med 26:749–56

Padhani A, Choyke PL (2006) New techniques in oncologic imaging. Taylor & Francis, New York

Padhani AR, Dzik-Jurasz A (2004) Perfusion MR imaging of extracranial tumor angiogenesis. Top Magn Reson Imaging 15:41–57

Padhani AR, Krohn KA, et al (2007) Imaging oxygenation of human tumours. Eur Radiol 17:861–72

Patterson DM, Padhani AR, et al (2008) Technology insight: water diffusion MRI–a potential new biomarker of response to cancer therapy. Nat Clin Pract Oncol 5:220–33

Payne GS, Leach MO (2006). Applications of magnetic resonance spectroscopy in radiotherapy treatment planning. Br J Radiol 79(Spec No 1):S16–26

Pope WB, Chen JH, et al (2008) Relationship between gene expression and enhancement in glioblastoma multiforme: exploratory DNA microarray analysis. Radiology 249:268–77

Prando A, Kurhanewicz J, et al (2005) Prostatic biopsy directed with endorectal MR spectroscopic imaging findings in patients with elevated prostate specific antigen levels and prior negative biopsy findings: early experience. Radiology 236:903–10

Provenzale JM, Mukundan S, et al (2006) Diffusion-weighted and perfusion MR imaging for brain tumor characterization and assessment of treatment response. Radiology 239:632–49

Robinson SP (2006) BOLD imaging of tumors. In: Padhani AR, Choyke P (eds) New techniques in oncologic imaging. Taylor and Francis, Boca Taton, FL, pp 257–72

Robinson SP, Rijken PF, et al (2003) Tumor vascular architecture and function evaluated by non-invasive susceptibility MRI methods and immunohistochemistry. J Magn Reson Imaging 17:445–54

Rock JP, Hearshen D, et al (2002) Correlations between magnetic resonance spectroscopy and image-guided histopathology, with special attention to radiation necrosis. Neurosurgery 51:912–9; discussion 919–20

Rollin N, Guyotat J, et al (2006) Clinical relevance of diffusion and perfusion magnetic resonance imaging in assessing intra-axial brain tumors. Neuroradiology 48:150–9

Tamada T, Sone T, et al (2008) Apparent diffusion coefficient values in peripheral and transition zones of the prostate: comparison between normal and malignant prostatic tissues and correlation with histologic grade. J Magn Reson Imaging 28:720–6

Tatum JL, Kelloff GJ, et al (2006) Hypoxia: importance in tumor biology, noninvasive measurement by imaging, and value of its measurement in the management of cancer therapy. Int J Radiat Biol 82:699–757

Thoeny HC, De Keyzer F (2007) Extracranial applications of diffusion-weighted magnetic resonance imaging. Eur Radiol 17:1385–93

Thoeny HC, Triantafyllou M, et al (2009) Combined ultrasmall superparamagnetic particles of iron oxide-enhanced and diffusion-weighted magnetic resonance imaging reliably detect pelvic lymph node metastases in normal-sized nodes of bladder and prostate cancer patients. Eur Urol 55:761–9

Thukral A, Thomasson DM, et al (2007) Inflammatory breast cancer: dynamic contrast-enhanced MR in patients receiving bevacizumab–initial experience. Radiology 244: 727–35

Tofts PS, Benton CE, et al (2007) Quantitative analysis of whole-tumor Gd enhancement histograms predicts malignant transformation in low-grade gliomas. J Magn Reson Imaging 25:208–14

Tofts PS, Brix G, et al (1999) Estimating kinetic parameters from dynamic contrast-enhanced T(1)-weighted MRI of a diffusable tracer: standardized quantities and symbols. J Magn Reson Imaging 10:223–32

Walker-Samuel S, Leach MO, et al (2006) Evaluation of response to treatment using DCE-MRI: the relationship between initial area under the gadolinium curve (IAUGC) and quantitative pharmacokinetic analysis. Phys Med Biol 51:3593–602

Wilkinson ID, Jellineck DA, et al (2006) Dexamethasone and enhancing solitary cerebral mass lesions: alterations in perfusion and blood-tumor barrier kinetics shown by magnetic resonance imaging. Neurosurgery 58:640–6; discussion 640–6

Willett CG, Boucher Y, et al (2004) Direct evidence that the VEGF-specific antibody bevacizumab has antivascular effects in human rectal cancer. Nat Med 10:145–7

Xu J, Humphrey PA, et al (2009) Magnetic resonance diffusion characteristics of histologically defined prostate cancer in humans. Magn Reson Med 61:842–50

Yabuuchi H, Matsuo Y, et al (2008) Parotid gland tumors: can addition of diffusion-weighted MR imaging to dynamic contrast-enhanced MR imaging improve diagnostic accuracy in characterization? Radiology 249:909–16

Yang D, Korogi Y, et al (2002) Cerebral gliomas: prospective comparison of multivoxel 2D chemical-shift imaging proton MR spectroscopy, echoplanar perfusion and diffusion-weighted MRI. Neuroradiology 44:656–66

Zakian KL, Sircar K, et al (2005) Correlation of proton MR spectroscopic imaging with gleason score based on step-section pathologic analysis after radical prostatectomy. Radiology 234:804–14

Zerhouni EA (2008) Major trends in the imaging sciences: 2007 Eugene P. Pendergrass New Horizons Lecture. Radiology 249:403–9

Zonari P, Baraldi P, et al (2007) Multimodal MRI in the characterization of glial neoplasms: the combined role of single-voxel MR spectroscopy, diffusion imaging and echo-planar perfusion imaging. Neuroradiology 49:795–803

The Potential of DW-MRI as an Imaging Biomarker in Clinical Trials

Andy Dzik-Jurasz and Phil Murphy

Andy Dzik-Jurasz, MD, PhD
Novartis Pharmaceuticals Corporation, One Health Plaza, East Hanover, NJ 07936-1080, USA
Phil Murphy, PhD
Oncology Medicines Development Centre, GlaxoSmithKline Research & Development, 1–3 Iron Bridge Road, Stockley Park West, Uxbridge, Middlesex UB11 1BT, UK

SUMMARY

Imaging is increasingly used to inform the drug development process, and provides valuable information from preclinical testing to clinical trials. The challenge is for imaging techniques to yield robust and reproducible measurements, which can indicate early treatment response or identify patients who are likely to respond to treatment. This allows timely decisions to be made, so that the development of the most promising drugs can be accelerated, while curtailing the development of treatments with doubtful clinical benefits. DW-MRI is one of a number of imaging methodologies which, when further developed and applied appropriately, could represent a major improvement over current imaging or other endpoints used to evaluate the success of therapy. In this chapter, we discuss the challenges faced by modern day drug development and review the process from concept to commercialization of drug therapies. The important role of imaging in this process is discussed, including the development of DW-MRI as a potential biomarker or surrogate study endpoint, and the challenges that need to be addressed to enable realization of such a goal.

16.1

Introduction

The cost of bringing a drug to market has recently been estimated to be in excess of $1 billion dollars with the costs only likely to rise (Adams et al. 2006; DiMasi and Grabowski 2007a, b). There is, however, little evidence to suggest that more drugs are being approved. Technological innovation is increasingly being seen as a means of improving the efficacy of new drug development, not only by reliably identifying efficacious drugs early but also by halting those that add no clinical benefit or result in unacceptable toxicity. Biomarker development is increasingly being seen as a strategy that will deliver this newly sought efficacy. The concept and theme of biomarkers is not new in health care and the terms are analogous whether used in clinical practice or drug development. They differ only in so much as a clinical biomarker is used to inform on patient management whilst in drug development, biomarkers provide insights into the efficacy and/or toxicity of a compound.

In recent years, there has been an explosion in the search for biomarkers, brought on in no small means by the increased understanding and emphasis of the molecular basis of disease. Imaging has and continues to play a substantial role in the non-invasive, serial visualization of tissue changes which reflect the underlying pathology. The impact morphological imaging has made on clinical practice is undeniable but the delay in detecting phenotypical changes in tumours using conventional imaging techniques is increasingly seen as an impediment to assessing drug efficacy in early clinical trials.

Since pharmacological activity occurs almost as an immediate response following a molecular drug-target interaction, a lag-time in the response in tumour size which occurs downstream to the drug action is inevitable. To improve early detection of drug effects, all imaging modalities have sought to detect physiological or molecular changes that occur prior to any change in the size of a tumour. In this respect, DW-MRI has been shown to be able to demonstrate changes prior to alterations in tumour size after drug treatment and has thus been proposed as a potential biomarker of early drug activity. This chapter briefly describes the drug development process, the concept of biomarkers and most importantly what it takes to develop and apply an imaging biomarker. DW-MRI is an exciting potential biomarker, which highlights the innovative way in which imaging is being used to probe the molecular basis of disease and targeted treatments, in the hope of improving the development of new therapies.

16.2

The Challenges Faced in Bringing New Drugs to Market

The pharmaceutical industry is continuously challenged to deliver novel, effective and safe medicines in an increasingly constrained financial market.

Consequently, efficient and streamlined drug development has never been more important. The overall challenge is to deliver low-cost medicines with an acceptable efficacy and safety profile. The current estimates of taking a drug from preclinical experimentation to regulatory approval are of the order of $800 million to $1 billion USD for small molecules and biopharmaceutical agents respectively (DiMasi et al. 2003; DiMasi and Grabowski 2007a, b).

The cost of any successful drug will necessarily include the cost of all the failed trials and compounds. Attrition therefore is an important metric by which the pharmaceutical industry assesses its productivity. DiMasi and Grabowski, for example, concluded that the probability of an anticancer drug reaching regulatory approval from first-in-human clinical studies is 26.1% (DiMasi and Grabowski 2007a). The cost of trials increases disproportionately with the size, complexity and phase of a trial. The probability of a Phase III clinical trial resulting in an approved drug has been calculated to be 57.1%, with higher success averaging at 68.4% for other (non-oncological) therapeutic areas. This finding is emphasized by Booth et al., who alluded that oncology projects are riskier than those in other therapeutics areas (Booth et al. 2003).

Despite these limitations, there is good evidence to suggest that the depth and breadth of drug development has never been greater. For example, the 2009 Pharma report (Report: Medicines in Development for Cancer) highlighted the extensive (>850) portfolio of cancer medicines in the industry pipeline (Pharmaceutical Research and Manufacturers of America 2009), with many of these programmes targeting novel cancer regulatory pathways (Booth et al. 2003). It remains to be seen what proportion of these compounds will show efficacy in the clinical setting, although it has been suggested that newer, targeted agents have a more favourable attrition rate (Walker et al. 2009).

Oncology presents unique challenges to the modern drug developer, including the heterogeneous range of solid and haematological malignancies presenting to the oncologist (Kamb et al. 2007); the high prevalence of combination treatments (Dancey et al. 2006) and the difficulty in determining response to evaluate drug efficacy (Weber 2009). The key challenges to drug development in the oncological setting are summarized in Table 16.1.

A clear framework which allows for efficient and speedy drug development is needed. Areas of focus in addressing this challenge include: (i) an early read-out of drug efficacy – ideally based on a rational under-

Table 16.1. Key challenges to drug development in oncology

Delivering a broad portfolio of medicines
Deconvolving complex molecular interactions in an inherently heterogeneous disease group
Escalating complexity and costs of global clinical trials
Implementation of acceptable endpoints for large, international multi-site trials
Developing powerful and sufficiently predictable endpoints for use in small trials

standing of a drug's biological mode of action; (ii) patient stratification – in the mid- to late stages of drug development, patients are selected to ensure the best chance of therapeutic success is closely balanced against unacceptable toxicity; (iii) address logistical complexities – late stage clinical trials are highly resource-intensive owing to their complexity, with many often unpredictable pitfalls conspiring against timely completion of project. As such, optimization of this stage of drug development still presents significant opportunities to reduce cost, increase speed and enhance data quality; (iv) optimize study endpoints – endpoints currently used in early clinical trials have varied success in predicting the outcome of subsequent larger-scale studies and would benefit from further refinement and optimization (DHANI et al. 2009; EL MARAGHI et al. 2008) and (v) development of novel biomarkers – the clinical trial framework represents a unique setting to develop the next generation of biomarkers, by studying large cohorts of patients/subjects stratified according to a predetermined phenotype. Such trials should provide a mechanism to collect samples, perform exploratory imaging and compare these to more established assessments of response. The key steps that may improve the process of modern drug development are summarized in Table 16.2.

Table 16.2. Solutions to improving the pathway of drug development

Early insight into the molecular mechanisms of drug action
Effective patient stratification
Address logistical complexities of studies
Optimize existing clinical trial endpoints
Transition exploratory biomarkers to robust clinical trial endpoints

16.3
The Process of Drug Development

The delivery of new drugs to the market place requires a coordinated effort involving multi-disciplinary teams to ensure scientific and operational success. An overview of drug development is presented, in order to better understand how a novel imaging methodology such as DW-MRI can be optimally integrated into clinical trials.

In this chapter, the term *drug development* refers to any or part of the process including the discovery, systematic testing, regulatory filling and life-cycle management of a drug product. In broad outline, the drug development process consists of three main phases: the discovery, preclinical and clinical phase. No individual phase should be viewed independently of another, and the progression from one phase to the next involves considerable overlap. The clinical phase is typically divided into three phases (Phase I, II and III) that take a medicine from the end of preclinical assessment through to regulatory filing (Fig. 16.1).

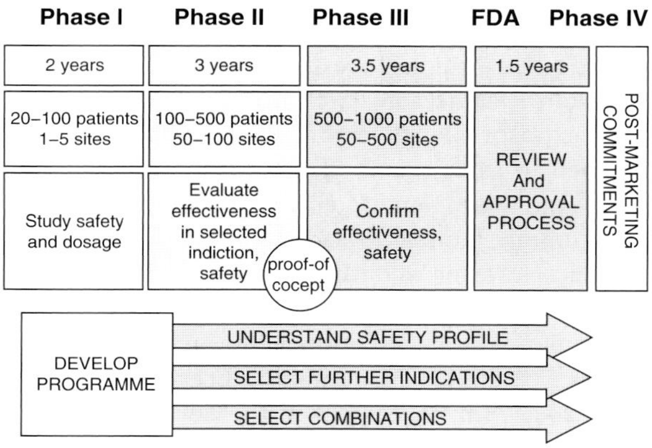

Fig. 16.1. The traditional phases of oncology drug development. The timescales and study metrics are only intended as a general outline. Each drug development programme (consisting of multiple studies) and each study will be unique. A key decision point, the so-called proof-of-concept is defined at the transition between Phase II and Phase III testing. This is the point at which data from the Phase II study is stringently evaluated to ensure there is confidence to commit to a costly Phase III programme. The programme as a whole may include multiple clinical studies at different phases intended to expand and improve the potential of an experimental medicine. In oncology in particular, multiple indications may be studied in parallel in addition to gaining efficacy by combining different agents

The discovery phase is focused on identifying and characterizing molecular targets and pathways with potential therapeutic exploitation. This phase is heavily reliant on the basic sciences, and has rapidly evolved with the support of laboratory technologies such as combinatorial chemistry (producing large numbers of organic compounds) and automated high-throughput screening (methods to express target proteins using in vitro systems thus enabling multiple micro-scale operations to be conducted). These innovations have dramatically accelerated and expanded the capabilities of the discovery process. Since rational drug design can result in multiple promising candidates, this stage of development is no longer considered as rate limiting. That being said, there are still many enhancements that can be made to the current drug discovery activities, with efforts increasingly being focused on effectively predicting clinical efficacy.

16.3.1
Preclinical In Vivo Studies

Following identification of promising drug candidates, investigations shift towards assessing in vivo pharmacokinetics, pharmacodynamics and toxicology. Toxicological studies can be extensive and aim to pre-empt serious clinical toxicity. Such studies will include dose-ranging investigations, as well as assessment of the acute, sub-chronic and chronic effects of drug exposure. Furthermore, considerable attention is given to assessments of mutagenicity, carcinogenicity and teratogenicity, employing a myriad of animal tumour models to ascertain drug toxicity and efficacy. However, as outlined by Kamb et al., disease models are suboptimal in their replication of clinical behaviour and are a factor in the unexpected outcomes of many investigational cancer drugs (KAMB et al. 2005). Improvements in the development and choice of such models and experimental design are likely to enhance the success at the clinical phases of drug development.

16.3.2
Phase I Clinical Trials

The conventional structure of clinical trials was designed to allow a step-wise progression towards establishing efficacy and safety whilst minimizing harmful exposure of subjects to potentially toxic formulations or combinations of drugs.

Phase I clinical trials are the first-in-human studies directed at recording drug pharmacokinetics and a first evaluation of safety across a range of doses. The studies are typically restricted to a few investigating centres and small subject cohorts. For many drugs, these Phase I studies are conducted on healthy volunteers. However, in life-threatening conditions where no alternative therapies exist such as cancer, patients are used at the outset. In addition to establishing the safety profile, the Phase I study in patients with cancer provides the opportunity to interrogate early indications of drug efficacy or apply biomarkers including imaging to evaluate mechanistic attributes of the drug to help optimize subsequent studies. However, in Phase I studies, the small cohort numbers and disease heterogeneity will remain an undeniable challenge to accurate prediction of efficacy.

16.3.3
Phase II Clinical Trials

Once a drug dose has been set and toxicity profile reviewed from analysis of Phase I data, a Phase II study will begin to gauge the efficacy of the drug in a target patient population. It also provides additional opportunity to gather more safety data. Multiple sites will be required in order to recruit adequate subject numbers to perform meaningful statistical analysis. The selected endpoints are required to define treatment efficacy despite limited exposure and numbers of patients. This presents a challenge which usually means that Phase II studies may overestimate or not sufficiently capture the efficacy of a compound (ADJEI et al. 2009). Successful Phase II studies aim to achieve a declaration of *proof-of-concept*, a stage at which patient benefit has been reasonably demonstrated and warrants continuation of the drug development process.

16.3.4
Phase III Clinical Trials

Phase III trials are considered *pivotal* as they are intended to evaluate the safety and efficacy of a drug within a large population for which drug administration is indicated. The data generated in such studies need to be sufficiently robust to withstand regulatory scrutiny. Typical trial designs include double-blind, parallel-arm studies comparing the experimental medicine with established standard of care. Evidence for efficacy in Phase III clinical studies is provided by robust and predetermined endpoints where a direct or strong indirect relationship between the endpoint and patient benefit is recognized. In cancer, time-to-event indices (such as progression-free survival or time to progression) are often employed because of their close association with overall survival advantage.

16.4

Biomarkers for Drug Development

The broadly accepted definition of a biomarker is "a characteristic that is objectively measured and evaluated as an indicator of normal biological processes, pathogenic processes, or pharmacologic responses to a therapeutic intervention" (ATKINSON et al. 2001) with a "surrogate marker" being a biomarker intended to substitute for a clinical endpoint (such as survival). A "surrogate" endpoint, on the other hand, is recognized as reasonably predicting clinical benefit based on epidemiological, therapeutic, pathophysiological or other scientific evidence. Substantial qualification data are required to transit a putative biomarker to a surrogate endpoint. However, this transition is not always necessary to provide substantial benefit to inform on the drug development process.

Biomarkers have a broad scope within drug development, whether in support of defining the mechanism of drug action, estimating optimal dose and scheduling, or identifying subjects most likely to respond to a given therapy. Applied judiciously, biomarkers may provide key supportive information. In the absence of a clear rationale, however, biomarkers will add to study cost, logistical complexity and at worst expose the subject to unwarranted risk (i.e. biopsy). That being said, the clinical trial framework represents an opportunity to accumulate data for biomarker development that may inform future studies. It is important, therefore, when choosing a biomarker for study to carefully consider whether: (i) the biomarker findings unambiguously contribute to drug development decision-making or (ii) if the biomarker is highly experimental then it should be integrated acknowledging the limitations of the exploratory findings.

Biomarkers were recognized as a key theme in the (USA) Food and Drug Administration's (FDA) Critical Path Initiative launched in 2004. In the report "Innovation Stagnation: Challenge and Opportunity on the Critical Path to New Medicines", multiple streams of focus were outlined to guide subsequent investment in order to improve the delivery of new medicines from manufacturing through to development (FDA 2004). It was acknowledged that biomarkers offer a promising opportunity to support drug development, with the provisos of (i) partnering the biomarker output to clinical outcome, (ii) assessing the performance of the biomarker during intervention/ drug trials using current outcome measures as comparators, (iii) identifying data gaps or remaining uncertainties and (iv) identifying ongoing clinical trials as test beds for assessing biomarker activity.

The ease with which blood can be sampled over performing a biopsy has been a strong motivator in the search for serum biomarkers, which analogously demonstrates the tremendous potential of imaging biomarkers.

The term "qualification" in drug development has been adopted to mean "the evidentiary process of linking a biomarker with biological processes and clinical endpoints" (WAGNER 2002). Wagner et al. have proposed a framework for biomarker development (WAGNER et al. 2007), which includes four distinct phases: (i) *Exploration* – limited, possibly in vitro evidence lacking strong clinical validation. Biomarkers in this phase could be applied to drug development only for generating hypotheses; (ii) *Demonstration* – some preclinical performance has been demonstrated. The biomarker could be used for decision-making but only as an adjunct to acceptable clinical endpoints; (iii) *Characterization* – linkage of biomarker observations to clinical outcome has been demonstrated in at least one study. Such a biomarker could be used for drug development decision-making including dose-finding; (iv) *Surrogacy* – the current clinical endpoint can be replaced by the new biomarker on the basis of multiple corroborating studies and could be included as endpoints in registration trials. Such frameworks are helpful in understanding how a biomarker could evolve from a concept towards application as an accepted tool in drug development. The framework also emphasizes the early need to identify biomarkers, in order to provide enough time for its development.

In order to facilitate the process of biomarker development the FDA committed to creating a concept paper on biomarker qualification (FDA 2006). The paper is intended to clarify the evidence necessary to support a range of regulatory uses of biomarkers. In addition, a framework will be developed to promote consistency in understanding biomarker development and application. Provision of such a framework will represent a milestone in establishing the role and scope of biomarkers in drug development.

16.5

Imaging in Clinical Trials

Imaging is used extensively in drug development, providing or contributing to primary or secondary study endpoints. Whilst imaging is used extensively across therapeutic areas, the basis of the majority of imaging studies is morphological. The true role of imaging as a functional or independent biomarker has yet to be realized. However, understanding the considerable challenges in delivering robust, timely and standardized anatomical imaging is a first step in understanding what DW-MRI needs to achieve to become a key study endpoint.

Figure 16.2 provides an overview of oncological imaging in drug development. The principal role of imaging is focused on the detailed assessment of disease burden. In some instances, endpoints such as dynamic contrast-enhanced MR imaging (DCE-MRI) or fluorodeoxyglucose-PET (FDG-PET) are incorporated as endpoints. However, these methods are often supplementary to the more established endpoints. The relationship between the imaging output and drug response in exploratory biomarker studies is often poorly understood and therefore it is also necessary to accept the limitations of any statistical analyses of the data.

Whilst standard imaging methods using more established tumour size measurement criteria will continue to contribute to study endpoints, it is likely that a broader application of novel methods will be witnessed. Robust qualification activities will be required to evolve current exploratory techniques to fully qualified endpoints. In order for DW-MRI to make this transition, (i) qualification activities are required to provide evidence that the read-out such as ADC has the intended clinical significance, (ii) pilot studies are required to establish the robustness of the technique across multiple centres with a focus on the rate of uninterpretability and methodological reproducibility and (iii) operational challenges need to be prospectively identified in order to implement and translate the technique globally.

16.6

Multi-Site Implementation of Imaging Techniques

As mentioned earlier, the challenges in establishing anatomically based read-outs for multi-site clinical trials are not inconsiderable and need to be borne in mind, given the central role for imaging in the interpretation of patient response (Fig. 16.3). The key challenges that should be recognized include:

- Standardization of imaging methodology across multiple scanning platforms, accounting for equipment availability and loco-regional variations in imaging practice.
- Controlling for reading/interpretation bias by appropriately implementing blinded, central review of imaging data.

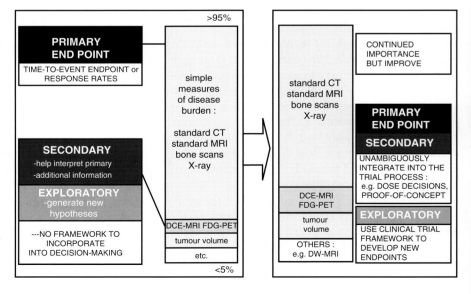

Fig. 16.2. An overview of how imaging currently contributes to study endpoints (*left*) in oncology trials and where the role of imaging may evolve towards (*right*). Currently, across all phases of development most imaging is performed for simple analyses of disease. If other imaging endpoints can demonstrate a more defined role in drug development it is likely they will contribute as either primary or secondary study endpoints

Fig. 16.3. A simplified model for performing centralized collection and review of imaging data in order to provide study results to the sponsor for statistical analysis (CRO = Contract Research Organisation; the sponsor is usually the pharmaceutical company in a commercial drug trial)

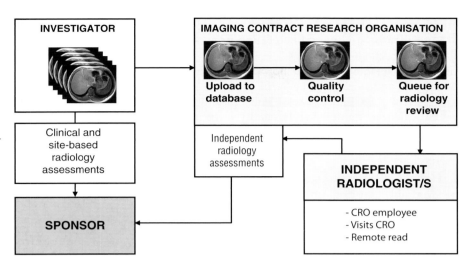

- Making imaging departments and personnel inclusive at initial study and site set-up.

16.6.1
Standardization of Image Acquisition

The challenges to standardizing a novel technique such as DW-MRI can better be appreciated if one considers all the known scanning parameters that need to be controlled even at the level of a mature technology such as CT (i.e. slice thickness, anatomical coverage, use and timing of contrast). Without methodological harmonization, techniques such as DW-MRI are likely to have limited if not deleterious impact on data interpretation. The lack of agreement on scanning platforms and discordant scanning techniques are common reasons for the varied results reported in the literature. The first step in standardization is to achieve methodological consensus, which has been initiated in fields such as DCE-MRI and [18]FDG-PET. Recently, consensus recommendations for standardizing DW-MRI were published (PADHANI et al. 2009). In general, the two resources most likely to facilitate successful implementation and management of multi-site imaging trials are:

- *Imaging CRO* – Using a Contract Research Organisation (CRO) with imaging expertise to implement acquisition guidelines and site training. A study sponsor will likely select this approach if the number of investigating sites exceeds five and/or the sites have limited experience of participation in clinical trials.

- *Network of expert centres* – with willingness to coordinate and the nomination of one centre as the primary imaging site. This is a particularly attractive model if the number of participating centres is limited and each centre has expertise in the scanning methodology.

A centre-based network will be attractive if there is a history of pre-existing collaboration between sites. However, the imaging implementation option selected must consider both the potential for subject recruitment and the need to harmonize imaging methodologies.

16.6.2
Quality Assurance and Quality Control

Ensuring data quality is particularly important if study sites with limited clinical trial experience have been recruited and novel techniques are being implemented. This is particularly true of DW-MRI where there may be study centres involved with less experience for the technique or multi-site trial work. Quality assurance processes will be required to deliver robust data and should include: (i) assessment of site capabilities including equipment availability; (ii) centralized assessment of phantom data to ensure optimal scanner operation and (iii) centralized review of test patient data to ensure that the site is acquiring data to a defined standard. Continuous quality control processes are then required to ensure study images remain of acceptable quality. Essential properties of the process include the ability to take corrective action if data do not meet the required needs.

16.6.3
Standardization of Image Review and Analysis

Centralized imaging review is now becoming more prevalent. This has been driven by the need to provide a consistent radiological assessment and/or image analysis, thereby minimizing variability in the endpoint, as well as the need to control for bias resulting from knowledge of a patient's clinical and treatment details.

For DW-MRI, centralized review would generally be favourable ensuring consistent analysis is applied to each dataset, including features such as reproducible outlines of the region of interest. An important role of a centralized review is to define the imaging requirements, implement a mechanism for data transmission and receipt, monitor data quality and provide image review.

Although the processes involved in site set-up, quality assurance/quality control and centralized review come at a price and added operational complexity, they do ensure protocol adherence and provide an objective basis for assessing trial data.

16.7
DW-MRI in Drug Development

The apparent diffusion coefficient (ADC), the commonly extracted DW-MRI parameter is a good example of an experimental biomarker. In the limited studies reported to date, DW-MRI has been implemented in parallel with conventional imaging studies and indicates potential use as a clinical prognostic and early treatment response output. In addition, preclinical studies have demonstrated its value by probing architectural modulation in tissues following administration of therapeutics. Each of these could translate into benefit in the development of a new medicine.

16.7.1
Prediction of Drug Efficacy

DW-MRI would be a valuable tool if it could "enrich" a trial by identifying subjects who are more likely to respond to therapy. In some studies, the baseline evaluation of a patient with DW-MRI has suggested a possible association of the baseline ADC measurement with subsequent therapeutic response. In a study of advanced rectal cancer, Dzik-Jurasz et al.

report that a lower baseline ADC value predicted for a greater reduction in tumour volume following chemoradiation (Dzik-Jurasz et al. 2002). By comparison, Hamstra et al. noted that in patients with high-grade glioma, the baseline ADC measurements did not predict for subsequent response to radiotherapy or chemoradiotherapy (Hamstra et al. 2005). To confirm the value of DW-MRI for the prediction of treatment response in clinical drug trials, considerably more data are required before DW-MRI can be considered as more than a promising experimental technique.

16.7.2
Early Assessment of Treatment Response

Early detection of treatment response refers to the ability to detect clinical response prior to conventional means (e.g. by size change using standard CT or MR imaging criteria). Such a capability could provide an alternative to the standard definitions of response or time-to-event endpoints currently employed in clinical trials. The study by Hamstra et al., suggested that early diffusion changes in patients with high-grade glioma were predictive of time-to-progression and overall survival (Hamstra et al. 2005). ADC changes were measured 3 weeks from baseline following a course of radiotherapy and chemotherapy. Despite the heterogeneity in treatment regimens, it was encouraging to see significant changes in diffusion parameters. Interestingly, the authors observed that since the ADC changes at 3 weeks post-treatment could predict for subsequent outcome, the DW-MRI response might be used to stratify subjects into an adaptive radiotherapy regimen. Furthermore, this study also suggested a means by which the degree of early responses could be used to optimize therapy (for example, by altering dose, changing drug or adding additional therapy or altering concomitant radiotherapy). In order to establish the use of such methods in, for example Phase II studies, further studies are needed to identify (i) variability in tumour response, (ii) drug class effects on diffusion measurements and ADC, (iii) optimal timing to capture significant changes using DW-MRI and (iv) determine clinically relevant thresholds for determining therapeutic effect.

It is clear from studies such as that by Hamstra et al. that early and significant changes are detectable using DW-MRI (Hamstra et al. 2005). Similar studies across other tumour types and therapies would establish the validity of these responses and can form the basis for establishing the role of the technique in drug development. Setting criteria that could be used to halt or continue with a trial would represent important output from future DW-MRI investigations. Until confidence in the technique can be established to support different drug development milestones, the technique can only be viewed as a valuable experimental imaging tool.

16.7.3
Evaluation of Drug-Response Characteristics

A change in the measured biomarker has an established relationship with drug dosage, drug scheduling or combination therapy. The establishment of an appropriate starting Phase II dose is an essential objective of a Phase I study. This is typically achieved by incrementally increasing drug dose until a predefined toxicity is reached. The *maximum tolerated dose* is used to define the highest dose of an administered drug that does not result in unacceptable side effects. Dose selection with this approach does not take into account how much drug is required to trigger a pharmacodynamic effect at the molecular level. However, this maximum tolerated dose, which is defined by the upper toxicity limit, may not be appropriate, for example, for alternative indications (e.g. patients with disease that compromises hepatic function in the context of drug which affects liver function) or the combination use with other drugs.

In order to appropriately evaluate dose-response, efficient read-outs are required to ensure subjects are not exposed to sub-therapeutic drug doses. Unfortunately, standard morphological evaluations by conventional imaging are unlikely to demonstrate visible changes soon after initiating therapy. DW-MRI, when optimized, could provide such a read-out enabling response at different dose levels to be evaluated within days of dosing. This is an opportunity that remains to be exploited by DW-MRI.

16.8
Role of DW-MRI in Preclinical Drug Development

Most large pharmaceutical companies provide for in-house or outsourced preclinical imaging programmes. The role of preclinical imaging is to gain insights into the in vivo behaviour of a drug candidate prior to entry into the clinical arena. Potential advantages include a better understanding of the behaviours of drugs in xenografts compared with the clinical setting. Thankfully, the modular aspect of many imaging protocols permits several imaging modalities to be implemented into a single in vivo experiment.

Several DW-MRI studies have been described for the assessment of novel anticancer agents using animal models. For example, in the study by Jordan et al. (2005), DCE-MRI and DW-MRI were applied in a mouse-bearing human xenograft model treated with agent PX-478 that inhibits hypoxia-responsive transcription factor. Significant changes in both DW-MRI and DCE-MRI parameters were observed. The complementary use of both techniques enabled a more informative assessment of the tumour micro-environment than either method alone. Such studies could provide insight into the optimal design and interpretation of analogous clinical studies. Similarly, DW-MRI was combined with DCE-MRI in the study by Berry et al., looking at the vascular response of a xenograft to a novel antibody targeted against vascular endothelial growth factor-A (VEGF) (BERRY et al. 2008). Viable tissue was characterized using DW-MRI, and this was used to define the DCE-MRI region of interest, enabling a more informative assessment of the tumour vascularity by accounting for tumour heterogeneity.

Assessments of established chemotherapeutic agents such as paclitaxel (GALONS et al. 1999) and docetaxel (JENNINGS et al. 2002) in disease models using DW-MRI have also been reported. Reports on the behaviour of established anticancer agents on tumour ADCs are equally important in defining the spectrum of DW-MRI responses and increases confidence in the interpretation of results.

Preclinical imaging therefore provides a platform to understand both the earliest in vivo behaviour of a drug and also to guide subsequent clinical imaging studies. Examples are beginning to emerge which define DW-MRI as an important component of preclinical studies. It is anticipated that the role of DW-MRI will increase as experience is gained in the behaviour of diffusion-based indices.

16.9
Current Status of DW-MRI for Drug Development

As discussed earlier, drug development consists of distinct phases designed to answer increasingly focused questions on the safety and efficacy of a

Table 16.3. Advantages and limitations of DW-MRI as a potential biomarker

Advantages
Broad applicability across clinical trials in solid tumours
Availability across multiple MR scanner platforms
Represents a downstream biomarker of cell death
Can be used as part of multi-parametric MR imaging evaluation, performed within a single scanning session (e.g. combining with morphological evaluation, DCE-MRI, spectroscopy)
Data analysis is not dependent on complex mathematical modelling

Limitations
Currently limited clinical site experience in using DW-MRI
DW-MRI reflects downstream cellular effects and will not provide direct evidence of receptor–ligand interactions
Industry has little experience of using the method for drug development purposes

potential drug. As a result, various tools are needed to support decision-making including the ability to predict clinical benefit. It is likely that DW-MRI will be one of a number of imaging methods that will complement other tissue or bio-fluid markers supporting the life cycle of a drug. Some key advantages and disadvantages of DW-MRI need to be taken into account in deciding whether to include the technique into a clinical trial. These are summarized in Table 16.3.

Currently, DW-MRI is used as an exploratory endpoint sometimes in combination with other techniques such as DCE-MRI. In such a setting, performance issues and potential ambiguity of results will not compromise the clinical trial success. The extensive use of MR imaging within clinical trials provides an invaluable platform to develop DW-MRI where collating exploratory DW-MRI data will support future use.

16.10

Conclusions

Drug development is challenged with delivering drugs cheaply and speedily to the pharmaceutical market. This needs to be achieved as efficiently as possible, enabling only successful medicines to consume the finite resources available. Given the current attrition rates for compounds, there exist many

deficiencies in the current drug development model. More informed decisions need to be made based on rational evaluation of drug effectiveness earlier in the life cycle of a drug and drug development. DW-MRI is one of a number of methodologies, which when further developed and applied appropriately, could represent a major improvement over current endpoints. However, there must first be focus on enabling DW-MRI as a standardized multi-centre method. Second, wide-scale implementation will enable data to be generated that will establish where the technique would be most valuable. If both of these are achieved, DW-MRI could in the future be used as primary or secondary study endpoints in drug trials, and can be used to complement existing morphological and functional imaging methods.

References

Adams CP, Brantner VV (2006) Estimating the cost of new drug development: is it really 802 million dollars? Health Aff (Millwood) 25:420–8

Adjei AA, Christian M, Ivy P (2009) Novel designs and end points for phase II clinical trials. Clin Cancer Res 15:1866–72

Atkinson AJ, et al (2001) Biomarkers and surrogate endpoints: Preferred definitions and conceptual framework. Clin Pharmacol Ther 69:89–95

Berry LR, et al (2008) Quantification of viable tumor microvascular characteristics by multispectral analysis. Magn Reson.Med 60:64–72

Booth B, Glassman R, Ma P (2003) Oncology's trials. Nat Rev Drug Discov 2:609–10

Dancey JE, Chen HX (2006) Strategies for optimizing combinations of molecularly targeted anticancer agents. Nat Rev Drug Discov 5:649–59

Dhani N, et al (2009) Alternate endpoints for screening phase II studies. Clin Cancer Res 15:1873–82

DiMasi JA, Grabowski HG (2007a) Economics of new oncology drug development. J Clin Oncol 25:209–16

DiMasi JA, Grabowski HG (2007b) The cost of biopharmaceutical R&D: is biotech different? Managerial Decision Econ 28:469–79

DiMasi JA, Hansen RW, Grabowski HG (2003) The price of innovation: new estimates of drug development costs. J Health Econ 22:151–85

Dzik-Jurasz A, et al (2002) Diffusion MRI for prediction of response of rectal cancer to chemoradiation. Lancet 360:307–8

El Maraghi RH, Eisenhauer EA (2008) Review of phase II trial designs used in studies of molecular targeted agents: outcomes and predictors of success in phase III. J Clin Oncol 26:1346–54

FDA (2004) Innovation stagnation: challenge and opportunity on the critical path to new medicines. FDA, USA

FDA (2006) Critical path opportunities initiated during 2006. FDA, USA

Galons JP, et al (1999) Early increases in breast tumor xenograft water mobility in response to paclitaxel therapy detected by non-invasive diffusion magnetic resonance imaging. Neoplasia 1:113–17

Hamstra DA, et al (2005) Evaluation of the functional diffusion map as an early biomarker of time-to-progression and overall survival in high-grade glioma. Proc Natl Acad Sci U S A 102:16759–64

Jennings D, et al (2002) Early response of prostate carcinoma xenografts to docetaxel chemotherapy monitored with diffusion MRI. Neoplasia 4:255–62

Jordan BF, Runquist M, Raghunand N, et al (2005) Dynamic contrast-enhanced and diffusion MRI show rapid and dramatic changes in tumor microenvironmentin response to inhibition of HIF-1alpha using PX-478. Neoplasia 7:475–85

Kamb A (2005) What's wrong with our cancer models? Nat Rev Drug Discov 4:161–5

Kamb A, Wee S, Lengauer C (2007) Why is cancer drug discovery so difficult? Nat Rev Drug Discov 6:115–20

Padhani AR, et al (2009) Diffusion-weighted magnetic resonance imaging as a cancer biomarker: consensus and recommendations. Neoplasia 11:102–25

Pharmaceutical Research and Manufacturers of America (2009) 2009 Report medicines in development for cancer

Rowinsky EK (2004) Curtailing the high rate of late-stage attrition of investigational therapeutics against unprecedented targets in patients with lung and other malignancies Clin Cancer Res 10:4220S–26S

Wagner JA (2002) Overview of biomarkers and surrogate endpoints in drug development. Dis Markers 18:41–6

Wagner JA, Williams SA, Webster CJ (2007) Biomarkers and surrogate end points for fit-for-purpose development and regulatory evaluation of new drugs. Clin Pharmacol Ther 81:104–7

Walker I, Newell H (2009) Do molecularly targeted agents in oncology have reduced attrition rates? Nat Rev Drug Discov 8:15–16

Weber WA (2009) Assessing tumor response to therapy. J Nucl Med 50(Suppl 1):1S–10S

Subject Index

List of Contributors

YASAMAN AMOOZADEH, MD
Joint Department of Medical Imaging,
University Health Network
Princess Margaret Hospital
University of Toronto
610 University Avenue,
Toronto, ON
Canada M5G 2M9

DAVID J. COLLINS, MInstP
CR UK – EPSARC Cancer Imaging Centre
Institute of Cancer Research & Royal Marsden Hospital
Downs Road
Sutton, SM2 5PT
United Kingdom

THOMAS L. CHENEVERT, PhD
University of Michigan
1500 East Medical Center Drive
Ann Arbor, MI 48109-0030
USA

MATTHEW BLACKLEDGE, MSc
CR UK – EPSARC Cancer Imaging Centre
Institute of Cancer Research & Royal Marsden Hospital
Downs Road
Sutton, SM2 5PT
United Kingdom

FREDERIK DE KEYZER, MSc
Department of Radiology
University Hospitals Leuven
Herestraat 49
3000 Leuven
Belgium

ANDY DZIK-JURASZ, MD
Novartis Pharmaceuticals Corporation
One Health Plaza
East Hanover
NJ 07936-1080
USA

JOHANNES M. FROEHLICH, PhD
Department of Diagnostic
Interventional and Pediatric Radiology
University of Bern, Inselspital
Freiburgstrasse 10, 3010 Bern
Switzerland

CRAIG J. GALBÁN, PhD
Department of Radiology
Center for Molecular Imaging
Biomedical Sciences Research Building
109 Zina Pitcher Place, Ann Arbor
MI 48109–2200
USA

MASOOM HAIDER, MD, FRCPC
Joint Department of Medical Imaging
University Health Network
Princess Margaret Hospital
University of Toronto
610 University Avenue,
Toronto, ON
Canada M5G 2M9

TOMOAKI ICHIKAWA, MD, PhD
Department of Radiology
University of Yamanashi
1110 Shimokato, Chuo
Yamanashi, 409–3898
Japan

Kartik S. Jhaveri, MD
Joint Department of Medical Imaging,
University Health Network
Princess Margaret Hospital
University of Toronto
610 University Avenue
Toronto, ON
Canada M5G 2M9

Ihab R. Kamel, MD, PhD
The Russell H. Morgan Department of Radiology
and Radiological Sciences
The Johns Hopkins Hospital
601 North Caroline Street
Baltimore, MD 21287
USA

Dow-Mu Koh, MD, MRCP, FRCR
Royal Marsden NHS Foundation Trust
Department of Radiology
Downs Road, Sutton
Surrey SM2 5PT
UK

Eleni Liapi, MD
The Russell H. Morgan Department of Radiology
and Radiological Sciences
The Johns Hopkins Hospital
601 North Caroline Street
Baltimore, MD 21287
USA

Ali Muhi, MD
Department of Radiology
University of Yamanashi
1110 Shimokato, Chuo
Yamanashi, 409–3898
Japan

Anwar Padhani, MD
Paul Strickland Scanner Centre
Mount Vernon Hospital
Rickmansworth Road, Northwood
Middlesex HA6 2RN
UK

Jignesh Patel, MD
Department of Radiology
New York University Langone Medical Center
560 First Avenue
New York, NY 10016
USA

Alnawaz Rehemtulla, PhD
Department of Radiology
Center for Molecular Imaging
Biomedical Sciences Research Building
109 Zina Pitcher Place
Ann Arbor
MI 48109–2200
USA

Brian D. Ross, PhD
Department of Radiology
Center for Molecular Imaging
Biomedical Sciences Research Building
109 Zina Pitcher Place
Ann Arbor
MI 48109-2200
USA

Taro Takahara, MD, PhD
Department of Radiology
Division of Radiology
Radiotherapy and Nuclear Medicine (RRN)
University Medical Center (UMC) Utrecht
Heidelberglaan 100, Utrecht
The Netherlands

Bachir Taouli, MD
Department of Radiology
New York University Langone Medical Center
560 First Avenue
New York, NY 10016,
USA

Harriet C. Thoeny, MD
Universitätsspital Bern Inselspital
Departement of Diagnostic,
Interventional and Paediatric Radiology
Freiburgstr 10, 3010 Bern
Switzerland

THOMAS C. KWEE, MD
Department of Radiology
Division of Radiology, Radiotherapy,
and Nuclear Medicine
University Medical Center Utrecht
Heidelberglaan 100, Utrecht,
The Netherlands

PHIL MURPHY, PhD
Oncology Medicines Development Centre
GlaxoSmithKline Research & Development
1–3 Iron Bridge Road
Stockley Park West
Uxbridge
Middlesex UB11 1BT
UK

NAKANISHI K, MD, PhD
Department of Diagnostic Radiology,
Osaka Medical Center for Cancer
and Cardiovascular Diseases
Nakamichi
Higashinari-Ku
537-8511 Osaka
Japan

ANDREAS GUTZEIT, MD
Department of Diagnostic and Interventional Radiology
Kantonsspital Winterthur
Brauerstrasse 15
Postfach 834
CH-8401 Winterthur
Switzerland

MEDICAL RADIOLOGY Diagnostic Imaging and Radiation Oncology

Titles in the series already published

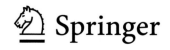

MEDICAL RADIOLOGY Diagnostic Imaging and Radiation Oncology
Titles in the series already published

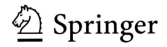 Springer

Printing and Binding: Stürtz GmbH, Würzburg